*f*P

THE HARVARD MEDICAL SCHOOL

GUIDE TO Taking Control *of*

Asthma

A Comprehensive Prevention
and Treatment Plan for
You and Your Family

Christopher H. Fanta, M.D.
Lynda M. Cristiano, M.D.
Kenan E. Haver, M.D.

THE PARTNERS ASTHMA CENTER
WITH
Nancy Waring, Ph.D.

FREE PRESS
NEW   YORK   LONDON   TORONTO   SYDNEY

𝑓P

FREE PRESS
A Division of Simon & Schuster, Inc.
1230 Avenue of the Americas
New York, NY 10020

First Free Press trade paperback edition 2003

FREE PRESS and colophon are trademarks
of Simon & Schuster, Inc.

For information regarding special discounts for bulk purchases,
please contact Simon & Schuster Special Sales at
1-800-456-6798 or business@simonandschuster.com

Designed by Amy Hill

Manufactured in the United States of America

5   7   9   10   8   6   4

Library of Congress Cataloging-in-Publication Data

Fanta, Christopher H.
The Harvard Medical School guide to taking control of asthma :
a comprehensive prevention and treatment plan for you and your family /
Christopher H. Fanta, Lynda M. Cristiano, Kenan E. Haver,
with Nancy Waring.
p.   cm.
Includes bibliographical references and index.
1. Asthma.   2. Asthma—Treatment.   I. Title: Guide to taking control of
asthma.   II. Title: Taking control of asthma.   III. Cristiano, Lynda M.
IV. Haver, Kenan E.   V. Harvard Medical School.   VI. Title.
RC591.F36   2003
616.2'3806—dc22   2003063145

ISBN 0-7432-2478-7

Acknowledgments

THE ORIGINS OF THIS BOOK can be found in the patient-education initiatives of the Partners Asthma Center. We believe strongly that the more our patients know about their asthma and its treatments, the better able they are to collaborate with their health care providers in keeping their asthma well controlled. Recognizing that our time spent together in the office is never sufficient to review all the information and skills needed for good asthma care, we created other means of communication. Partners Asthma Center publishes a quarterly patient-education newsletter, called *Breath of Fresh Air,* and distributes an introductory booklet on asthma, called *Partners Asthma Center's Guide to Asthma.* Much of the content of this book was originally prepared for one or the other of these Partners Asthma Center publications.

With this book we have been given the opportunity to expand and update this information and to share it with an audience that reaches far beyond our medical practices.

We are grateful to **Anthony Komaroff, M.D.,** editor in chief at Harvard Health Publications, for his suggestion that we write this book, his direction on how best to shape it, and his perseverance in helping us bring it to fruition. Without his guidance and support there would have been no book.

Nancy Waring, Ph.D., writer and editor, is the other person without whose tireless work this book would never have come about. She turned our conversations, notes, and preexisting materials into chapters, edited our words, helped us find our writing "voice," interviewed our patients for their "asthma stories," and researched extra material to supplement our content. She did all this with unfailing enthusiasm and good spirit.

An editorial coordinator at Harvard Health Publications, **Christine Junge,** proved an invaluable resource. She kept us coherent, relatively on time, and organized.

Many other people contributed their time and talent to the development of this book. Among them are **Elaine Carter, R.N., BSN,** Partners Asthma Center nurse educator; **Donna Champagne, LICSW,** leader of the Partners Asthma Center support group; **David Christiani, M.D.,** Pulmonary and Occupational Medicine at the Massachusetts General Hospital and member of Partners

Asthma Center; **Kay Coady,** administrative assistant in the Pulmonary and Critical Care Division at Brigham and Women's Hospital; **Ellie Goldberg,** educational rights specialist; **Susan Korrick, M.D.,** Occupational Medicine at Brigham and Women's Hospital; **Robb Scholten,** information officer, Osher Institute, Harvard Medical School; **Elisabeth Steib, R.N.,** Partners Asthma Center nurse educator; **Marie Trottier,** university disability coordinator and disability compliance officer, Harvard University; **Linda Walsh, R.N., BSN,** director of clinical services, Newton Health Department, Newton, Massachusetts; **Rosalyn Wright, M.D.,** Pulmonary and Critical Care Medicine at the Beth-Israel Deaconess Medical Center; and **Jean Zotter,** director, Boston Urban Asthma Coalition.

Perhaps most important, we wish to express our immense appreciation to all of our patients, who constantly teach us about asthma and about caring for patients with asthma by allowing us to participate in their care. We especially acknowledge our gratitude to the patients who generously shared their experiences with asthma for the patient stories that appear in this book (their names have been changed to protect their privacy). Their eloquence speaks volumes.

Finally, behind every physician-author stands a supportive and highly tolerant family. With our deepest love and appreciation, we thank our family members:

Charlotte and Eugene Fanta
Carol Hardy-Fanta
and our beloved children, Allison and Carly

Adelaide and John F. Cristiano
Daniel J. Rizika and our precious daughters,
Lauren Cristiano Rizika and Alexa Cristiano Rizika

Thomas and Barbara Haver
My wife, Linda Wang, and our wonderful daughters,
Hana and Serena

Christopher H. Fanta, M.D.
Lynda M. Cristiano, M.D.
Kenan E. Haver, M.D.
March 2003

Contents

PART III
Caring for Your Asthma

Preface

HERE, AT THE START OF THE TWENTY-FIRST CENTURY, we find ourselves witnessing two seemingly contradictory trends in the world of asthma care. We find asthma becoming more common and more severe in our country and in many of the Westernized nations of the world. More people are developing asthma. More people are being hospitalized for treatment of severe flare-ups of asthma, and more fatal episodes of severe asthma are occurring. At the same time, our understanding of the underlying processes that make asthmatic air passageways behave the way they do has grown enormously, and better, easier-to-take treatments have made their way to our pharmacies. New, highly effective, and convenient therapies for asthma are widely available.

It wasn't very long ago—20 to 30 years ago—that asthma was conceived of primarily as a disease of episodic spasm of the involuntary muscles that surround the breathing tubes, a concept understood by the Roman physician Galen nearly 2,000 years earlier. Many physicians didn't consider asthma to be a terribly serious disease. A famous physician, Sir William Osler (1849–1919), commented: "Asthmatics don't die, they just pant into old age." We sometimes still hear of the asthmatic tendency being attributed, erroneously, to emotional stresses and difficult child-parent relationships. Our treatments have focused on medications that cause the bronchial muscles to relax—"bronchodilators." Even today, our schools and playgrounds are filled with asthmatic children who carry medication inhalers to deliver bronchodilator treatments when they are feeling short of breath or tight in the chest.

Our medical understanding of asthma has advanced dramatically over these past 20 to 30 years. We now understand asthma to be a chronic inflammatory condition of the bronchial tubes. The type of inflammation characteristic of asthma has the appearance of an allergic response. Great strides have been made in identifying what cells and chemicals in the body participate in this allergic-type reaction, and what stimuli produce it, in susceptible individuals. We now see that contraction of the muscles surrounding the breathing tubes is a manifestation of chronically inflamed asthmatic airways. The inflammation and the susceptibility to spasmodic narrowing of the breathing tubes persist even when someone with asthma feels well—that is, totally free of symptoms.

In people with more than very mild asthma, treatment now focuses on suppressing the allergic inflammation of the breathing tubes. Safe and effective medicines, taken once or twice daily, can reduce asthmatic inflammation, inhibit contraction of the bronchial muscles, and *prevent* narrowing of the air passageways. For a time, the best medicines available to treat asthma included theophylline, a not-so-distant relative of caffeine. Imagine taking—or giving to your asthmatic child—a caffeine-like substance just before bedtime to maintain comfortable breathing overnight! There was also a time, as we started to focus on treating inflammation of the bronchial tubes, when we asked some of our patients to inhale anti-inflammatory medicines in doses of 6 to 12 sprays at a time. Now it is a rare patient who needs more than two inhalations twice daily to keep asthma under good control.

Because of the tremendous advances in understanding and treating asthma, our book has good news to share, and also carries a message of great optimism for the future. The vast majority of people with asthma can achieve good control of their illness with currently available medications. Only a small minority cannot.

But a small part of a very large number—say, for example, 1 percent of the estimated 15 million Americans with asthma—is still a large number of people with persistent, difficult-to-control asthma. For this group there is also reason for optimism, because we stand on the threshold of a new age of asthma therapies with the emergence of biotherapeutic drugs specifically designed to interrupt individual steps in the allergic response. In our chapter on new and future asthma therapies, we also consider the emerging field of pharmacogenetics, which is likely to yield information that will make it possible, before a prescription is written, to predict your response to different antiasthmatic medications based on analysis of your unique genetic profile.

A parallel revolution in medicine over the last 20 to 30 years that is relevant to asthma has to do not with scientific knowledge or new medical breakthroughs but with the fundamental human interaction at the heart of the delivery of medical care: the patient-doctor relationship. Patients have become more active participants in their own care, making informed decisions under the general guidance of their physicians. Nowhere is this collaborative interaction between patient and physician more appropriate than for a chronic condition with potential, often unpredictable flare-ups, such as asthma. Again and again in studies conducted in the last two to three decades, educational programs teaching asthma comanagement skills have been shown to improve health outcomes and patient satisfaction.

The more you know about asthma and its treatments, the better the choices you make in caring for your own or your child's asthma. It is a good feeling to understand what is going on in your body, to know how to respond to signals that your body sends, and to breathe better again as a result of your actions. As you will hear in the voices of our patients throughout this book, feeling in control of your asthma—rather than feeling overwhelmed or frightened by it—builds confidence and a greater sense of security. This book is intended to share with you the knowledge and skills you need to gain control over your asthma, so that you can participate with your health care provider in making sound judgments about your asthma management.

This book is organized into three sections. The first section reviews what asthma is, how it is diagnosed, and how you can judge its severity. It also explores potential explanations for the rising prevalence of asthma in our communities. The second section describes in detail the medications and other forms of treatment available to treat asthma. It emphasizes practical details, including how to take your medications effectively, what short-term and long-term side effects to expect, and what relative advantages and disadvantages each medicine has. The third section guides you through strategies for managing your asthma, both on a day-to-day basis and when faced with flare-ups of your symptoms (asthmatic "attacks"). It includes information about managing asthma under special circumstances (for example, in very young children, in the elderly, and during pregnancy) and what to consider if your asthma isn't getting better. Toward the end of the book, we encourage you to develop—with your physician—your own asthma "action plan."

Medicine is both art and science. This book contains many opinions as well as factual information. These opinions reflect the views of the authors, who take responsibility for any errors or omissions this book may contain. At the same time, our views and practice patterns did not form in a vacuum. They have been shaped by our reading of the medical literature, by our experiences in the practice of medicine, and by our discussions with our colleagues. We are privileged to practice at an academic medical center surrounded by outstanding allergists and pulmonologists (and other related specialists) skilled in the treatment of asthma. We practice at the Partners Asthma Center, a center for excellence in asthma care that is part of the Partners Healthcare System in Massachusetts.

In 1989 allergists and pulmonary specialists at Brigham and Women's Hospital in Boston began a collaboration in asthma clinical care, to complement a long history of collaboration in asthma research. When the Brigham and Women's and Massachusetts General Hospitals formed a partnership in 1994, called Partners Healthcare, we expanded our collaboration to include allergists and pulmonologists at both hospitals. As a result, our expertise extended to children as well as adults, and we became the Partners Asthma Center. Over the years additional hospitals have joined the Partners Healthcare network. Asthma specialists at Faulkner Hospital, Newton-Wellesley Hospital, and North Shore Medical Center have joined with us in an expanded Partners Asthma Center that now comprises approximately 50 physicians, together with asthma nurses, nurse-practitioners, and respiratory therapists.

The stated mission of the Partners Asthma Center is:

> To provide optimal medical care for persons with asthma and related diseases, to develop new knowledge about asthma and its management through state-of-the-art medical research, to train medical students and graduate physicians in the specialized skills of asthma care, and to promote improved understanding about asthma and related diseases through educational programs and materials for our patients, for other health care providers, and for the community.

We are grateful for the opportunity to further our mission at the Partners Asthma Center with the publication of this book. We invite you to communicate with us directly at asthma@partners.org and to visit our Web site at www.asthma.partners.org. And we wish you healthy breathing.

Christopher H. Fanta, M.D.

Lynda M. Cristiano, M.D.

Kenan E. Haver, M.D.

July 2003

PART I

Understanding Asthma

CHAPTER 1

What Is Asthma?

WHAT ASTHMA FEELS LIKE

"I can't swim across the pool underwater, and it took me three tries to blow out all of my birthday candles."
— DANIEL, 6

"Even if you talk about it with people, they can't grasp the depth of asthma. Most people are preconditioned: 'Oh, asthma is all in your head; oh, you can do this and you can do that.' They don't realize that this is your lung involved, this is your heart, everything you've got is involved in asthma trying to breathe. People don't understand unless they have it or are directly affected by it."
— HAZEL, 56

"It feels like someone has their hands around your lungs and is squeezing them very tightly and you are trying to break that grip. You can't breathe, and you can't get away from that fierce set of hands around your lungs."
— MARGARET, 60

THE EXPERIENCE OF ASTHMA varies greatly among people who have asthma, mainly because of its variable severity. For some people it is a minor annoyance, a tickle of a cough felt high in the throat after exercise. For others it is the cause of restless nights with frequent awakenings due to cough and labored breathing. For still others asthma manifests as severe attacks, characterized by a suffocating sensation and the sense that the next breath may be the last. Some people with asthma are Olympic athletes, able to compete at the highest levels of physical strength and endurance. Others find themselves frequently in and out of the local emergency room, unable to plan routine daily activities because of unpredictable episodes of difficult breathing.

The loved ones of people with asthma often share much of the emotional burden—if not the direct experience—of asthma. It can be exceedingly difficult to watch someone struggle with his or her breathing and feel unable to help. No one is likely to feel this distress more deeply than the parent of a child with asthma, especially a small child still too young to verbalize what he or she is going through. How can you keep your child safe, you wonder, through this respiratory tract infection, through the day at school, the soccer game, or the summer away at camp? You try to find the right balance between safety and restrictive limitations. Many children and parents express complaints about the unpredictable nature of asthma. They say that never knowing when they will have an "episode" and if that episode will be severe makes having asthma so stressful. This is reflected in asthma surveys that show many families suffer disrupted plans and activities because of the disease.

Whatever your experience with asthma, you are not alone. In a recent national survey, an estimated 15 million Americans reported asthma symptoms during the preceding 12 months, including approximately 3.5 million children under the age of 15 years.

Nearly 27 million Americans have at one time in their lives been diagnosed with asthma by a physician. People of all ages have asthma; it occurs in all countries and among all populations around the world. Most strikingly, over the past 20 years asthma has become increasingly common in many parts of the industrialized world. We are in the midst, some physicians would say, of an asthma epidemic.

Asthma is an ancient disease. Greek physicians like Hippocrates in 460 B.C. wrote of asthma. They used the word ασθμα, meaning to pant or breathe hard. A description by the Greek physician Aretaeus from the second half of the first century A.D. vividly captures the struggle to breathe characteristic of a severe asthma attack:

> They go into the open air, since no house suffices for their respiration; they breathe standing, as if desiring to draw in all the air they can possibly inhale; and, in their want of air, they also open the mouth as if best to enjoy more of it. Pale in countenance, except the cheeks, which are ruddy; sweat about the forehead and clavicles; cough incessant and laborious; expectoration small, thin, cold, resembling the efflorescence of foam; neck swells with the inflation of the breath.

For most people, difficulty breathing is the most overwhelming but not the only symptom of asthma. Shortness of breath is often accompanied by a sensation of tightness in the chest that can make you feel as if you had a wide rubber band bound tightly around your torso. Wheezes—musical whistling sounds heard especially with breathing out—are a trademark symptom of asthma. Cough, often worse at night, is also common.

To give you just a few specific examples of the variable nature of asthma, one of our patients, a 15-year-old girl who competes in high school athletics, experiences brief bouts of coughing and shortness of breath usually only after a demanding track meet or basketball game. Another patient, a man in his forties, is aware of a slight wheeze most of the time and has been hospitalized many times because of his asthma. He has multiple allergies that cause his asthma to flare up, including allergy to furry pets and sensitivities to cigarette smoke and strong fragrances, and finds himself out of breath merely climbing a single flight of stairs.

The majority of our patients fall somewhere in between these extremes. But wherever you are on the continuum, you share with these patients—and with everyone who has asthma—a tendency for your breathing passageways, the bronchial tubes, to narrow abnormally in response to certain stimuli.

As shown in the pictures below, your lungs are built to bring oxygen into your body and to release a gas called carbon dioxide (CO_2) out of your body. Oxygen is essential to supply energy to your cells, and CO_2 is a waste product made by your cells.

Narrowing of the bronchial tubes of your lungs leads to the symptoms of

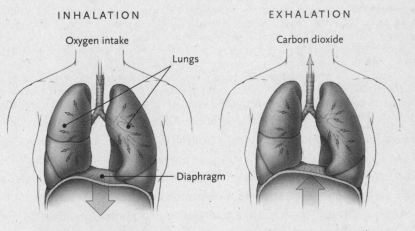

INHALATION

Oxygen intake

Lungs

Diaphragm

Diaphragm pulls downward,
helping lungs expand with air

EXHALATION

Carbon dioxide

Diaphragm returns upward,
forcing lungs to expel carbon dioxide

FIGURE 1: WHAT HAPPENS AS YOU BREATHE
As you breathe in, your diaphragm descends, expanding your rib cage and lungs. As you exhale, your diaphragm moves upward and your lungs expel gas, including carbon dioxide.

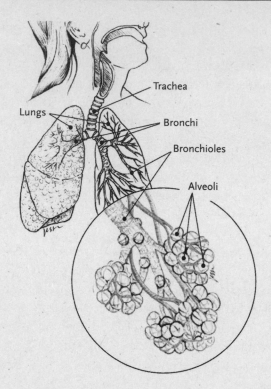

FIGURE 2: HOW THE INSIDES OF THE LUNGS WORK
Healthy lungs are like balloons that inflate and deflate, taking in oxygen-rich air and expelling carbon dioxide (CO_2) waste. But unlike balloons, the lungs aren't hollow. Instead, they're filled with millions of microscopic sacs, called alveoli, in a configuration that resembles a bunch of grapes. The air we inhale passes through the trachea, which branches into the two bronchi that feed the right and left lungs. These main bronchi divide into smaller and smaller branches throughout both lungs, ultimately narrowing into small stems (called bronchioles) that terminate in alveoli.

When we inhale, the air passageways dilate and the alveoli expand to admit air, providing oxygen to networks of tiny blood vessels in the alveoli walls. These capillaries also transport CO_2 back to the alveoli. When we exhale, the alveoli shrink, forcing CO_2 into the bronchioles, back through the bronchi and trachea, and out of the body. Asthma involves the bronchi and bronchioles throughout both lungs.

asthma. Difficulty breathing results from the extra work involved in having to move air through these narrowed tubes, and wheezing sounds are produced by air rushing through them. Cough results from irritation of nerves in the walls of the breathing tubes, and in some cases it's the body's attempt to remove excess secretions.

Having asthma does not mean that your airways are always constricted. It means that you always have the *potential* for your airways to narrow abnormally. Much of the time your airways are fully open, and at those times you

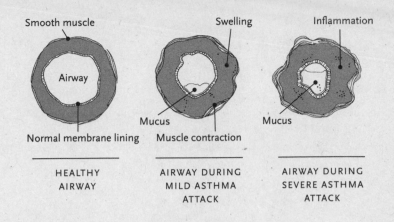

FIGURE 3: NORMAL AIRWAYS, AND AIRWAYS NARROWED BY ASTHMA
In a healthy airway (left), the passageway is unrestricted and airflow is normal. During a mild asthma attack (center), the airway walls thicken with inflammation, and muscles in the walls contract, narrowing the airways. The airways also may begin to fill with mucus, which further interferes with the flow of air. Wheezing and coughing develop as airflow deteriorates. During a severe asthma attack (right), the combination of muscle spasms, wall thickening, and increased mucus in the airways can block airflow severely.

can breathe normally. At other times your breathing may be very labored, as though you were trying to breathe through a straw with a great weight on your chest. This variability in the diameter of your breathing passages is characteristic of asthma and distinguishes it from many other lung diseases, such as emphysema and chronic bronchitis that result from cigarette smoking. With these diseases, breathing limitation tends to be permanent and unchanging, day in and day out. (For more on emphysema and chronic bronchitis, see Chapters 2, 14, and 15.) This variable narrowing of the breathing tubes that can come and go over a period of minutes to hours or days is called reversible airway narrowing and is one of the hallmarks of asthma.

TRIGGERS AND TWITCHY AIRWAYS

The concept of reversible airway narrowing is good to keep in mind because it is so central to our understanding of asthma. Another, less medical-sounding term that you will want to have in your asthma vocabulary is *twitchy*, which is used to describe the hypersensitive airways of people with asthma. Having twitchy airways doesn't mean that they *feel* twitchy—they don't. Twitchiness in the airways refers not to a sensation but to an underlying tendency for the airways to react by narrowing when they encounter certain stimuli—such as air pollutants or cold air. The very same stimuli will have no such effect on your

Asthma Triggers

COMMON, NONALLERGIC TRIGGERS	COMMON ALLERGIC TRIGGERS	UNIQUE TRIGGERS
Exercise, particularly in cold air	Dust mites	Aspirin
Viral respiratory tract infections	Cockroach debris	Sulfites
Irritants (air pollution, tobacco smoke, other forms of smoke, strong fumes)	Cat and dog (and other furry animal) dander	Menstrual periods
Certain medications (beta-blockers)	Bird feathers	
Emotional stress	Seasonal pollens	
	Mold	

partner, friend, or sister who does not have the twitchy airways of asthma. Medical terms used to describe this fundamental property of asthmatic airways are *hyperresponsiveness* and *hyperreactivity*.

If you have asthma, the word *trigger*—in its medical sense—may already be in your vocabulary. Triggers are those stimuli that set off airway narrowing in people with asthma, causing their symptoms to flare up. You may have found that if you go for a jog on a cold winter day, you begin to cough and breathe heavily afterward. Perhaps if you are around cigarette smoke or strong perfumes, you experience tightening in your chest and need to use your asthma medications. If a simple head cold settles in your chest, you may begin to wheeze and become seriously short of breath. You may even find that your asthma is sensitive to weather changes, particularly changes in humidity and barometric pressure.

Certain medications can also be asthma triggers. Aspirin is an asthma trigger for about 1 in 20 adults. (The effect of aspirin and related medications on asthma is discussed in greater depth in Chapter 11.) Everyone with asthma should avoid the group of medicines called beta-blockers, which are used to treat heart disease, high blood pressure, glaucoma, migraine headaches, and some forms of thyroid disease. One of the side effects of these medications, unique to people with asthma, is narrowing of the airways.

Food allergy can cause severe and potentially life-threatening reactions, typically involving the lips, throat, and tongue, and sometimes precipitating a very severe, generalized reaction called anaphylaxis (low blood pressure due to dilation of blood vessels throughout the body). However, food is very rarely the cause of an isolated allergic reaction involving the bronchial tubes (that is, an asthmatic reaction). (Still, if you notice a connection between eating certain foods and worsening of your asthma, by all means avoid those foods.) There is one exception: we know that the sulfites used to preserve certain foods and beverages can cause some people's asthma to flare up. Sulfite preservatives are found in processed potatoes and shrimp, and in many dried fruits, beers, and wines. (For more on food allergies, see Chapters 4 and 15.)

Our overview of asthma triggers wouldn't be complete without a brief word about the roles of stress and strong emotions. There was a time when asthma was thought to be caused by your emotions. Ulcers, colitis, and back pain were also at one time or another blamed on the psyche. We now know much more about the biology of asthma (and of these other illnesses) and can say with certainty that your strong emotions do not cause you to have asthma. They may be one of your asthma triggers and may cause some (generally mild) airway narrowing if you have asthmatic airways. They do not, however, cause you to have asthma in the first place. If you have asthma, it's not your fault!

Having lived with asthma, you can probably identify most of the things that make your asthma worse. Knowing as best you can what these things are is important, because you can then often avoid these "triggers." Sometimes avoidance is relatively easy, like staying away from the cat at your neighbor's house. At other times it involves hard work, like removing mildew from the bathroom or reducing dust accumulation in the bedroom. The payoff is better breathing and fewer attacks of asthma. (See Chapter 4 for guidance on minimizing your exposure to your asthma triggers.)

Now that you know about triggers and twitchy, or hyperresponsive, airways, you can understand why the experience of asthma is different for different people. For one thing, you may react to a specific allergic trigger whereas another person with asthma, who does not have that particular allergic sensitivity, will not. For example, if you are allergic to cats, you will probably develop symptoms of your asthma when sitting on the cat's favorite chair, but your friend with asthma who does not share your sensitivity to cat dander can sit in the very same chair without any adverse effect on his or her asthma. Furthermore, the extent of your reaction to an asthma trigger will depend on the degree of twitchiness of your airways. Two people with asthma who are sensitive to the same asthmatic trigger may react differently to it, depending on how sensitive their bronchial tubes are. A person with very sensitive airways may develop a severe asthma attack when entering a smoke-filled room. A person with only mildly sensitive airways will likely have a more minor reaction under the same circumstances.

Your particular asthma triggers and the degree of sensitivity of your airways also explain why your asthma gets better or worse at different times. The twitchiness of your airways can vary over time. It can worsen, for example, during the late summer and early fall in New England, if you are sensitive to ragweed pollen, and then lessen after the first frost. It may be the case that during your allergy season, exercise that previously caused no symptoms now precipitates cough and wheezing. Similarly, being around paint fumes now leaves you breathless and feeling constricted across your chest. The reason is that once ragweed pollen has irritated your sensitive airways, they become extrasensitive to all your asthma triggers (not just to ragweed allergen). When the pollen exposure is over, your airways gradually become less sensitive again and your asthma quiets down.

WHY DO THE BREATHING TUBES NARROW?

One cause of airway narrowing is contraction of the muscles that form a ring around our breathing tubes. These are "involuntary" muscles, like the muscles that constrict the pupils of our eyes or move food through our intestines. When exposed to an asthma trigger, they can contract quickly—in less than one minute—squeezing the bronchial tubes and causing them to become narrow. These muscles can also relax relatively quickly (in just a few minutes), either on their own or in response to medication. The terms used to describe these processes are *bronchoconstriction* or *bronchospasm* (for narrowing of the tubes) and *bronchodilation* (for their opening wider).

Inflammation is the other cause of airway narrowing in asthma. Inflammation is a medical term used to describe how our bodies react to various injuries, irritations, or infections. Inflammation generally involves some swelling (leakage of fluid from the blood vessels) and an influx from the blood of cells not normally present in that part of the body.

In asthma, inflammation involves special inflammatory cells that come out of the blood and take up residence in the walls of the bronchial tubes. These inflammatory cells contain powerful chemicals that can cause swelling of the walls of the bronchial tubes and can also stimulate the production of extra mucus. Mucus is also called phlegm. In medical dictionaries, mucus that is coughed up is called sputum, although most people use *phlegm* and *sputum* interchangeably. The mucus can plug the tubes, leaving little room for air to move in and out. Anyone who has had a head cold (all of us!) knows the effect that swelling of the nasal passageways and increased nasal mucus can have on efforts to breathe through one's nose. Similarly, difficulty breathing in asthma can be the result of swelling and excess mucus in the bronchial tubes. Unlike contraction of the muscles of the bronchial tubes, the swelling of the walls of the bronchial tubes and excess secretions within them take many hours or even days to subside.

Remembering these two different causes for narrowing of the breathing tubes is important. Medications used to treat asthma focus on these two mechanisms. They are designed to relax the muscles surrounding the airways, to reduce the inflammation of the breathing tubes, or both. Also, the speed with which asthma medications take effect depends on their site of action: bronchodilators (see Chapter 5), which relax the muscles surrounding the airways, can have a rapid effect; anti-inflammatory medications (see Chapters 6, 7, and 8) act more slowly.

WHAT CAUSES THE BRONCHIAL TUBES TO BE "TWITCHY"?

By now you may be wondering what causes the bronchial tubes to become twitchy (hypersensitive), or prone to abnormal narrowing, in the first place. In other words, what causes asthma? No one is certain of the answer to this question, and there may be not one but many different causes.

An important medical discovery made several years ago was that some inflammation is present in the bronchial tubes of people with asthma even when they feel well and when their breathing is normal. Medical researchers performed experiments in which small pieces of the walls of the bronchial tubes were sampled by biopsy. The samples were taken at times when the subjects were feeling well, free of symptoms of asthma. In the samples, scientists found evidence of persistent inflammation of the bronchial tubes.

Airway inflammation in asthma is chronic, at least to some degree. The inflammation may be so mild that it does not cause narrowing of the bronchial tubes. But the persistent presence of this inflammation is probably a major reason that the bronchial tubes are twitchy, or capable of narrowing abnormally. Medically speaking, persistent airway inflammation is an important (and treatable) cause of airway hyperresponsiveness.

DOES ASTHMA EVER JUST GO AWAY?

It is well known that children often "outgrow" their asthma. Particularly around early adolescence, asthma symptoms often go away, at least temporarily. However, up to two thirds of children with asthma continue to suffer from the disorder through puberty and adulthood.

Exactly what happens biologically to cause this change is uncertain. Part of the equation is probably simply growing bigger: as we grow, our lungs enlarge, and so do the bronchial tubes. To some extent, this makes us less prone to critical narrowing of the breathing tubes and to asthma. Another part of the equation may have to do with changes in our immune systems, particularly as they come under the influence of the sex hormones (estrogen and testosterone), although this remains speculation.

If you had asthma as a small child, and now as a young adult you are free of symptoms, you may not be entirely out of the woods. Recurrence of asthmatic symptoms in early adulthood is a common experience. The property of twitchy airways, characteristic of asthma, may stay with you, although in a milder form. Then, under the right conditions (for example, you get a pet cat or move to a new city), the sensitivity of your airways again increases and you once again experience the consequences: cough, tightness in your chest, and intermittent wheezing.

If you are an adult with asthma, the prospect that you will yet outgrow it is slim. Its severity may wax and wane, but only infrequently (less than 10 percent of the time) does asthma simply disappear for good. Better to plan to live well with asthma than simply wish it away . . . at least for now, until an asthma cure is found.

WHAT DO ALLERGIES HAVE TO DO WITH ASTHMA?

As you know from our discussion of asthma triggers, and perhaps also from your own experience, not all asthma is allergic. People with no allergic sensitivities can have asthma triggered by exercise, respiratory infections, air pollutants, and other nonallergic stimuli of asthma. Nonetheless, for many people (especially children), asthma involves an allergic sensitization of the breathing tubes and, consequently, allergic reactions in these tubes.

The idea of an allergic reaction in the bronchial tubes may seem strange. When we think of someone's allergies, we're likely to think of sneezing and a runny or stuffy nose; red, itchy, watery eyes; or perhaps dry, red, itchy skin. In fact, allergic rhinitis (allergies of the nose), allergic conjunctivitis (allergies of the lining of the eyes), and allergic dermatitis (allergies of the skin, also called eczema) frequently occur together in various combinations both in individuals and in families, and they often occur together with asthma.

The reason is that these conditions share a common mechanism; they result from a specific type of allergic reaction. The tendency for this specific type of allergic reaction is called atopy, and people who have this tendency are said to be "atopic." Asthma accompanied by allergies is often referred to as atopic asthma, or extrinsic asthma. When no tendency toward these allergic reactions can be found, asthma is said to be nonatopic, or intrinsic. Approximately 75 percent of all children and perhaps half of all adults with asthma have the atopic variety.

In asthma, allergens are inhaled substances that cause a characteristic (allergic) reaction in the bronchial tubes of susceptible people. Common allergens include animal dander; house dust; pollens of grasses, trees, and common weeds; and spores of various molds. Some people encounter allergens in the workplace, such as the baker who becomes allergic to flour dust and develops so-called baker's asthma. Other substances that we commonly breathe in, including air pollutants, appear to be the wrong size and shape to function as allergens. Although they may further irritate already sensitive airways and make your asthma flare up, they do not cause true allergic reactions.

THE ALLERGIC IMMUNE RESPONSE

Although we all breathe in allergens such as house dust, not everyone's bronchial tubes have the allergic tendency to recognize the particular allergen and react to it. If you have asthma and house dust allergy, you make a special kind of protein, called an antibody, that is precisely shaped to recognize and attach itself firmly to house dust allergen. This antibody belongs to the family of immune defenders called immunoglobulins. Those that are specifically designed to recognize allergens are referred to as immunoglobulin E, or IgE (pronounced eye-gee-ee) for short.

If your genes program your body to make IgE antibodies when you are exposed to house dust, you typically make IgE antibodies to this allergen within your first few years of life. Thereafter, whenever you breathe in house dust, these antibodies are waiting and ready to grab onto the house dust particles inhaled into your breathing tubes. You may also make other IgE antibodies, shaped slightly differently, that recognize cat allergen, or seasonal pollens, or any of scores of different allergens to which the human body produces allergic reactions. We don't know why some people make these antibodies and others do not. However, the tendency (atopy) appears to be passed on in the genes from one generation to the next.

The IgE antibodies do not roam freely in your breathing tubes but are firmly attached to immune system cells called mast cells. Mast cells are located mainly in parts of the body that regularly encounter substances from the outside world: our skin, our intestinal tract, the lining of our eyes (conjunctivae), our nose, and our breathing tubes. In people with allergies, the surfaces of their mast cells are coated with firmly attached IgE antibodies. All remains quiet until the IgE antibodies recognize and attach themselves to an allergen. Then, within seconds, an explosive reaction takes place. The mast cells are stimulated to release a barrage of chemicals that carry out the inflammatory reaction. These chemicals include histamine—which you may be aware of if you are familiar with antihistamines for treating allergies—leukotrienes (about which we will talk more later), and many others. Together, these inflammatory chemicals cause blood vessels to leak fluid, producing swelling in the breathing tubes. They stimulate the walls of the breathing tubes to secrete

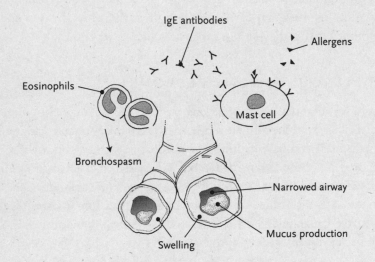

FIGURE 4: ASTHMA—AN INFLAMMATORY RESPONSE

1. Immune system cells called B lymphocytes make IgE antibodies.

2. One end of the IgE antibodies attaches to several types of cells, particularly mast cells. Mast cells live in the lining of the breathing tubes (and other parts of the body).

3. The other end of the IgE antibodies lies waiting for a particular allergen (for example, cat dander) to come into the lungs. The shape of that end of the IgE antibodies is such that it can attach to that particular allergen.

4. The allergen enters the lung. The ends of the IgE antibodies catch the allergen. When this happens, a signal is sent to the inside of the mast cells. That signal causes the mast cells suddenly to release chemicals that cause narrowing of the airways:

   • The muscles that ring the airways contract, causing the airways to narrow.

   • Excess mucus flows into the airways, making it even harder for air to pass through.

   • Fluid leaks from the blood to the walls of the airways, causing them to swell.

   • Eosinophils are attracted from the blood to the walls of the breathing tubes. There they release additional inflammatory chemicals.

Imagine This Scenario

You shuffle across the not-so-recently vacuumed bedroom carpet and lie down on the old mattress you've been meaning to replace, releasing house dust allergens into the air. You breathe the house dust allergens into your lungs, and there, waiting on the surface of mast cells in your bronchial tubes, are antibodies that recognize this allergen and attach themselves to it. The mast cells then release an explosion of inflammatory chemicals that cause the muscles surrounding your bronchial tubes to contract. These chemicals attract other inflammatory cells out of the bloodstream and into the bronchial tubes; they cause fluid to leak out of the blood vessels and into the bronchial walls, making them swell; and they stimulate the mucous glands to release mucus into the bronchial tubes. You can see that the stage is set for an asthma attack.

mucus. They also make the muscles surrounding the breathing tubes contract, causing narrowing of these passageways.

As if that weren't enough, mast cells also call in reinforcements, other cells involved in allergic inflammation that travel from the blood to the site of the allergic reaction and make things worse. The most important of these reinforcements are blood cells called eosinophils. People with asthma characteristically have eosinophils in the walls of their breathing tubes, where these cells linger, even when asthma is quiet. When asthma flares, more eosinophils accumulate. Like mast cells, they release chemicals that cause airways to narrow.

WHAT CAUSES ASTHMA?

As we've noted, no one knows exactly the cause or causes of asthma, and we can't even say for sure if it is one disease or a group of diseases with very similar manifestations. (A wise lung doctor once said, "Asthma is like love. Everyone knows what it is, but no one can agree on its definition.")

Still, much has been learned about the root causes of asthma. We know that asthma probably results from a combination of genetic susceptibility (for more on genes and asthma, see Chapter 8) and exposure to things in the environment. We inherit a tendency to develop asthma from one or both of our parents. However, even if we are born with the genes for asthma, we may never go on to develop the disease. We know this from studies of identical twins, who share the same genetic information. When one twin has asthma, the chance that the other twin will also develop it is only about one in three. Clearly, something in the environment must also be responsible for asthma.

Genes linked to asthma have recently been discovered. It's almost certain that not just one gene but a complex combination of genes accounts for the predisposition to asthma. Within the next few years we will probably learn which genes these are: We can then study how the proteins made under their direction interact to cause asthma and allergies, and perhaps explain how their interaction with stimuli in the environment has come to cause, in recent years, more frequent asthma.

We do not know exactly what in our environment contributes to the development of asthma in people with a genetic predisposition. It may involve breathing particles they are allergic to, cigarette smoke, air pollution, viruses or other germs, or some combination of these and possibly other factors.

Strange as this may seem, *not* being exposed to enough of certain stimuli such as bacteria and toxins early in life may make a person more likely to develop allergic diseases like asthma (see the "hygiene hypothesis," discussed in the next section). When considering the environmental causes of asthma, it is worth remembering that most asthma begins in early childhood. Compared with older children and adults, young children naturally tend to spend more time closer to the ground. It is to that environment, rich in both allergens and bacteria, that researchers must turn their attention in their search for the exposures that cause asthma.

WHY ARE INCREASING NUMBERS OF PEOPLE SUFFERING FROM ASTHMA?

You may have noticed that in recent years more people are carrying inhalers filled with asthma medications, and that more children miss school and more colleagues miss work because of asthma. If so, your observations are borne out by scientific studies showing that asthma has become increasingly common. Community surveys conducted in the 1960s and then repeated in the same communities 25 years later found that significantly more people had asthma and allergies at the time of the second survey. In the United States the annual prevalence of asthma increased from 3.1 percent in 1980 to 5.5 percent in 1996, a 74 percent increase.

In the United States and other Westernized countries, such as Western European nations, Australia, and New Zealand, between 5 and 7 of every 100 people are now estimated to have asthma. In rural Africa and Asia, on the other hand, less than 1 percent of the population has the disease. The higher prevalence of asthma in urban versus rural environments, and in Westernized versus developing countries, has made researchers wonder if something about our Westernized lifestyles is contributing to the modern epidemic of allergies and asthma.

Air pollution would seem an obvious culprit, but this popular explanation for the increase in asthma does not hold up under close examination. When Germany became a unified country again in 1990 after the fall of the Soviet Union, researchers compared asthma prevalence in the former East Germany and West Germany. The expectation was that asthma would be more common among people living in the highly polluted East German cities. In fact, just the opposite was true: asthma turned out to be more common in West Germany, indicating that something other than air pollution must be responsible.

Two other intriguing theories, both having to do with early childhood, are worth considering. According to one theory, modern urban life is exposing us at an early age to more common household allergens and making us more susceptible to allergy-related asthma. As a rule, we're much more likely than our ancestors to live in the city, which means we're indoors more of the time, in close quarters with dust mites, cockroaches, and animal hair (both pets' and pests'). Add to this the fact that in recent decades, television, computers, and video games have seduced us and our children into staying inside even more, and you can see that we spend a lot more of our time in the company of indoor allergens than our grandparents did. Also, in response to the energy crisis of the 1970s, home insulation was upgraded, and our houses and apartments tended to be more tightly sealed. The result was far less circulation of fresh air and, consequently, exposure to higher concentrations of allergens.

The second theory—called the hygiene hypothesis—has to do with how our immune system is challenged in the early years of life. According to this hypothesis, the immune systems of children who are exposed to lots of important infections and toxins early in life tend to ignore less serious challenges, such as those from allergens like pollen and dog dander. On the other hand, when children are exposed to relatively fewer serious infections, as has been the case in the developed nations over the past 50 years, the immune system has more "free time" to direct its attention against harmless allergens. Stated another way, the good news of the past 50 years is that serious infections such as tuberculosis and whooping cough are much less common. The bad news, according to this theory, is that our immune systems are more likely to react in a way that causes allergic diseases, including asthma.

There is growing evidence for the hygiene hypothesis: several major studies supporting it have been published in recent years. For example, one recent large study found that infants who go to day care and/or have older siblings are less likely to develop asthma later in childhood than those who don't attend day care or have siblings. Because they were more frequently exposed to other children, the infants who went to day care and had older siblings were naturally exposed to more germs. It may be that their developing immune systems learned to focus on germs and to ignore allergens, thereby decreasing the likelihood of allergies and asthma later in childhood. Another study, conducted in rural communities in Europe, observed that higher amounts of certain bacterial toxins found in children's mattresses were protective against the development of asthma and allergies. If your immune system is exposed to these nonliving parts of germs at a young age, it seems to become tolerant to other aspects of the natural environment, including pollens and animal dander. In parts of the world where children grow up in close proximity to farm animals and their droppings, the prevalence of asthma tends to be low.

Yet another theory about the increase in asthma has to do not with our immune system but with our weight. We all know that obesity is a common medical problem in the United States and that it has been linked to heart disease and diabetes, among other diseases. Findings from several studies suggest that we can add asthma to the list of obesity-related illnesses. In one study, researchers looked at more than 7,000 children, age 4 to 17, and found that those who were overweight were almost twice as likely to develop asthma as normal-weight children. The exact connection between asthma and obesity is unknown, but it may be that the pressure of excess weight on the chest can contribute to constriction of the airways. We have some supportive evidence for these various theories, but not enough to consider any of them fact.

One thing we are sure of, though, is that the burden of asthma is not shared equally throughout this country. African-Americans in the United States are hospitalized at least three times more often for asthma than white people, and the gap has widened over the last decade or two. The highest rates of asthma hospitalizations occur among Hispanics and African-Americans living in our inner cities and, more specifically, within the poorer neighborhoods of our inner cities. The racial differences in asthma severity probably relate mostly to poverty. Being poor and living in the inner city typically mean worse housing conditions, greater exposure to air pollutants and indoor allergens such as debris from cockroaches, less access to medications and preventive medical care, and more medical, social, and psychological conditions that interfere with good asthma care. One of the greatest challenges facing modern asthma care is achieving an equitable distribution of the available asthma therapies to people of all racial and ethnic backgrounds, regardless of socioeconomic status. (For more on inner-city asthma, see Chapter 11.)

CAN ASTHMA AND ALLERGIES BE PREVENTED?

Our inquiries about what causes asthma and why it is becoming more prevalent suggest the obvious follow-up question: Can asthma and allergies be prevented? The answer is "Not yet, not with any certainty."

Here are some things you *can* do. Children born to mothers who smoke cigarettes are more likely to develop asthma. Teenagers and adults who smoke cigarettes are themselves more likely to develop asthma. For these and innumerable other reasons, you can improve your own health and that of your children by not smoking.

Children born of atopic parents more often develop asthma if they grow up in homes with high levels of dust mite or cockroach allergens than children of such parents who have less allergic exposure during early childhood. If you have asthma and allergies and you worry that your child will develop asthma, keeping a clean home makes good sense. We cannot make the same claim about a pet-free house. Recent evidence does not support the idea that having a cat at home will predispose your child to developing asthma and allergies later in life. In fact, just the opposite may be true under certain circumstances.

Finally, we hear a lot about breast-feeding and immune protection, which raises the question of whether or not breast-fed babies are less likely to develop asthma. Although we can say for sure that breast milk is the best nutrition for babies, it is hard to know whether breast-feeding helps protect against the development of asthma. Breast milk is full of nutrients and maternal antibodies and hormones that help protect infants from infections. As to whether breast milk protects against asthma, the research findings are inconsistent. One recent large study suggested that breast-feeding an infant for at least four months after birth protects against childhood asthma, whereas another study found a potential connection between breast-feeding and increased likelihood of childhood asthma, but only if the mother had asthma.

More definitive recommendations about the primary prevention of asthma will need to await better understanding of the cause(s) of asthma. Studies are under way to test anti-inflammatory medications as a means of preventing the development of asthma in children as young as 2 to 4 years old who were judged to be at increased risk. We have to await the results of these studies. In the meantime, it is probably best not to rearrange your life or lifestyle based on speculation and theory (with a notable exception: don't smoke cigarettes!).

Although the possibility of preventing asthma is still pretty "iffy," the probability of controlling it and preventing disabling episodes is excellent, with careful attention to avoiding the things that cause flare-ups, and close adherence to a medication plan tailored to your particular needs. We began this book with the observation that if you have asthma, you have plenty of company. That company includes many people who lead, or have led, active, successful lives. Among them are John F. Kennedy, the 35th president of the United States, and Theodore Roosevelt, the 26th president. Other famous people said to have asthma are the actresses Liza Minnelli and Elizabeth Taylor, the singer Judy Collins, and the saxophonist Kenny G. A number of Olympic athletes have asthma, including swimmers Tom Dolan, Amy Van Dyken, and Nancy Hogshead and track-and-field star Jackie Joyner-Kersee.

Asthma needn't prevent you from leading an active life, including participation in intense physical activities. If you work closely with your doctor to control your symptoms, you can probably be symptom-free and fully active most of the time. Our purpose throughout this book is to help you achieve this goal. Don't settle for anything less.

CHAPTER 2

Diagnosing Your Asthma

"I found out I had asthma when I was in third grade. It started during a Little League game, when I was running home really fast. I couldn't breathe. I started freaking out and thinking maybe I was going to die. Everyone was wondering what was wrong. I went to the doctor and found out it was asthma. Then I was worried that maybe I couldn't play sports anymore, but the doctor said I could."
— DON, 18

"I was always 'bronchial' as a child. I got a lot of colds that settled in my chest, and missed a lot of school. I wasn't affected so much as a teenager. I'm surprised I wasn't diagnosed sooner, but I wasn't diagnosed until I was 24. I had another bad cold, with wheezing and difficulty breathing. I went to my primary care doctor, and he said, 'It sounds like you have asthma.' "
— MARGARET, 60

SOMETIMES THE DIAGNOSIS OF ASTHMA is straightforward. A young child who is generally healthy but develops noisy, whistling breathing and a persistent cough every time he or she goes out to play in the cold winter air—and has the same trouble when around a pet cat—probably has asthma. You don't need an asthma specialist to tell you that your child has asthma; your mother-in-law, neighbor, or child's schoolteacher has probably already suggested it.

The diagnosis is straightforward in this example because all the clues are there. First, there are the characteristic symptoms. Coughing, wheezing, and shortness of breath are typical of asthma. Other sensations may include tightness across the chest, the sense that something prevents you from taking a full, deep breath in, or occasionally a tickle under the chin (although without the bumps or redness that suggest a skin rash). Second, in this example, symptoms are triggered by stimuli (exercising on a cold day and exposure to a furry animal) that are also typical for asthma. An allergic sensitivity to a cat, in which the sensitivity causes narrowing of the breathing tubes, is in most instances asthma.

Then there is the fact that these symptoms come and go. The narrowing of the breathing tubes varies over time in asthma. The symptoms of asthma may last for minutes, hours, or days, but they are not permanent. People often describe an "attack" of asthma: when the symptoms abate, the attack is over and they feel better again.

This brings us to the fourth characteristic feature of this story: in between episodes of coughing, wheezing, and shortness of breath, the child feels perfectly well, without any respiratory symptoms. For someone with asthma, days, weeks, or months may go by without any chest symptoms until some trigger sets off another round of asthma symptoms. The symptoms of asthma are intermittent, even though the tendency for narrowing of the breathing tubes is persistent (present even when symptoms are not).

One of the biggest sources of confusion has to do with this last observation. It is easy to believe that you have asthma when you are coughing, wheezing, and short of breath, and then to believe that your asthma has gone away when you are well again. In truth, the *manifestations* of your asthma come and go— and the narrowing of your breathing tubes comes and goes—but your asthma is there all the time. As discussed in Chapter 1, asthma is the tendency of the breathing tubes to narrow abnormally in response to certain stimuli. That tendency is present even when you are feeling well. Understanding this fact is more than a matter of terminology. It allows you to take actions when you are well that will prevent the next "attack" of asthma symptoms.

THE DOCTOR'S ROLE IN DIAGNOSING ASTHMA

The doctor will ask you questions about your (or your child's) respiratory symptoms in more detail. If you are coughing, are you coughing up clear mucus (also called phlegm or sputum)? That is common in asthma. Or do you have a fever, and are you coughing up dark, discolored mucus? That would be unusual for asthma but common in a respiratory tract infection, such as bronchitis or pneumonia. Do the symptoms awaken you or your child (or both!) at night? Asthma often worsens in the early-morning hours, but so do other respiratory diseases. If your child is very small, you may be asked to be a particularly careful observer: How many breaths does the child take in one minute (his or her breathing rate)? Do the nostrils flare open with each breath in, and do the spaces between the ribs and the indentation at the front of the neck above the breastbone get sucked inward with each strained inhalation? These are signs of labored breathing that may indicate an asthma attack. Do your child's lips and skin turn blue when he or she is struggling to breathe? This is a serious finding, suggesting low oxygen in the blood.

The doctor will also want to know about all the things that make your breathing—or your child's breathing—worse, and better. Some may be non-specific and as likely to occur in any condition that, like asthma, causes breathing difficulties. For instance, many people complain that they find it hard to breathe in very hot and humid weather or in smoke-filled rooms. A person with asthma might well mention these reactions, but so too would someone with emphysema or heart failure or cystic fibrosis. These complaints are not specific to asthma.

On the other hand, if working in the horse barn or dusting at home or spray-painting automobiles at work brings on coughing and wheezing and shortness of breath, the doctor will strongly suspect asthma based on these highly characteristic triggers of your symptoms. Along these same lines, does taking aspirin, ibuprofen, or Aleve provoke your symptoms? Does wine, beer, or food containing sulfites cause you to have your symptoms? Have you recently started any new medications (such as a beta-blocker for your heart or for high blood pressure)? Has your house been overrun by roaches or mice? Any of these characteristic triggers of asthma symptoms might explain your recent symptoms and point to a diagnosis of asthma.

Another consideration will be the age at which symptoms of asthma begin. Approximately 75 percent of all people with asthma experience symptoms for the first time by age 7. Adults are often first diagnosed with asthma in their twenties and thirties, but in retrospect they can usually find some clues to asthma beginning at an earlier age: the frequent bronchitis as a child, the coughing and wheezing that lingered for weeks after each cold, the excessive shortness of breath when playing sports with other children. Their asthma actually began in early childhood but was not diagnosed until early adulthood. The onset of asthma at age 60 or 70 is uncommon. We search long and hard for another explanation for coughing and wheezing at this age. Some other illness mimicking asthma is usually the correct diagnosis. (See Chapter 14 for a discussion of asthma in the elderly.)

Other questions from your doctor may provide some circumstantial evidence for or against asthma, as this diagnostic case is being built. Is there any history of other allergic diseases—hay fever, hives, or eczema, for example? These conditions point to an allergic tendency (called atopy) that would weigh in favor of an allergic disease of the bronchial tubes (that is, asthma). Similarly, a strong family history of allergies and asthma would weigh indirectly in favor of your symptoms being due to asthma. On the other hand, if you have smoked cigarettes for more than 10 to 20 years, your doctor will begin to wonder whether emphysema and chronic bronchitis, rather than asthma, is the cause of your wheeze, cough, and shortness of breath.

Certainly, your doctor (or other health care provider) will want to examine you (or your child) and, in particular, listen with a stethoscope to your lungs. The wheezes of asthma have a characteristic musical quality. They can be heard throughout the chest, and they tend to be particularly prominent (and perhaps exclusively heard) when you breathe out. During a breathing cycle (that is, one breath in and one breath out), the bronchial tubes throughout the lungs always narrow more when you breathe out, and widen more when you breathe in.

At the same time, your doctor knows that "not all that wheezes is asthma." Other illnesses can cause a musical sound during breathing. For example, as suggested above, sometimes the wheezing sounds due to chronic bronchitis and emphysema closely mimic the wheezing of asthma. (See Chapters 14 and 15 for more on chronic bronchitis and emphysema.) At other times the wheeze is clearly distinguishable, as in a swelling of the upper airway (for example, epiglottitis, an infectious swelling of the tissue at the back of the throat just above the vocal cords), when the sound is low-pitched and heard mainly on inspiration. Another example is a "focal wheeze," heard primarily at one location in the lungs, suggesting the narrowing of a single bronchial tube (possibly caused by a tumor or an aspirated peanut—in other words, a peanut that has "gone down the wrong tube" and been inhaled into the lungs).

Equally important, your doctor will know that the absence of wheezes does not exclude a diagnosis of asthma. The chest can sound perfectly clear to the stethoscope in someone with asthma if you listen at a time when the breathing tubes are not narrowed or narrowed only a little. You or your child may have asthma but be free of symptoms at the moment that you are in the doctor's office. If the doctor could only listen to your lungs when you are coughing at three o'clock in the morning or when you develop a chest cold! Given the story of your symptoms, the doctor may still suspect asthma even if no wheezing is heard during your examination.

DIAGNOSTIC TESTING

What further tests can your doctor perform to rule asthma in or out for certain? Isn't there some simple blood test for asthma? The answer is no, there is no blood test for asthma. There are blood and skin tests for allergies (for further discussion of these tests, see Chapter 4), but whether or not there is evidence that you have allergies will not answer the question, "Do I have asthma?" People with allergies revealed by blood or skin testing may have hay fever or eczema without having asthma; and people with no detectable allergies at all may still have asthma.

Sometimes, when considering a diagnosis of asthma, the doctor will send a blood sample to be tested for the number of eosinophils or the amount of immunoglobulin E antibody (IgE). Lots of eosinophils or high levels of IgE antibody in the blood point to an allergic predisposition and weigh somewhat in favor of an allergic disease such as asthma. (IgE and eosinophils are discussed in more detail in Chapters 1 and 8.) But, like having a strong family history of asthma, this blood test result offers only circumstantial evidence in favor of a diagnosis of asthma. It is far from proof.

Would a chest X ray help diagnose asthma? No, but we would recommend one anyway. The narrowing of the bronchial tubes cannot be seen with a chest X ray, so a chest X ray in asthma is almost always normal. But we find it useful in order to exclude alternative diagnoses. Some of the diseases that can be mistaken for asthma will show up on a chest X ray. For example, in young children the X ray can reveal congenital abnormalities, cystic fibrosis, and small objects that have accidentally been breathed into the lungs. In young adults the chest X ray can reveal sarcoidosis (an inflammatory condition of the lungs) and Hodgkin's disease. In older adults the X ray can reveal advanced emphysema, congestive heart failure, chronic respiratory infections, and lung cancers. (For more on other diseases and conditions that can be mistaken for asthma, see Chapters 14 and 15.)

DIAGNOSIS BY "THERAPEUTIC TRIAL"

Suppose that just by listening to the story that you tell, your doctor believes that you or your child has asthma. He or she may hear wheezes on listening to the chest, or you may report hearing wheezes that you recognize as asthmatic. Everything seems to fit well for a diagnosis of asthma, and alternative diagnoses seem unlikely given the information at hand. The odds favor a diagnosis of asthma: statistically speaking, asthma is a very common illness of childhood. Other causes of intermittent wheezing, coughing, and shortness of breath occur much more rarely.

At this point your doctor may ask you to begin treatment for asthma. Depending on your age and the perceived severity of your asthma, the treatment may be one or more medications taken once or more each day. The doctor will want you to begin to feel better quickly and will tailor your treatment accordingly.

On the other hand, if you are feeling well during your office visit and if the diagnosis of asthma is not entirely certain, your doctor may prescribe a medication, usually a quick-acting bronchodilator (see Chapter 5), to be taken when your symptoms occur. In an adult, the medication is delivered from an inhaler device. Depending on age, a child may be given one of the following to use: an inhaler with a holding chamber (with or without a mask); a bronchodilator given by nebulization; or medication in the form of a liquid or chewable tablet.

As part of this therapeutic trial, your doctor will instruct you to take the medicine when you develop the symptoms that are suspected of resulting from asthma. If the coughing, wheezing, shortness of breath, and chest tightness go away within minutes of taking the medication—because it has successfully opened the bronchial tubes more widely by causing the muscles surrounding these tubes to relax—a diagnosis of asthma is likely. If the medication provides absolutely no relief and the symptoms continue despite taking it, there is a good chance that something other than asthma is the cause. Further testing will be necessary.

In some instances this approach may be sufficient, but it is not perfect. It may be hard to be certain that the medication caused the symptoms to go away; maybe it was just the act of resting quietly for five to ten minutes that brought relief. Or perhaps the symptoms go away only partially after using the medication: Is the correct diagnosis asthma with inadequate treatment, or is it some other illness helped only a little by a bronchodilator medication?

MEASURING YOUR BREATHING: PULMONARY FUNCTION TESTS

At our asthma center, and in many physicians' offices, equipment is available to measure how fast you can force air from your lungs. The equipment is called a spirometer and the test is called spirometry (*spiro* derives from the Greek word for "breath"). It is the most commonly performed test in the pulmonary function testing laboratory of any hospital. The question of how fast you can force air from your lungs is the key one because it reflects in large measure how wide open (or narrow) the bronchial tubes are. If these air passageways are wide open (like a garden hose), the air can flow out rapidly. If the air passageways are narrowed (like a straw) because of asthmatic constriction, the air will flow out slowly.

Here's a fine point: *air* is a mixture of gases in our atmosphere, mostly nitrogen, with approximately 21 percent oxygen. The gas that you breathe out is a different mixture, with a little less oxygen and nitrogen and considerably more carbon dioxide than contained in air. Strictly speaking, you breathe in air and breathe out a different gas mixture. But unless you are speaking with a physician at a very intellectual cocktail party, you can probably skip the distinction, as we have throughout this book.

Spirometry is painless and takes five minutes or less to perform. Seated in a chair, you are asked to breathe into a recording device. A soft plastic clip like a clothespin will pinch your nostrils together so that all of the air coming out of your lungs will pass through your mouth and into the recording equipment. You will be asked first to inhale the largest breath that you can, then quickly and forcefully empty all the air that you can from your lungs in a steady, continuous effort until there is no more air to expel. It takes at least six seconds of blowing out hard to get every last ounce of air out. When you are done and have rested a moment or two, you will be asked to repeat the test a second time, then usually a third time as well. The best of the three efforts will be recorded as your spirometry result.

Spirometry records how much air you can exhale and how fast it exits your lungs. The amount exhaled is referred to as your vital capacity. The speed at which the air was exhaled is best characterized by the amount of air that came out in the first second of exhalation. The speed at which you can force air out of your lungs is described in liters per second. The amount of air that you forced from your lungs in the first second of exhalation is, for obvious reasons, referred to as the one-second forced expiratory volume and is abbreviated as FEV_1 (pronounced eff-ee-vee-one). It is a measure of the rate of flow: liters in one second.

The computerized spirometer has been programmed with the normal values for FEV_1 and vital capacity for a person of your gender, age, and height. "Normal" is based on the results from testing healthy people who never smoked cigarettes, have no respiratory symptoms, and have no history of heart or lung disease. Healthy people of your gender, age, and height will have a range of values, some higher than average, some lower than average. Your test results will be compared with that normal range: Are the FEV_1 and vital capacity within the normal range for a healthy person of your gender, age, and height, or is the FEV_1 below normal, with a normal vital capacity? The latter pattern is seen in asthma.

Asthma is not the only disorder that can cause this pattern, which is called obstructive because the flow of air out of the lungs is "obstructed" or abnormally slow. Other diseases have an obstructive pattern that is indistinguishable on spirometry from that of asthma. These include emphysema and chronic bronchitis (the cigarette-smoking-related lung diseases), bronchiectasis (the lung disease of cystic fibrosis), and bronchiolitis (a narrowing of the very smallest bronchial tubes, called bronchioles). A simple chest cold (an acute bronchitis) will not cause your spirometry to change significantly.

What good is this test, then, if it cannot distinguish asthma from other related lung diseases? It is a very good test, for the following reasons. First, if you are young and have never smoked cigarettes, far and away the most common cause of an obstructive pattern on spirometry is asthma. The other diseases are far less likely to be the cause because they occur much less frequently. Second, if you want to know how severely narrowed your bronchial tubes are, spirometry is the best test. The test results may not only point to a diagnosis of asthma but also inform your doctor as to how severe the bronchial narrowing is at this moment in time. This information will help him or her choose the appropriate intensity of treatment.

The third reason may be the most convincing. There is a second phase to spirometry that can help clinch the diagnosis of asthma. If your breathing tests have an obstructive pattern, you will routinely be asked to take a quick-acting asthma medication while still in the office or pulmonary function testing lab, then repeat the spirometry test. Most often the medication administered is an inhaled bronchodilator that acts to relax the muscles surrounding the bronchial tubes. If the obstructive pattern is due to asthma, it will to a large extent, and perhaps entirely, disappear within five to ten minutes of taking this medication. On the repeat test, the air will empty much faster from your lungs than on the first test. Specifically, on post-bronchodilator testing, the FEV_1 will increase by at least 15 percent. In this way one can demonstrate the reversible airway narrowing that is characteristic of asthma.

At last, we have come up with a test to diagnose asthma with great certainty. If your doctor suspects that you have asthma and orders spirometry, if the spirometry shows an obstructive pattern, and if there is a big improvement after the administration of a quick-acting bronchodilator medication (and especially if the obstructive pattern disappears on the repeat spirometry test), you have asthma. Period.

With young children, if they say that they can hold their breath underwater, we find they can manage the maneuver involved with spirometry. In general, children can give a reliable test performance around age 6. Testing is best done in an office or laboratory that is experienced in pediatric pulmonary function testing. To help capture the child's interest and cooperation, computer software is available that displays candles being blown out on a birthday cake or a hot air balloon being kept aloft with the force of the exhalation while the child is blowing into the spirometer.

WHAT IF SPIROMETRY IS NOT AVAILABLE TO ME?

As valuable as spirometry is in helping evaluate asthma and other breathing conditions, it is *not* available in most physicians' offices. The cost of the equipment and associated technical support and the expertise needed to interpret the results stand in the way of its routine use in most general medical practices. Also, your doctor and you may decide that it is too much trouble and too expensive for you to go to your local hospital to have your pulmonary function tested. In this case, the peak flow meter is a simpler alternative.

As you will learn throughout this book (see Chapters 3, 10, 11, 12, 13, 16, and 17), we consider the peak flow meter an exceedingly valuable tool for monitoring the condition of your asthma. Like a spirometer, a peak flow meter can measure how fast air can be forced from the lungs, an indicator of how

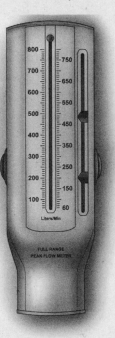

FIGURE 5: PEAK FLOW METER
When you breathe forcefully into a peak flow meter, it measures the maximum speed with which air can be pushed out of your lungs through the system of breathing tubes. It's a valuable tool for monitoring your asthma.

Normal Peak Flow Values for Adult Women and Men, in Liters/Minute*

WOMEN

Age	Height				
	4 FT. 7 IN.	5 FEET	5 FT. 5 IN.	5 FT. 10 IN.	6 FT. 3 IN.
20	390	423	460	496	529
25	385	418	454	490	523
30	380	413	448	483	516
35	375	408	442	476	509
40	370	402	436	470	502
45	365	397	430	464	495
50	360	391	424	457	488
55	355	386	418	451	482
60	350	380	412	445	475
65	345	375	406	439	468
70	340	369	400	432	461

MEN

Age	Height				
	5 FEET	5 FT. 5 IN.	5 FT. 10 IN.	6 FT. 3 IN.	6 FT. 8 IN.
20	554	602	649	693	740
25	543	590	636	679	725
30	532	577	622	664	710
35	521	565	619	651	695
40	509	552	596	636	680
45	498	540	583	622	665
50	486	527	569	607	649
55	475	515	556	593	634
60	463	502	542	578	618
65	452	490	529	564	603
70	440	477	515	550	587

*People of any given age and height with normal lung function will have a *range* of values. The numbers given in these charts are the average values from the middle of this range of normal values. The range of normal values extends approximately 100 liters/minute below the average numbers given for men, and approximately 85 liters/minute below the average numbers shown for women. Thus, a 20-year-old man who is 5 feet tall and has a peak flow of 520 liters/minute has a peak flow 34 liters/minute below the *average* value for a healthy person of his same age and height, but his peak flow is within the range of normal values.

much obstruction there is in your airways. Unlike with spirometry, the peak flow meter does not record how much air can be emptied from your lungs, the vital capacity. As a result, it cannot distinguish diseases like asthma (which reduce the peak flow because of narrowing of the bronchial tubes) from diseases like lung scarring or pneumonia or collapse (which reduce peak flow because the lungs contain less air). It cannot indicate to your doctor that the problem causing your coughing or wheezing or chest tightness is one characterized by an *obstructive* abnormality. It is neither as detailed nor as sensitive an instrument as the spirometer.

Still, it is relatively inexpensive (as little as $20 to $30 for individual-use devices) and useful in several ways. First, a normal peak flow value is reassuring: there is no sign of serious asthma at that time. Second, a result indicating a reduced peak flow can be followed by administration of a bronchodilating medication. If the peak flow increases within minutes by approximately 20 percent, the results support a diagnosis of asthma. Third, a peak flow value can be readily recorded at every visit to the doctor. Keeping track of the trend in your peak flow values is, in our opinion, an important part of your asthma care.

Measuring your peak flow requires a rapid expiratory burst of only about one second. The results depend critically on the strength of the effort; you need to give a hard, rapid blast with your respiratory muscles. The results are recorded in liters per minute. Like FEV_1, normal peak flow varies with age, height, and gender. Normal reference values have been compiled, based on measurements made in healthy, nonsmoking people. Tables containing the normal values for peak flow are widely available, like the one on page 30. (Normal peak flow values for children are given later in Chapter 12.) Each time you are tested, you should make at least three efforts at achieving your best value. The highest of the three is considered to be your actual peak flow.

DIAGNOSING ASTHMA WHEN YOUR BREATHING TESTS ARE NORMAL

Asthmatic narrowing of the breathing tubes comes and goes. When you are having your breathing tested, you may be feeling well and have normal lung function. (If your breathing feels poor but your breathing tests are normal, the cause of your symptoms is probably something other than asthma.) How can your doctor be sure that the symptoms you report are due to asthma if at the moment of your visit your chest examination and breathing tests are normal?

Three options are available. First, you can return when you're not feeling well. Your asthmatic symptoms will probably return at some point, and at that

How to Test Your Peak Flow

1. Slide the indicator down as far as it will go. This sets the meter to zero.

2. Hold the meter in one hand. Keep your fingers away from the numbers so that you won't interfere with the movement of the indicator.

3. Sit upright or stand up. Take a full breath in, as big as you can. Close your lips firmly around the mouthpiece of the peak flow meter. Blow out as fast and hard as you can. You need only blow out for one to two seconds, but it needs to be a quick and forceful exhalation from the very start. Be careful not to put your tongue in the hole of the mouthpiece.

4. The indicator will go up and stay up. Find the number where the marker stopped. This number indicates your peak flow on this first effort. Set the indicator back down to zero to repeat the measurement.

5. Repeat the peak flow measurement two more times, being sure to first set the indicator back to zero and making a note of your peak flow number.

6. Write down the *best* of your three tries on a piece of paper or on your peak flow chart. The best of the three tries is your peak flow at that moment.

time your doctor can examine and test your lungs. Like the auto mechanic trying to explain an odd knocking sound in your car's engine, your doctor will have an easier time being certain as to the diagnosis if the symptoms are present at the time of the visit. The disadvantages to this approach are probably obvious. You may want to fend off serious symptoms of asthma before they recur, rather than waiting to react to their presence. And it may not be easy to get an immediate appointment with your medical provider when your symptoms do occur.

The second approach takes advantage of self-measurement of your lung function at home (or at school or work). You can obtain a peak flow meter for home use; they are plastic, lightweight, and easily portable. Measure and record your peak flow when you feel well, then again when you develop that troublesome cough or chest tightness. Peak flow values that remain unchanged with each test, both when you are feeling well and when you are having symptoms suggesting possible asthma, argue against a diagnosis of asthma. Peak flow values that fall by approximately 20 percent or more during symptomatic periods and that recover to normal when you are feeling well point strongly to a diagnosis of asthma. You will want to bring the written record of your peak flow values to your next doctor's appointment for his or her review and interpretation.

This approach can be combined very effectively with the therapeutic trial described above. Your doctor may give you a quick-acting bronchodilator to use when you develop symptoms. Check your peak flow when symptomatic, then again after taking the bronchodilator. A big improvement (more than 20 percent) in peak flow after using the bronchodilator, together with symptomatic improvement, is strong evidence for a diagnosis of asthma.

Your doctor can write a prescription for a peak flow meter to be obtained at your local pharmacy. You can also purchase one by mail. One national vendor is National Allergy Supply, 1-800-522-1448.

The third approach is the most precise, but also the most labor intensive and most costly. It involves a more detailed pulmonary test, called a bronchoprovocation challenge, which is conducted under close supervision in the pulmonary function testing laboratory. The idea is to find out whether a stimulus applied to the bronchial tubes will provoke their narrowing (as in asthma) or not. A similar concept underlies a test with which you may be more familiar: the exercise stress test. In someone with a significant coronary blockage, exercise brings out the problem that was not evident at rest: the patient may experience chest pain while walking on the treadmill, and the electrocardiogram now gives evidence of lack of blood supply to an area of the heart.

So too, in a carefully monitored setting, it is possible to demonstrate the sensitivity of the bronchial tubes to a provocative stimulus. The purpose of the bronchoprovocation challenge test is to try to bring out bronchial tube narrowing in a person with asthma—in effect, to cause a minor asthma flare-up. If the subject does not have asthma, the stimulus has no significant effect on his or her breathing.

To test for bronchial tube narrowing, repetitive breathing tests (that is, spirometry) are performed. In many pulmonary function laboratories, the provocative stimulus is a chemical called methacholine. Odorless and tasteless, methacholine is derived from a normal nerve transmitter in the body (acetylcholine). It is a nonspecific stimulant for contraction of the bronchial tubes; it does not depend on whether you have allergic or nonallergic asthma or on any other special characteristics of your asthma. Methacholine is given by inhalation in minute quantities at first. If no reaction is observed (the rate of airflow out of the lungs, as measured by FEV_1, remains unchanged), then the next higher dose is given. If no significant change is observed, then a still higher dose of methacholine is inhaled, and so forth. If at any point the patient experiences coughing, wheezing, or tightness in the chest and the FEV_1 falls by 20 percent or more, the test is stopped and a bronchodilating medication administered.

If a relatively small dose of methacholine triggers significant narrowing of the breathing tubes, asthma is likely. If the FEV_1 does not fall by 20 percent even after the highest dose of the stimulus, a diagnosis of asthma can be excluded. Methacholine is just one of a number of possible provocative stimuli. In children, exercise or possibly rapid breathing of cold air is also commonly used. Typically, just one "dose" is administered.

Bronchoprovocation challenges are specialized tests not available at every medical facility. At our asthma center, where they are available, we tend to reserve their use for special circumstances, such as when a therapeutic trial combined with home peak flow monitoring has been inconclusive, when previous evidence for asthma has been ambiguous, or when for some reason an immediate answer regarding the diagnosis of asthma is needed, rather than an assessment based on observations made over a period of time.

CONSULTATION WITH AN ASTHMA SPECIALIST

Most often the diagnosis of asthma will be made by your primary care physician, whether a pediatrician, family physician, or internist. You may have had previous experiences with asthma. Perhaps it runs in your family, and you may suspect the diagnosis and call your physician's attention to it. What sounds like asthma, comes and goes like asthma, and responds to medications like asthma is in all probability asthma.

It is in those other situations, where there is uncertainty about the diagnosis, that an asthma specialist can be helpful. Perhaps some aspects of your story are typical for asthma but others are not. Perhaps your major complaint is only recurrent coughing: Could it be asthma, or is it some other lung disease? Perhaps you have tried asthma medications and found that they don't work for you. Are you using the medicines incorrectly, or is the diagnosis of asthma wrong? If you or your doctor—or both—are puzzled about a diagnosis of asthma, consultation with a specialist is warranted.

An asthma specialist will have the advantage of being able to focus on this one medical problem and to spend time talking to you and examining you carefully with the diagnosis of asthma in mind. He or she will be familiar with the many diseases that can mimic asthma and will have access to methods of testing often not available to your primary physician. You may also find your asthma specialist and his or her staff to be a wonderful resource for one-on-one teaching about asthma and related diseases and for educational resources that you can review at home.

Most asthma specialists are either allergists or pulmonary medicine specialists (pulmonologists)—or, in rare instances, both. Allergists come to asthma with an in-depth understanding of allergies and the immune system. Pulmonologists train in diseases of the chest, with a strong background in assessment of pulmonary function. At our asthma center, allergists and pulmonologists practice side by side and share a common understanding of asthma and its treatments. We place little emphasis on the differences in our specialist training and pursue a shared and collaborative approach to our patients.

Still, we have to acknowledge that you may encounter differences between allergists and pulmonologists in their thinking about asthma. To characterize these differences in very broad terms, allergists have more expertise in performing and interpreting allergy tests and are more inclined to recommend allergen immunotherapy (see Chapter 4) to treat asthma and other atopic diseases. Pulmonologists have more expertise in pulmonary function tests, including bronchoprovocation challenges, and are skilled at invasive procedures such as bronchoscopy (examining the inside of the windpipe and bronchial tubes with a flexible, lighted tube). In the end, it is likely that the choice between consultation with an allergist or a pulmonologist will depend mostly on the resources available in your medical community, the referral patterns already established by your primary physician, and the reputation of the individual specialists whom you are considering.

ONE LAST POINT

What we describe in this chapter about the diagnosis of asthma assumes an orderly process (whether very straightforward or quite complex) that unfolds over one or more visits to the doctor. In the case of a very young child it may even involve waiting a season or two to see if the child's wheezing recurs. However, sometimes this process is short-circuited. On occasion, the first manifestation of asthma is a sudden, severe asthma attack that lands the patient in the hospital emergency department. In this instance, the diagnosis of asthma is probably immediately obvious to the treating physician because of the severity of symptoms and the dramatic findings on physical examination, and treatment begins immediately.

Asthma that announces itself so dramatically might seem to suggest a severe case. Although severe asthma may be heralded in this way, it is also possible to have a single, severe episode of asthma followed by mild disease over the ensuing months and years. Even people with mild asthma can have severe flare-ups.

Naturally, the first thing that every adult, child, or parent of a child diagnosed with asthma wants to know is, "How serious is my asthma?" That is the question we answer in the next chapter.

CHAPTER 3

Judging the Severity of Your Asthma

For both you and your doctor, knowing how severe your asthma is will help in adjusting the intensity of your treatment. In asthma treatment, one size does not fit all. Not everyone with asthma receives, or should receive, the same treatment. Choosing a treatment appropriate for you will depend on an accurate assessment of how severe your asthma is. (For a fuller discussion about matching appropriate treatment to asthma severity, see Chapter 10.) And because your symptoms may vary over time, from week to week or from month to month, you will need to report accurately to your doctor your experiences with asthma. When you visit your doctor, he or she gets a "snapshot" of the severity of your asthma based on how you are doing at that moment. What the doctor needs is more like a motion picture, based on your experiences with asthma 24 hours a day, 7 days a week. You can provide that motion picture by the way you describe your symptoms since you last saw the doctor.

While paying close attention to your asthma symptoms is always important, accurately assessing their severity when you are having an asthma flare-up is crucial. Something has set off your asthma, and you are having trouble with your breathing. You may suddenly develop bad coughing spells; you may become breathless after walking up one flight of stairs. Sleeping may be difficult because of tightness in your chest, so you may find yourself more comfortable sitting in a lounge chair all night. Is it safe to wait until morning to call the doctor, or should you seek emergency help immediately? Is this flare-up dangerous, or just annoying? How you respond to an attack will depend on how serious you perceive it to be. Accurately judging the severity of an asthma flare-up can be lifesaving, either for you or for your child with asthma. We will have more to say about this important subject later in this chapter, and in Chapters 12, 16, and 17.

SETTING GOALS

A reasonable starting point in a discussion of the severity of asthma is agreement on what good asthma control should look like. At present, asthma cannot be cured, but it can be controlled. What are reasonable expectations for well-controlled asthma? To answer this question, we will draw on the collective opinion of a group of national experts who considered this and other questions about asthma diagnosis and management in a systematic way. When they had arrived at a consensus, they compiled their recommendations in a document widely distributed to health care providers around the country (www.nhlbi.nih.gov/guidelines/asthma). Because their work has been instrumental in setting national standards for asthma care, it is worth taking a moment to review its origins.

Under the auspices of the National Heart, Lung, and Blood Institute of the National Institutes of Health, numerous groups with an interest in asthma came together in the late 1980s in a collaborative effort initially called the National Asthma Education Program and now called the National Asthma Education and Prevention Program. A centerpiece of this program was the creation of a set of standards for assessing and treating asthma based on the best scientific knowledge available, as interpreted by experts in the field. An expert panel was assembled, chaired by Dr. Albert Sheffer, an allergist at the Brigham and Women's Hospital and a member of Partners Asthma Center. The panel brought together allergists and pulmonary physicians, internists and pediatricians, nurses, family physicians, and health educators. Other asthma experts around the country reviewed its recommendations. The final document was published in 1991 as *Expert Panel Report: Guidelines for the Diagnosis and Management of Asthma.*

This report, often referred to simply as the *Guidelines,* had a huge impact on asthma management in this country. It was a touchstone for all health care providers, offering a recommended approach to care that was widely accepted as the best available. Since then, many local quality-improvement initiatives in medical practices throughout the nation have judged the quality of asthma care by how closely it adheres to these national guidelines. In 1997, in response to newly available asthma treatments and new medical understandings about the biology of asthma, a revised set of guidelines was released by the National Institutes of Health, called, predictably, *Expert Panel Report II: Guidelines for the Diagnosis and Treatment of Asthma.* Most recently, *Update on Selected Topics 2002* has been added to this body of knowledge and clinical recommendations.

The *Guidelines* set out the following goals for well-controlled asthma:

- Prevent chronic and troublesome symptoms (for example, coughing or breathlessness in the night, in the early morning, or after exertion)

- Maintain normal or near-normal pulmonary function

- Maintain normal activity levels (including exercise and other physical activity)

- Prevent recurrent exacerbations of asthma and minimize the need for emergency department visits or hospitalizations

- Provide optimal pharmacotherapy with minimal or no adverse effects

- Meet patients' and families' expectations and ensure their satisfaction with asthma care

CRITERIA FOR JUDGING ASTHMA SEVERITY

In one sense, judging the severity of your asthma can be based on how far from these goals of good control your asthma is. If you are having frequent asthmatic symptoms, are limited in your ability to exercise because of asthma, have impaired lung function, and often experience attacks that require emergency care, your asthma is severe and out of control. If the opposite is true— you rarely have any symptoms of your asthma, you can exercise without limitation because of asthma, your lung function is almost always normal, and you never suffer severe flare-ups—then you have well-controlled asthma. If you don't need any regular medication to keep your asthma well controlled, you certainly have mild asthma.

Let's take this concept of asthma severity one step further by comparing two people who have good asthma control: one takes no regular medications; the other requires three different medications every day to achieve good control. We would say that the first person has asthma that is intrinsically mild. The bronchial tubes are wide open and not particularly sensitive to the stimuli of asthma in the world around us. The second person has asthma that is intrinsically more severe. Only with the help of several medications are his or her bronchial tubes open and the twitchiness of the bronchial tubes kept in check. Without these medications, this individual's bronchial tubes would narrow and become increasingly sensitive to his or her triggers of asthma.

Why does one person have intrinsically more severe asthma than another?

Like so many aspects of our health, some combination of our genetic makeup and what we are exposed to in the environment probably explains the differences (see Chapters 1 and 8 for more on this subject). Research into the genetic basis of asthma advances year by year, and undoubtedly in the near future we will know not only which genes predispose us to develop asthma, but also what specific combination of asthma-producing genes makes one case of asthma more severe than another.

As for the environment, we know now that any stimuli—particularly inhaled substances—that cause inflammation of the bronchial tubes will create more severe asthma. If you are allergic to dogs, and your family decides to bring a puppy into the house, your asthma may go from mild to severe. If you are allergic to mold, and you move into a damp, musty basement apartment, your asthma may worsen. In these examples, repetitive exposure to something you are allergic to causes the bronchial tubes to become increasingly inflamed and, as a result, hypersensitive. Consequently, the medications (and other interventions) needed to control your asthma may need to be stepped up.

JUDGING ASTHMA SEVERITY BEFORE BEGINNING REGULAR ASTHMA TREATMENT

Let's turn things around for a moment. Imagine that you have been newly diagnosed with asthma. You have not yet been prescribed any treatment. You have been relying on an over-the-counter bronchodilator such as Primatene Mist or borrowing your child's prescription inhaler, albuterol. Your asthma is not well controlled, and you are hoping that some treatment plan recommended by your doctor will bring sustained relief. Your doctor's task is to judge the severity of your asthma in order to prescribe the right intensity of asthma medications.

Your doctor will enlist your aid in estimating the severity of your asthma by asking you questions about the course of your asthma over the last two to four weeks. In keeping with the recommendations of the expert panels of the National Asthma Education and Prevention Program, he or she can draw upon the following specific criteria in considering the severity of your asthma:

1. **The frequency of routine asthma symptoms.** How often in a day or in a week do you have coughing, chest tightness, or wheezing? How often in the course of a month do you wake from your sleep with asthmatic symptoms? You will need to share an accurate record of your asthma symptoms with your health care provider. If your memory of events

more remote than last night's supper tends to be as vague as ours, the best method may be to keep a diary recording your (or your child's) symptoms on a calendar.

2. **The frequency with which you need to use medication to relieve your asthma symptoms.** Virtually everyone with asthma will carry a quick-acting bronchodilator medication (such as albuterol) for prompt relief of asthmatic symptoms. How often do you reach for this quick-relief inhaler? Every day? More than once a day? How long does one rescue inhaler last for you? (If you have multiple rescue inhalers—one at home, one at work, one in the car—this last question won't work for you.)

3. **What is your lung function measurement, or peak flow?** This is a number that we can easily put on a scale from normal to very low, from 100 percent to less than 50 percent (compared with healthy people without asthma). It is true that your peak flow (as measured with your peak flow meter) may vary over time. We are interested in your usual or average peak flow, as well as in the extent to which it varies from one time of day to another. A peak flow that is steadily normal will obviously reflect better control of asthma than a value that is sometimes normal and sometimes 30 percent or 40 percent lower than normal. Reliable information about lung function is difficult to obtain in children younger than about 6.

4. **How often do you experience an asthma attack or flare-up?** It is somewhat difficult to define precisely what we mean by an attack, as opposed to just the occurrence of asthma symptoms. Mild symptoms can be part of everyday asthma; severe symptoms requiring emergency attention are not part of everyday asthma. For the purposes of this discussion, we would define an asthma attack or flare-up as symptoms that are more severe than your usual ones and that are not fully relieved by one or two doses of your quick-relief bronchodilator medication, or symptoms that cause you to seek urgent, unscheduled medical care.

From this information a picture of your asthma over time emerges, in terms of how much trouble it is causing you and how narrowed your breathing tubes are compared with normal (and therefore how limited your breathing capacity is likely to be). In one sense, you might say that no two people with asthma are exactly alike with respect to the severity of their asthma. There are probably an infinite number of variations in precisely how people experience asthma, and a continuous spectrum from very severe to very mild asthma. Nonetheless, it has proved useful to create different categories of asthma severity and to assign people with asthma to one of these categories. It is thereby possible to make general recommendations for care among people with asthma who fall into the same category of severity.

At the recommendation of the second Expert Panel of the National Asthma Education and Prevention Program in 1997, four categories of asthma severity have been defined: mild intermittent asthma, mild persistent asthma, moderate persistent asthma, and severe persistent asthma. They are based on symptoms and lung function at a time when you are using only your quick-acting bronchodilator inhaler—taken as needed for relief of symptoms, before beginning any regular, preventive medication you might need. Which category fits you?

• **Mild intermittent asthma:** Symptoms of asthma occur infrequently, no more than twice a week. Nighttime awakenings because of asthma occur no more than twice a month. Your peak flow is within the normal range (more than 80 percent of the average normal value for a person of your age, height, and gender) and varies relatively little (less than 20 percent over the course of a day). Asthma flare-ups are relatively brief (lasting less than an hour) and infrequent.

• **Mild persistent asthma:** Symptoms of asthma occur several times each week (more than twice a week but less than every day). You wake from your sleep with asthma more than twice a month (but less than every week). Your peak flow is usually within the normal range (more than 80 percent of the average normal value for you), but it may vary by as much as 30 percent throughout the day. Asthma attacks may interfere with your normal activities.

• **Moderate persistent asthma:** You experience symptoms of asthma every day. You use your quick-acting bronchodilator for relief of these symptoms every day. More than once a week you wake from sleep because of asthma symptoms. Your peak flow is reduced, as low as 60 percent of normal, and may vary by more than 30 percent throughout the day. Exacerbations may occur two or more times each week and may last for days.

• **Severe persistent asthma:** You have continual symptoms of asthma; you are almost never free of symptoms. Nearly every night your asthma wakes you from sleep. You use your bronchodilator inhaler so often that it does not last a full month. Your breathing tests (peak flow) are less than 60 percent of normal and vary by more than 30 percent over the course of the day. Asthma flare-ups are very common, perhaps several times a day.

Classification of Asthma Severity:
Clinical Features Before Treatment*

STEP	SYMPTOMS**	NIGHTTIME SYMPTOMS
STEP 4 Severe persistent	Continual symptoms Limited physical activity Frequent exacerbations	Frequent
STEP 3 Moderate persistent	Daily symptoms Daily use of inhaled quick-acting bronchodilator*** Exacerbations affect activity Exacerbations more than 2 times a week; may last days	More often than 1 time a week
STEP 2 Mild persistent	Symptoms more than 2 times a week but less than 1 time a day Exacerbations may affect activity	More often than 2 times a month
STEP 1 Mild intermittent	Symptoms no more than 2 times a week Asymptomatic and normal peak flow between exacerbations Exacerbations brief (lasting a matter of minutes); intensity may vary	No more often than 2 times a month

* If you have any one of the features listed in a category, you are considered to belong in that, most severe category. As noted, the severity of asthma changes over time, so your classification into one of these categories may also change.

** Regardless of category of severity, you may suffer exacerbations that vary from mild to severe. Even patients with mild intermittent asthma are at risk for severe and life-threatening attacks.

*** Refers to use of your quick-acting bronchodilator *for symptoms*, and not to its *preventive* use, such as before exercising.

Adapted from National Institutes of Health material

As you consider these categories of asthma, you may find that your asthma has features that belong in more than one category. Here are two examples:

• You may experience symptoms of asthma no more than once or twice a week (as in mild intermittent asthma) but find that your best peak flow after taking your quick-acting bronchodilator medication is only 70 percent of normal (as in moderate persistent asthma).

- You may sleep soundly without ever waking up due to asthma (mild intermittent asthma), but during the day you have episodes of coughing and chest tightness and need to use your quick-acting bronchodilator medication several times each week (mild persistent asthma).

In assessing the severity of your asthma, the most appropriate category for you will be based on the *most severe* feature of your asthma, whether it is daytime symptoms, nighttime symptoms, peak flow, or frequency of asthma attacks. That being the case, in the two examples given here, the categories of asthma severity would be moderate persistent asthma for the first, and mild persistent asthma for the second.

Your doctor will tailor the intensity of your treatment to the severity of your asthma, with the goal of keeping your asthma well controlled with the least amount of medication necessary. As you will learn in Part II of this book, some actions (such as the avoidance of allergens and bronchial irritants) are appropriate for everyone with asthma. Other interventions, specifically the choice of medications, will vary according to how severe your asthma is.

Three Key Points to Remember

- **Asthma severity can change over time.** A child who enters a new classroom with a furry classroom pet may go from having mild intermittent asthma to having moderate persistent asthma. The child's sleep may now be frequently disturbed because of asthmatic symptoms, and he or she might need to use rescue medication more often. Moved to a different classroom environment without the pet, the child's asthma severity would probably lessen again, usually in a matter of a few days.

- **Even people with severe persistent asthma can achieve the goals of well-controlled asthma.** With modern asthma therapies, these goals can usually be reached with a minimum of medication side effects, and often no side effects at all.

- **Even people with mild intermittent asthma can suffer severe asthma flare-ups.** Having mild asthma does not mean that it cannot on occasion become suddenly severe, requiring an emergency department visit or even overnight hospitalization. That is why it is so important to be vigilant against asthma triggers, even if your asthma is mild.

YOUR DOCTOR'S ROLE IN JUDGING ASTHMA SEVERITY

As we have discussed, your doctor will rely in large measure on the information you provide about your symptoms of asthma and your measurements of your peak flow to judge the severity of your asthma. The more accurate the information, the better your doctor's judgment will be. Providing anything less than the most accurate information you have about your child's asthma is not a good idea. Insufficient medication can lead to poorly controlled asthma. Poorly controlled asthma can interfere with a child's sleep, school performance, self-esteem, and ability to participate in sports; it can also isolate children from their peers and set the stage for severe worsening of their asthma.

Along with listening to your (or your child's) symptoms, your doctor will listen to your lungs with a stethoscope. Hearing wheezes tells the doctor that your airways are narrowed and your asthma is not well controlled, but it does not help the doctor determine *how narrow* your airways have become. This is not something a doctor can judge well just from listening—even though some doctors think they can.

Among older children and adults, we encourage measurement of your breathing at each office visit for your asthma. A breathing test may be as sophisticated as spirometry or as simple as a peak flow measurement. The latter takes no more than 30 seconds, is painless, and is usually free of charge. A peak flow measurement in a doctor's office provides the same information that you acquire with your home peak flow meter, but it is performed under supervision, ensuring proper technique and an accurate reading. No blood test or X ray can substitute for this information. In fact, just as no blood test or X ray can diagnose your asthma (see Chapter 2), no blood test or X ray can indicate to your doctor how severe your asthma is.

ASSESSING HOW SEVERE A SUDDEN WORSENING OF YOUR ASTHMA IS

Asthma flare-ups can be categorized as mild, moderate, or severe. Being able to recognize a severe asthma attack is extremely important. It is one of the crucial skills that we hope you will have after reading this book. Without meaning to be overly dramatic, we emphasize that the ability to recognize—and respond to—severe asthma flare-ups can be lifesaving. (For more on recognizing and responding to severe asthma attacks, see Chapters 12, 16 and 17.) Failure to appreciate the seriousness of severe asthma flare-ups too often results in their progression to dangerous, life-threatening narrowing and blockage of the airways. The potential exists for the attack progressively to worsen, to the point of suffocation. You need to be alert to the telltale signs of a severe attack—whether in your child or in yourself.

Your child is having a severe asthma flare-up when he or she appears breathless even while at rest. An infant will stop feeding normally; an older child will want to sit bolt upright. A verbal child will be only able to speak individual words, needing to pause to catch his or her breath between each word or two. The child will appear agitated and may be wheezing loudly; his or her nostrils may flare with each breath in. You may see a tugging inward at the base of the neck in front of the windpipe when the child breathes in, along with inward retraction of the skin and muscle between each rib.

The rate of the child's breathing is particularly useful information. The younger your child, the more rapid his or her *normal* breathing rate is. Counting rapid breathing rates will take some care and is most easily accomplished by two adults. One person keeps track of the second hand of a watch or clock while the other counts each rise and fall of the chest. One full cycle—breath in followed by breath out—counts as one breath. Count the number of breaths in 30 seconds, then multiple by 2 to get the respiratory rate (breaths per minute). In the table below, we list the normal breathing rates for children of different ages. If when at rest your child is breathing faster than the normal rate for his or her age, he or she is probably having trouble breathing.

On rare occasions, a severe asthma attack may progress to become life-endangering. Clues to this dire emergency include the following: drowsiness,

Normal Respiratory Rates in Children of Different Ages

AGE (YEARS)	RESPIRATORY RATE
0–1	31
1–2	26
2–3	25
3–4	24
4–5	23
5–6	22
6–7	21
7 or older	20 or less

confusion, or loss of consciousness; skin and lips turning blue (cyanosis) due to low blood oxygen; shallow, ineffective breathing; and a heart rate that goes from rapid to very slow (fewer than 60 beats per minute). The best response to any of these ominous signs is to call for emergency help, such as by dialing 911 on your telephone.

MEASURING THE SEVERITY OF AN ASTHMA FLARE-UP: USING YOUR PEAK FLOW METER

In Chapter 2 we discussed how you should use your peak flow meter to measure how well you are breathing. In an older child or an adult, measurement of peak flow is a very direct way to determine the severity of an acute exacerbation. If you have measured your peak flow when you are feeling well, you know what your best value is (called your "personal best" peak flow value). If your peak flow falls to less than half of your personal best value, you are having a severe attack.

At one time, physicians routinely encouraged their patients to check their peak flows every day. We no longer find this procedure necessary for most patients. For one thing, it is an added burden in already busy lives. For another, it is not clear that daily peak flow recordings will alert you to asthma flare-ups before your symptoms will.

Still, having a peak flow meter at home is very useful when it comes to assessing the severity of your asthma symptoms. We advise patients to keep a peak flow meter at home and to think of it like a thermometer. If you are sweaty or chilly and feel feverish, you will probably find it useful to take your temperature with a thermometer. If you find that your temperature is 104 degrees, you will likely respond differently than if it is only 99 degrees.

Similarly, if you were to develop persistent coughing and wheezing, it would be useful to check your peak flow. A good example is when you develop a chest cold. Imagine that you have a sore throat and stuffy nose, cough and chest congestion. You feel tired and out of breath, and you are not sure how much of your discomfort you can blame on the respiratory tract infection and how much on your asthma.

It is all too easy to fool yourself, to minimize the severity of the symptoms, to believe that you will feel better by morning if you can only get a good night's sleep. It is better to measure your breathing. If the results on testing your peak flow are not much different than your usual, your asthma is still under control and your chest symptoms are indeed primarily due to the cold. At the other extreme, if your peak flow is less than half of your usual value, the problem is not just a cold; you are having a severe asthma attack. You will need to take action, promptly, to deal with the flare-up.

Knowing your peak flow under these circumstances is also enormously useful for communicating by telephone (or perhaps e-mail) with your doctor or other health care provider. If you can specify what your peak flow is (and how it compares with your personal best value), your doctor will be able to give you advice that is appropriate to the severity of your condition. Measuring your flow takes less than a minute.

PERMANENT AIRWAY NARROWING IN ASTHMA: "AIRWAY REMODELING"

As we have tried to communicate, asthma is a dynamic condition of your airways. At one moment your airways function normally, but at another moment they are constricted and partially blocked. With treatment, troublesome asthma can be brought under good control, and an asthma attack goes away. Even after the worst possible asthma flare-up, the airways typically recover fully and breathing is restored to normal. This is not the case with emphysema and chronic bronchitis, which are characterized by a permanent impairment of lung function.

For some people with asthma, however, the asthmatic inflammation of the airways leads to permanent structural changes of the bronchial tubes. In these people, the chronic inflammation in the airways leads to scarring, and scars represent permanent changes. The bronchial tubes become permanently narrower and less flexible, without the possibility of a return to normal. The term used to describe these changes in airway wall architecture is airway remodeling.

The consequence of this permanent airway remodeling is reduced lung capacity, even when you are at your best. You feel well, without coughing or wheezing, and the doctor hears no wheezing when examining your chest. Yet your breathing tests show a decreased capacity to expel the air from your lungs. If the permanent narrowing is severe, even simple activities like climbing a flight of stairs can become an effort.

No one knows why airway remodeling happens in some people with asthma and not in others. Our impression is that it is most common in people with severe and long-standing asthma, especially asthma that has not been treated with anti-inflammatory medications. Studies suggest that people with mild asthma tend to continue with mild asthma and are unlikely to develop permanent loss of lung function. Furthermore, children with mild asthma who don't outgrow their asthma tend to become adults with mild asthma.

How can you be sure that you are not developing a permanent loss of lung function over time? Keep track of your lung function over the years. You can check it periodically at home, and you can ask your doctor to measure it in the office or pulmonary function testing laboratory. If your lung function does not decline over the years (except for age-appropriate changes), it will provide reassurance that, like most people with asthma, when you are well your lung function is approximately normal. And "normal" for a person with asthma means what "normal" does for any healthy, nonsmoking person—just plain normal.

PART II

Treatments for Asthma

CHAPTER 4

Nonpharmacological Therapies:
Taking Action Against Your Asthma Triggers

IN THIS SECTION OF THE BOOK, we turn our attention to modern-day treatments available for your asthma and allergies, consider complementary and alternative therapies, and take a look at potential therapies that may become available in the near future. We want to emphasize that even for the most severe asthma, highly effective, safe, and convenient medications are available; we will examine these in detail in Chapters 5 through 8. However, we begin this discussion of treatments for asthma not with medicines, but with another important strategy for feeling better: avoidance of your asthma triggers—both those triggers that cause your bronchial tubes to narrow for a short time and those that lead to increased asthmatic inflammation of the bronchial tubes. As was discussed in Chapter 1, more asthmatic inflammation means twitchier, more reactive airways and more asthmatic symptoms.

The inflamed bronchial tubes of asthma have been compared to a scraped knee after a fall on the pavement (without the pain!). Irritants and allergens breathed into these sensitized airways are like harsh chemicals poured onto scraped skin: they make the irritation and swelling worse and they prevent healing. If you can avoid them, or lessen your exposure to them, the swelling and sensitivity in your airways lessen. You will gradually notice less coughing, fewer nighttime awakenings, easier breathing, and less frequent need for medications to relieve the symptoms of asthma.

WHAT TRIGGERS THEIR ASTHMA

"Some of the things that aggravate my asthma are dust in the wind, pollen, a really bad cold, cigarette smoke, and strange odors like ammonia, or some strong food odors that smell like old oil, and exhaust fumes from cars. Seems like I'm always discovering something new that doesn't agree with me. You have to be really careful because you have to avoid

certain areas and certain stores even. You learn, by elimination; you may get sick, but you learn where not to go and what not to do."
—HAZEL, 56

"My asthma only attacks when I'm playing basketball or running laps or have bad colds. Then I sometimes start coughing and feel like I can't breathe and my lungs hurt."
—ANDREA, 10

"I was quite a child to deal with. There was my asthma, and then there was an anxiety thing attached to the asthma. Getting scared and anxious can trigger stuff. If you get nervous that you're going to have an asthma attack, sometimes you do."
—TANYA, 17

Some triggers of asthma, such as exercise or beta-blocker medications, do not worsen asthmatic inflammation. They cause the bronchial muscles to contract and the airways to narrow, but when the muscles relax and the episode is over, there is no leftover effect, no change in the underlying sensitivity of the airways. Other triggers of asthma, such as allergens, not only stimulate the bronchial muscles to constrict but also worsen the inflammation of the airways. In other words, they trigger constriction of the bronchial muscles and at the same time make the airways more irritable. A single exposure to an allergen you are sensitive to can make your bronchial tubes more twitchy for hours or days thereafter. The good news is that by avoiding the things that cause asthmatic inflammation, you can reduce the severity of your asthma; you can make your bronchial tubes less asthmatic.

Because of the importance of allergens in causing asthmatic inflammation (in both adults and children) we begin with consideration of the questions, How can I tell if I am allergic, and to what might I be allergic?

ALLERGY TESTING

It may be possible to sort out your allergic sensitivities simply by careful detective work. Keeping a diary of when your asthma worsens and of what events and exposures precede your asthmatic symptoms may suffice. You may find, for example, that your asthma gets better whenever you are away from home (and your pet dog) for several days, or that you have trouble breathing whenever you spend time in the damp, moldy basement. However, even after careful self-monitoring, you may be left wondering about possible allergic triggers. If that is the case, allergy testing may help.

There are two types of tests your physician can recommend to help identify your allergic sensitivities. One is a blood test that measures immunoglobulin E (IgE) antibodies in your blood to specific allergens to which you may be sensitive. People without these allergic sensitivities will not have these specific allergic antibody proteins in their blood. This blood test is called RAST (for radioallergosorbent test), referring to the chemical process by which these antibodies are identified in the blood.

Allergy skin tests are another way to test for allergic sensitivities. A particular allergic sensitivity is tested by pricking (or scratching or injecting) into the skin a small amount of the substance to which you may be allergic. Normally (in the absence of allergies), the body doesn't react to this substance. However, if you are allergic to it, the skin produces a localized red, itchy reaction, a hive. The hive appears within minutes of the allergy skin test and lasts up to approximately 24 hours.

Skin tests have several advantages over the RAST: they are more accurate, less expensive, and provide immediate visual feedback as to the presence of any allergic sensitivities. Witnessing your skin swell and redden, and feeling it become itchy following the introduction of just a tiny amount of the allergen, can provide strong motivation to try to avoid that allergen in the future! The disadvantages of skin testing (which are not shared by RAST blood tests) are the small risk of a major allergic reaction and the need to stop antihistamines before testing. Also, when a skin disease such as psoriasis or eczema is present where the allergen is to be introduced (usually the forearm or the back), allergy skin tests can't be done.

If you think about it, neither of these two tests answers exactly the question we would like answered. We would like to know if *breathing in* certain substances causes asthma to worsen. The most exact test would be to measure your breathing before and after inhaling a small amount of the particular substance in question. However, such a test, which is done in certain experimental settings and is called an inhalation challenge, is time-consuming, potentially dangerous (it could provoke a severe asthma flare-up), and tests only one substance at a time.

RASTs and allergy skin tests are used as a substitute for inhalation challenges. The assumption—which mostly holds true—is that if you have asthma and have allergic antibodies in your blood to a certain allergen or react with a hive when that allergen is injected into your skin, then if you were to breathe that allergen into your bronchial tubes, you would have an allergic reaction there, causing narrowing of your bronchial tubes and asthma symptoms. With RASTs and allergy skin tests, you can have your allergic sensitivities to multiple allergens tested all at one time. At our asthma center, our usual panel of allergy skin tests assesses 20 substances, including cats and dogs, house dust mites, cockroaches, common molds, and pollens from regional trees, grasses, and weeds.

An important distinction to keep in mind is that while allergy testing can identify what you are allergic to, it is not useful in *diagnosing* asthma. You can have asthma but negative skin tests (no reactions to common allergens found), and you can have many positive skin test reactions but no asthma. Someone with hay fever and nasal allergies might have many allergic reactions but not have asthma.

Also, allergy skin tests only identify your sensitivity to one type of asthmatic stimuli, allergens (particularly inhaled allergens). Other, nonallergic triggers, such as aspirin or sulfites (chemicals often used to preserve foods and beverages such as beer, wine, processed potatoes, dried fruits, and shrimp), cannot be tested in this way. Many people are interested in whether certain foods might make their asthma worse. Allergy testing is generally not very helpful for this purpose. A hive reaction to a small amount of strawberry injected into your skin is not an accurate predictor of whether eating strawberries might make your asthma worse.

Despite these limitations, the results of allergy skin testing can be helpful in clarifying your allergic sensitivities. For example, you may have suspected that your asthma is made worse by dust, based on your experience with housecleaning and use of a forced hot air heating system in the winter. A hivelike reaction to house dust mite allergen during allergy skin testing confirms your suspicion. If the dust mite antigen is breathed in (such as when you stir dust into the air with a dry mop or when the furnace blows dust from the vents in your floors), the same type of allergic reaction that you witnessed taking place on your forearm during the skin test will probably also take place in your bronchial tubes, causing worsening of your asthma. That worsening may take the form of an asthma "attack," or it may simply mean that your bronchial tubes have been made more sensitive, more "twitchy," so that the next time you exercise, breathe cold air, or encounter cigarette smoke, your bronchial tubes will react more intensely.

In this example, confirmation of your sensitivity to dust mites can lead to action. As we discuss below, there are many steps you can take to reduce your exposure to dust mites. Equally helpful, if your skin tests show that you do *not* have dust mite allergy, you can save yourself the time and effort involved with these preventive measures, since they are unlikely to help your asthma.

MODIFYING YOUR EXPOSURE TO INDOOR ALLERGENS

The more scientists have learned about the allergens in the air we breathe, the better we have become at identifying ways to reduce exposure to them. Some specific examples, with practical advice regarding methods to reduce your exposure, follow. We begin with the indoor allergens.

DUST MITES

If dusting or vacuuming makes your asthma worse, you are probably allergic to a particular protein found in the droppings of the dust mite. The dust mite is a microscopic living creature that thrives in warm, moist environments worldwide and feeds on human scales (sloughed skin) and animal dander. (*Dander* refers to tiny scales that peel off an animal's skin, hair, or feathers and float in the air.) Dust mites collect in pillows, mattresses, and box springs, in carpeting and upholstered furniture, and wherever house dust accumulates (along blinds and curtains, on books, stuffed animals, and other knickknacks, and on counters and shelves). The allergen from dust mites is found in the highest concentration in our bedrooms.

That being the case, the bedroom is a good place to start making inroads against the dust mite. First, cover your mattress, box spring, and pillows in zippered, allergy-proof plastic wraps. As an added protection, tape over the zippers to eliminate the escape of mite particles. Wash your sheets and pillowcases weekly in hot water to kill mites that accumulate on their surfaces.

Recently, the value of dust mite allergen–impermeable mattress covers was investigated in a study of more than one thousand adults with asthma, of

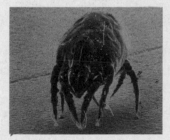

FIGURE 6: THE DUST MITE, A LIVING CREATURE (MAGNIFIED VIEW)
You may be surprised to learn that dust mites, the source of one of the most common allergic triggers of asthma, are microscopic creatures that thrive in warm, moist environments and feed on sloughed human skin and animal dander. Dust mites like to collect in pillows, mattresses, and box springs, in carpeting and upholstered furniture, and anywhere else that dust accumulates.

whom two thirds proved to be dust mite allergic. One group of patients was randomly assigned to use the special "dust proof" covers while the other group used standard polyester-cotton covers. The results were discouraging. At the end of one year, the concentration of dust mite allergen vacuumed from the surfaces of the mattresses using the special covers was no different than prior to use of the covers, and lung function and need for asthma medications were indistinguishable between the two groups. How is one to interpret these results? Clearly, as a single intervention, the dust mite allergen–impermeable covers were a failure. Their value, if any, must be as part of a more comprehen-

Will a HEPA Vacuum Cleaner or Room Air Purifier Make Your Asthma Better?

HEPA stands for "high efficiency particulate air." Devices such as vacuum cleaners and room air purifiers equipped with HEPA filters can trap some of the allergens that might otherwise wind up in the air and, ultimately, your airways, where they can worsen asthma.

Let's start with vacuum cleaners. One of the reasons for vacuuming is to get rid of allergens. But vacuuming, alas, can actually distribute allergens such as dust mites into the air. Allergenic particles from these microscopic creatures are small enough to pass through most conventional filter bags, and can be blown out the exhaust end of the vacuum cleaner. So where does that leave you? You can buy a special vacuum cleaner equipped with a HEPA filter that will trap dust mite particles and other allergens much more effectively than a regular vacuum. (You can't just add a HEPA filter to your old vacuum, however, because these filters require vacuum cleaners with stronger-than-ordinary suction.) The downside is that HEPA vacuum cleaners are pricey—upwards of $300. A less expensive, but perhaps not quite as effective, option is to stick with your old vacuum and use special small-pore vacuum filter bags that are available to fit most vacuum cleaner brands.

As for air purifiers, some people find that their allergy-related asthma symptoms lessen with the use of a room air purifier (the bedroom is a good spot for one of these) equipped with a HEPA filter. These free-standing units come in various sizes (to accommodate rooms of various sizes) and can reduce the level of allergens such as pollens and animal dander in the air. Like HEPA vacuums, these too may cost several hundred dollars. If you are considering an air purifier equipped with a HEPA filter, you might want to rent one and try it out for a few months to see if your allergy symptoms diminish.

Don't forget, though, that while HEPA filters can reduce allergens, they won't eliminate them altogether. When possible, it's best to eliminate the source of allergens, which may mean, for example, finding a new home for your child's pet hamster.

sive program of dust mite allergen avoidance. In addition, they may prove to be more effective in dust mite allergic children, whose asthma is not yet as well established.

Carpets are a reservoir of the dust mite allergen. The best solution is to take up the carpeting. As an alternative, vacuum it—or better yet, have someone else vacuum it—using special, small-pore vacuum filter bags to trap the mite allergen inside the vacuum cleaner. Another option is a vacuum cleaner equipped with a HEPA filter, or high-efficiency particulate air filter. When dusting, use a damp cloth to minimize dispersal of dust mite particles into the air.

You can help keep the growth of dust mites in check by maintaining the indoor humidity at less than 50 to 60 percent. A device called a hygrometer is available at hardware stores to measure indoor humidity. Despite the comfort a humidifier provides, we would advise against running one during cold winter months, since dust mites thrive in humid conditions. Also, remember that dust mites feed on animal dander as well as on human scales, so indoor cats and dogs contribute to the growth of dust mites. It's a good idea to keep your pet cat or dog out of the bedroom, even if you aren't allergic to the animal.

Stuffed animals, too, are dust collectors and are best kept out of the bedroom if your child has asthma. If stuffed animals are a must, washable ones are preferable. For children, the bedroom is often a playroom as well as a place to sleep: because your child is likely to spend so much time there, it's especially important that the bedroom be as dust-free as possible.

A word of encouragement, if all this seems like a lot of effort: one study showed that when these measures were taken in the home, and especially in the bedroom, children with dust-mite-allergic asthma had fewer symptoms, needed their quick-acting bronchodilator less often, and in general became less sensitive to all their asthma triggers.

COCKROACHES

The unloved cockroach is another creature known to trigger asthma flare-ups. Cockroach excrement and the debris from decomposing cockroach bodies are just the right size to be lifted into the air, breathed into the bronchial tubes, and recognized by some people's immune systems as a signal to mount an allergic reaction.

Recently, a major federally funded research project looked for allergy-producing substances in the homes of hundreds of children with asthma living in cities across the United States. The researchers measured the amount of cat, dust mite, and cockroach allergen in the bedrooms of these children, aged 4 to 9 years. The results were quite striking.

The most important allergen in these inner-city homes came from cock-

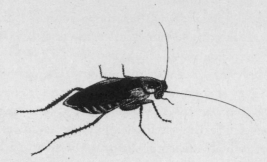

FIGURE 7: THE UNLOVED COCKROACH (MAGNIFIED VIEW)
Here's how the cockroach fits into the story of allergies and asthma. It turns out that cockroach excrement and the debris from decomposing cockroach bodies are of just the right size to be lifted into the air, breathed into the bronchial tubes, and recognized by the immune system—in certain people—as a signal to mount an allergic reaction. In the bronchial tubes, the allergic reaction is asthma.

roaches, and the worst asthma was found in those children who had both the allergic tendency to react to cockroach allergens and exposure to high concentrations of these allergens in their homes. Half of the children's bedrooms had high levels of cockroach dust, and approximately 20 percent of the children had both allergic sensitivity to cockroaches and high-level exposure.

If your immune system reacts to cockroach debris, it is especially important to keep your home free of these insects. Cockroaches are often found in paper bags, newspapers, and cardboard boxes, so don't leave any of these around. Be sure to keep food and garbage in closed containers and to take out the garbage regularly. Take special care to wash dirty dishes promptly and make sure that counter surfaces, shelves, and floors are free of crumbs and spills. Cockroaches like damp places, so watch for puddles of water around the house, especially in the kitchen and bathrooms. Wash out glass bottles and cans before putting them in the recycling bin.

Consider boric acid roach traps rather than sprayed pesticides for ridding your home of these pests, since sprayed pesticides may be irritating to your airways. If you do use a spray, make sure the house is well ventilated, have a professional exterminator or someone else apply the pesticide in your absence, and return home only after the odor is gone.

PETS

Cats come to mind as the pets most likely to cause allergic reactions, and rightly so. Cat allergen is one of the most potent stimuli for allergic responses. Humans worldwide make allergy antibodies to antigens associated with cats, especially to proteins in their saliva. The fastidious cat licks its fur constantly, distributing this allergenic material over its entire body and wherever it deposits its fur. The allergen is hardy, able to elicit an allergic response for many months, and is readily airborne, ideal for inhalation into asthmatic airways.

Dogs, too, cause their share of sneezing and wheezing. Our patients who would like to have a dog often ask us if some dogs are "safer" than others. Some people tell us that certain breeds of dogs make their asthma flare up but other breeds do not. However, we can't predict whether any particular breed of dog is more or less likely to set off your asthma. Unfortunately, there is no such thing as a hypoallergenic dog, short- or long-haired.

In fact, there are no hypoallergenic warm-blooded animals, furry or feathered. The dander, skin flakes, saliva, and urine of fur-bearing animals are all culprits in causing allergic responses in sensitive people. Consequently, rodents too—whether pests or pets, such as your child's hamster or gerbil— can trigger asthma, as can the classroom bunny rabbit at your child's school. The same is true of birds, as well as products, such as pillows, filled with feathers, or winter clothing insulated with down.

If you can't bear to give up your cat or dog, even if you know that being around the animal makes your asthma worse, at least try to keep the pet out of the bedroom. Bathing cats (admittedly hard to do without risk of personal injury!) and dogs once a week may help reduce the amount of allergic material on their fur. Regular vacuuming will decrease the amount of pet hair that collects in your home. Animal hair and other allergens settle in rugs, so the fewer rugs in your home, the better. (In carpeted homes, the allergen from a cat is still detectable for up to six months after the cat's removal from the home.) Remember, people can have allergic reactions to any furry or feathered animal but not to fish or reptiles. Consider the possibility of a pet turtle, fish, iguana, or even a snake!

If you have allergies to furry animals or birds and you are visiting a friend who has one or more of these creatures, you can try to minimize your reaction by pretreating with antiallergy medications and your quick-acting bronchodilator (see Chapter 5 for a detailed discussion of bronchodilator use).

INDOOR MOLDS

At one time or another you have probably seen mold growing on old bread, ceiling tiles, carpeting, or wallpaper. You recognize it by the characteristic discoloration it causes and by its musty smell. Mold is a hardy plantlike microscopic organism that can grow on many different surfaces. Molds propagate by sending out tiny spores, which function like seeds. As it happens, these mold spores are the perfect size to become airborne and inhaled into our airways. Molds thrive in damp places, such as a damp basement, in the tile grout in your shower stall, and in the cabinet under your sink. Don't be surprised if you also find them behind the wallpaper or along damp ceiling tiles. In cold climates, condensation on north-facing walls can promote mold growth. In schools mold may be found around the water fountain, below sinks, and in carpeting laid over cement floors. Occasionally, ventilation systems in homes and workplaces can become contaminated with mold.

Washing mildewed surfaces with diluted bleach (mixed half-and-half with water) will kill the mold. But the key to ridding your home of indoor mold is moisture control. Fixing leaky roofs, pipes, and faucets and eliminating other water sources associated with mold growth will help, as will keeping your kitchen, bathroom, and basement well aired. Dehumidifiers, air conditioners, and exhaust fans can help keep the indoor humidity low (between 30 and 60 percent).

You may wonder if it is necessary to have the ventilation system in your home, apartment building, or workplace cleaned. The answer may be yes, if there is visible mold growing on the interior surfaces of the ducts. For more information about this question and about the general subject of indoor mold and asthma, a useful Internet resource can be found at the Environmental Protection Agency's Web site on indoor air quality: www.epa.gov/iaq/pubs/moldresources/html.

MODIFYING YOUR EXPOSURE TO OUTDOOR ALLERGENS

OUTDOOR MOLDS

Mold grows on dead and decaying plant life, contributing to the cycle by which plants decompose and become part of the soil. From spring until the first frost, mold spores are spread by the wind and become part of the air we breathe. In a recent study of more than 1,000 adults with asthma across three continents, skin test sensitivity to outdoor molds (specifically, *Alternaria* and *Cladosporium*) was associated with more severe asthma symptoms.

The major emphasis on avoiding mold exposure should be your indoor environment. Outdoor mold is everywhere. If you are allergic to mold, one of the best things you can do is to take your medications faithfully during summer and early fall, the peak times for outdoor molds. (Of course, being faithful to your medication schedule is important year-round to protect yourself against asthma flare-ups.) Avoid working with peat, mulch, hay, or dead wood. Try to persuade someone else to rake and bag the fallen leaves this autumn. If you must do these tasks yourself, wear a face mask and avoid hot, humid days.

If you have a computer or have access to one, you can keep track of the results of air testing for mold spore (and pollen) concentrations online. One Internet site is provided by the American Academy of Allergy, Asthma, and Immunology: www.aaaai.com (click on "Pollen Counts").

SEASONAL POLLENS

For people with seasonal allergies, the pollens of grasses, weeds, and trees are among the most notorious culprits. Pollens are a fine powder released by all flowering plants and carried by the wind to fertilize other plants of the same species. One ragweed plant is said to be capable of making a billion pollen grains each season, and it is estimated that throughout North America 100 million tons of ragweed pollen are produced each year. Ragweed is only one of the many plants whose pollen causes allergic reactions. Among the others are Russian thistle, wormwood, pigweed, plantains, timothy, Kentucky bluegrass, orchard grass, alders, poplars, birches, oaks, beeches, elms, and maples. Plants that we cultivate for their flowers also produce pollens, but their pollens are mostly transported from flower to flower by bees and other insects, and less is released into the air where it is available to be breathed into our lungs or deposited on our eyes.

In susceptible people, seasonal pollens typically cause the runny nose, sneezing, and nasal congestion, along with watery, itchy eyes, that we know as hay fever. Interestingly, these pollens are less likely to worsen asthma. The pollen grains are mostly too large to make their way down into the system of bronchial tubes in the lungs. They tend to be filtered out by the nose and throat. In the large study noted above, in which sensitivity to mold spores was associated with more severe asthma, among adults with asthma who had skin test sensitivity to pollens no association was found between pollen exposure and worse asthma control.

An interesting exception has been discovered in the mini-epidemics of asthma known to occur after a thunderstorm. It appears that thunderstorms create exactly the right climatologic circumstances to fracture ryegrass pollen grains into smaller granules of a breathable size and concentrate them in the air at ground level. These findings have helped researchers in England and Australia explain why patients with asthma needed emergency department care more frequently in the hours and days following local thunderstorms.

Generally speaking, pollination is a seasonal phenomenon. Tree pollens are most likely to be bothersome in early to midspring, grass pollens during late spring and early summer, and pollens from weeds during late summer and early fall. The farther north, the later the pollen season. In the southern part of the United States, pollination may be a year-round fact of nature.

If you have seasonal allergies and asthma, you may have a pretty good idea about when the pollen count is high without hearing a meteorologist's report. Still, it's a good idea to listen to news reports of pollen (and mold spore) counts before you go outside, and perhaps to modify your outdoor activities accordingly. Pollen levels tend to be highest between five and ten in the morning (when the dew dries and the wind first blows) and lowest in the late afternoon or after a rain. If possible, keep your windows and doors closed and use air conditioning to cool your home (or car) and to filter the pollens from the air. Avoid window and attic fans. Better not to hang sheets and clothes outside to dry when pollen counts are high; an automatic drier is preferable.

SOME COMMON SENSE ABOUT AVOIDING ALLERGENS

A word of common sense about all of our allergen-avoidance recommendations: life cannot be lived in an allergen-proof bubble. We live complex lives with many competing demands on our time and energy. On the one hand, good breathing for you and your children is a priority, and anything you can do to improve your environment to help achieve that goal is desirable. On the other hand, the aim of modern medical care for asthma and allergies is to leave you free to live your life without restrictions as to when you can leave the house, where you can travel, or what you can do.

It is up to you to make choices that improve your asthma while not compromising your quality of life. Washing sheets in hot water, exterminating cockroaches, and taking up the damp carpet from the basement floor will probably not restrict your desired lifestyle. Trying to vacuum twice daily and never going for a walk in the woods in the fall are probably excessive. For most people, moderation is the best choice. Don't rely solely on medications to control your asthma; don't expect to be asthma-free by strictly reducing allergen exposures. Work toward a common goal using both approaches.

Finally, remember that our allergen avoidance recommendations apply only to people who are sensitive to these allergens. Many people, especially adults with asthma, have nonallergic asthma; reducing allergen exposures would not be expected to improve their asthma.

ALLERGY SHOTS (ALLERGEN IMMUNOTHERAPY)

"Should I (or my child) get allergy shots?" The practice of injecting small amounts of allergen for the purpose of desensitizing people who are sensitive to that allergen has been going on for more than 90 years. After all this time, debate still rages in the medical community over the merits of allergy shots in the treatment of asthma. Although generalizations must be made with caution, because there are many exceptions, as a general rule allergists treating asthma are more inclined to encourage this practice, while pulmonologists treating asthma are more likely to discourage it. And as we listen to our patients describe their experiences, we hear a mixed bag of reactions: some patients feel they have derived benefit from their allergy shots, others have abandoned them because they haven't helped, and still others have experienced severe reactions that made them consider the practice harmful.

Allergy shots (properly called allergy desensitization injections or allergen immunotherapy) can be lifesaving when used to treat severe reactions to stinging insects (for example, throat swelling or loss of consciousness after bee or wasp stings). Furthermore, many studies have shown them to be effective in the treatment of seasonal allergies of the nose and eyes to plant pollens (hay fever). But in the treatment of asthma, controversy abounds. A recent report describing the results of a trial of immunotherapy in children (about which we will speak more below) included the following summary of our state of knowledge: "Injections of allergens are widely prescribed for patients with asthma, but little is known about the effectiveness of immunotherapy."

The idea behind this practice is straightforward: if the immune system is exposed to very minute quantities of a substance to which it makes allergic reactions, it may gradually grow tolerant of that substance and stop making harmful reactions to it. For example, if you repeatedly receive injections under the skin of small amounts of the allergic substance in cat dander, you might gradually lose your allergic sensitivity to cat dander (that is, become desensitized to cat dander). It seems that the body's immune system can be directed to make other, non-allergy-related antibodies (immunoglobulin G) against the allergen, and less of the allergic antibody IgE.

Although the basic principle is simple, the practice is complicated. For one thing, you have to be sure that you are allergic to cats (or mold or dust mites or ragweed) and that this allergen is the major culprit causing your asthma symptoms. It would do no good to become desensitized to cats while you continue to smoke cigarettes, live in a dusty home, and keep a parrot.

In addition, caution must be taken to make sure that you receive just the right amount of cat antigen; too much may trigger an asthma reaction. Also, because the antigen is injected under the skin, a reaction could occur throughout the entire body, including low blood pressure, itching, and wheezing—a potentially life-threatening reaction called anaphylaxis. Each injection poses some risk, although small, of a harmful allergic reaction to the injection.

Finally, the effectiveness of allergy shots depends on the ability of medical companies to isolate and purify the chemical component of cat dander (or other allergens) to which you are allergic. For some allergies, the substances are well characterized and purified; for others, this is not yet the case. Thus, there may be variations between one manufactured batch of allergen and another, and between one allergist's preparations and another's.

The potential promise of allergy shots is that they may lead to fewer asthmatic symptoms, reduce the need for daily medications, and correct the basic allergic mechanisms in the body. Some doctors believe that the potential benefits from allergy shots justify the risks and costs, as well as the inconvenience of weekly doctor's visits for the initial few months, followed typically by visits every two to three weeks for up to three to five years. Other doctors believe that routine medical treatments for asthma are safer and more effective than allergy shots.

All this being said, the fundamental question remains: Do allergy injections really *work* for the treatment of asthma? Do they add anything to a treatment approach based on allergen avoidance and use of antiasthmatic medications? A landmark study published in 1997 attempted to answer this question in a carefully designed medical experiment. Researchers at Johns Hopkins University School of Medicine enrolled approximately 120 children between the ages of 5 and 12 years in this study. All of the children had reactions on allergy skin testing to at least two of the common allergens tested. Most had what would be categorized as moderate persistent or severe persistent asthma.

Half the group was assigned at random to receive allergen immunotherapy (treatment for up to seven allergens per child); the other half received placebo injections (shots with no active ingredient—in this case, shots containing no allergens). The doctors managing the children's asthma were not told which treatment their patient was assigned to receive. According to a written plan, the doctors tried to reduce the asthma medications that the children were receiving to the minimum necessary. The investigators wanted to determine whether the children receiving allergy shots could have their medications reduced more than those given the placebo.

The experiment continued for slightly more than two and a half years. In the end, both groups were able to have their medications reduced somewhat, but there was no difference between the group receiving allergy shots and the placebo group. Likewise, the two groups did not differ in their need for medical care, their symptoms of asthma, and their measured peak flow values.

Thirty-one percent of the children receiving allergy shots were said to experience a partial or complete remission of their asthma—in other words, their symptoms were said to partly or completely go away. But the percent of children in the placebo-treated group whose symptoms lessened or went away was the same. Wondering if any subgroups might benefit more than the study population as a whole, the researchers analyzed the results further and found that children younger than 8½ and children with mild asthma were able to reduce their medications more with the help of allergy shots than with placebo injections. Adverse reactions to allergy shots did occur, and about half of these reactions were sufficiently serious to require treatment. The rate of harmful reactions in the group treated with allergy shots was 2.6 per 100 injections.

Our interpretation of these results is the same as that of the researchers who conducted the study. Allergy shots were of no detectable additional benefit in allergic children with year-round asthma who were, at the same time, receiving appropriate medical treatment.

AIRBORNE IRRITANTS

Allergens are not the only substances we breathe in that can stimulate inflammation of the bronchial tubes. Imagine that you are a firefighter with asthma, breathing in smoke from burning buildings or forest fires. Imagine that you live in a first-floor apartment near an outdoor bus depot, where diesel exhaust from idling bus engines constantly wafts into your window. Or imagine that during school recess, when your child gets to run around the playground, air pollution levels exceed the standards for healthy air quality.

Smoke, diesel exhaust, and air pollutants such as ozone are not allergens. They do not cause the body's immune system to make an allergic reaction with its IgE antibodies and allergy cells to their specific components. They do not discriminate between allergic and nonallergic asthma; they can make both worse. Like allergens, these irritants can provoke symptoms of asthma and also make the bronchial tubes more twitchy, more sensitive to all the various triggers of asthma. In effect, they make your bronchial tubes more asthmatic. The practical consequence is more breathing trouble, more days lost from school and work, more emergency department visits for asthma—unless you can avoid these sorts of nonallergic irritant exposures.

Sometimes irritant exposures are relatively brief and are more annoying than disease producing. For example, fumes from new carpeting, fresh paint, nail polish remover, fabric softener, cedar chips, bleach, strong perfumes, and dyes may bother your asthma for a time. When you move away from them, within a short while—with or without a dose of your quick-acting bronchodilator medication—you feel better again. Exposure to other irritants tends to be more prolonged, leading to more airway inflammation and a generally increased sensitivity of your airways. Here we focus on two particular examples of this type of exposure: air pollutants and tobacco smoke.

INDOOR AND OUTDOOR AIR POLLUTION

The air pollution produced by the machinery of our modern world is good for no one's lungs and is especially bad for the lungs of people with asthma and other respiratory problems. Emissions from cars, trucks, power plants, and factories are major sources of air pollution and are evident in the smog (the word comes from the combination of the words *smoke* and *fog*) we see blanketing the air in our major cities. (Ozone, formed when chemicals emitted in fuel combustion come into contact with sunlight, is a major component of smog.)

If you live in a big city, where air pollution is likely to be heavy, you are probably accustomed to hearing radio and television warnings about poor air quality, especially on hot, humid summer days. Heeding these warnings and limiting outdoor activities when possible may prevent you from having an asthma attack triggered by ozone and other pollutants. While breathing rapidly during aerobic exercise, you expose your airways to a greater volume of air pollutants than when you are breathing quietly at rest, so if you are a runner who has access to a gym, it's a good idea to confine your running to an indoor track or treadmill when pollution levels are high.

People living in the inner city may heat their apartments with their gas-burning stoves, which emit the gaseous irritant nitrogen dioxide. If you live in the country, you may heat your house with a wood-burning stove or fireplace, releasing a mixture of gaseous and particulate irritants into the air, both indoors and outdoors. You can protect yourself somewhat by using an airtight stove and maintaining a highly efficient fireplace chimney. Also, be sure to avoid chemically treated wood, since smoke from this wood contains more pollutants than smoke from natural wood.

TOBACCO SMOKE

As we all know, the list of well-documented and serious health hazards from cigarette smoking is long. For people with asthma, cigarette smoking poses a kind of double jeopardy. On top of the allergic-type inflammation typical of asthma, cigarette smoke stimulates further swelling and narrowing of the breathing tubes and the excess production of phlegm—leading to the smoker's cough. And of course, having asthma is no protection against the development of cigarette-smoke-induced emphysema.

The dangers of "passive smoking," or inhaling the smoke from other people's lit cigarettes, including increased risk for lung cancer, have also become well recognized in recent years. With approximately 24 percent of American adults still smoking cigarettes, it is estimated that as many as 15 million children and adolescents are exposed to secondhand cigarette smoke in their homes. In the multicity study mentioned above that involved children with asthma living in our inner cities, 39 percent of households had at least one cigarette smoker. In this instance, the sins of the parents are truly visited on their children. Children with asthma who are exposed to cigarette smoke have more asthmatic symptoms and more frequent need for emergency department care for their asthma than children in smoke-free homes.

Before leaving the topic of environmental exposures that worsen asthma—both in the short and the long term—it is important to note how poverty comes into play as a cause of more severe asthma. People living in the inner cities have more severe asthma and are more likely to die from an overwhelming attack of asthma . . . if they are poor. Cigarette smoking, poor housing conditions, cockroach infestation, exposure to automobile exhaust and local industrial pollution, lack of air-conditioning units (with their built-in air filters), and inability to modify living conditions are all more common among inner-city residents living in poverty. Many other factors also come into play, such as lack of access to good, preventive medical care and affordable medications. But the underlying cause of severe asthma probably originates in the everyday unfavorable living (and working) conditions. (For more on inner-city asthma, see Chapter 11.)

VIRAL RESPIRATORY INFECTIONS

We conclude this chapter with a discussion of viral respiratory infections, still the most common cause of severe asthma flare-ups in both children and adults. It is a common story that we hear: my son (or daughter or other relative or coworker) had a cold and then I came down with it. First there were the chills and generalized achiness, then a sore throat, runny nose, perhaps a low-grade fever, and a hoarse voice. Everyone else (without asthma) quickly got over the cold, and my cold symptoms, too, got better, but then I started to develop coughing and chest congestion, tightness across my chest, and difficulty breathing. Last night I had to spend much of the night sitting up because of my coughing and wheezing.

Not only can viral infections trigger severe asthma flare-ups, they also tend to make bronchial inflammation worse for several days to a few weeks after the infection. Well-controlled asthma can become unstable—due to increased bronchial irritability—during this period. The exercise workout that was well tolerated now triggers your asthmatic symptoms; you find yourself more sensitive to smoke, fumes, or other chemical irritants.

For most of us, the chances of avoiding at least one such viral respiratory infection during the winter months are slim. In fact, it's not unusual for children to have as many as six to ten colds in a single year. That being said, you (and your child) can reduce the likelihood of "catching" these germs by avoiding close contact with others who have a cold or the flu. Frequent hand washing also helps. Most viruses are spread from nasal or oral secretions onto surfaces, are picked up by hand contact, and are then spread from your hands to your nose and mouth. So wash your hands frequently, particularly after having shaken hands with someone who appears to have a cold, or playing with a child who has been rubbing his or her runny nose.

You can protect yourself (and your child) from the flu by getting a flu shot. Lest you are concerned that flu shots might not be safe for people with asthma, a recent research study sponsored by the American Lung Association found no worsening of asthma symptoms in a large group of adults and children with asthma who were given the flu vaccine.

CHAPTER 5

Asthma Medications: The Quick Relievers and How to Inhale Them

AT ONE TIME OR ANOTHER, everyone with asthma needs medication to continue breathing comfortably. In this chapter and the next three, we review the different medications used to treat asthma. We discuss their purpose, anticipated effects, potential side effects, and the forms in which they can be taken. In subsequent chapters on the management of asthma (Chapters 10 through 16), we address the broader issues of which medications are appropriate for which people with asthma, and how and when these medications are best used.

In a general sense, antiasthmatic medications have two potential aims: 1) to prevent or reverse contraction of the bronchial muscles (bronchoconstriction), and 2) to reduce inflammation of the walls of the bronchial tubes. Medications that address bronchoconstriction are called bronchodilators; medications that target inflammation are referred to as anti-inflammatory medications. These two types of medications work on very different timetables. The muscles that surround the breathing tubes can be made to contract in minutes—as you know if you suddenly have asthma symptoms after running to catch the bus on a cold winter day—and likewise can be made to relax (with bronchodilator medicines) within minutes. Inflammation of the bronchial tubes comes on more slowly (in the days after a respiratory tract infection or during your allergy season) and takes days to respond to anti-inflammatory medications. Bronchodilators can be used intermittently for fast relief of coughing and chest tightness brought on, for instance, during a soccer game. Anti-inflammatory medications need to be taken regularly (daily) over many days, and perhaps indefinitely.

In recent years we have come to categorize asthma medicines as "quick relievers" and "controllers" (controllers are the focus of Chapters 6 and 7). These terms reflect how the medications are meant to be used, rather than emphasizing the mechanism of airway narrowing they target (contraction of the bronchial muscles or inflammation of the bronchial walls). This division of asthma medications into quick relievers and controllers came about because some newer asthma medications seem to have both bronchodilator and anti-inflammatory effects, and because some newer bronchodilators are prescribed for daily use to prevent asthma symptoms. All of the controller medications— not just the anti-inflammatory medications—should be taken every day, whether you have symptoms of asthma or not. As noted above, quick relievers can be taken as needed whenever you have uncomfortable symptoms of asthma. Virtually everyone with asthma should have a quick reliever handy at all times, just in case.

About Generic and Brand Medication Names

All medications have two names: the generic name, which is the name of the chemical, and the brand name, created by the manufacturer. In this book, the generic name is followed by one or more brand names in parentheses. For the short-acting beta-2 agonists, the generic and brand names are:

Albuterol (Proventil, Ventolin)

Metaproterenol (Alupent, Metaprel)

Pirbuterol (Maxair)

Terbutaline (Brethine)

WHAT ARE THE "QUICK RELIEVERS"?

"Quick relievers" are the medications to turn to for fast relief of asthma symptoms. They are also known as quick-acting bronchodilators, since they dilate, or open up, the bronchial tubes. The most frequently used quick relievers are called beta-agonist bronchodilators and are described in detail later.

When taken by inhalation—usually by a puff or two from your bronchodilator inhaler—the quick relievers begin to work within a minute or so and typically provide relief for approximately four to six hours. They relax the muscles surrounding the bronchial tubes so the tubes open wider. When the muscles relax, the bronchial tubes can usually open fully, and breathing is usually restored to normal. We say "usually" because sometimes the bronchial tubes are swollen and filled with mucus. Quick-reliever bronchodilators cannot reduce swelling of the bronchial tubes or mucus blockage. As noted above, the anti-inflammatory medications (see Chapter 6) treat these aspects of asthma.

Besides using your quick reliever to stop symptoms that have already started, you can also use it 10 to 15 minutes before a predictable exposure to something that typically sets off your asthma—exercise, for example (see Chapter 11 for information on treating exercise-induced asthma), or the cat at your neighbor's house. Quick relievers can often prevent tightening of the bronchial tubes that would otherwise occur. If your asthma symptoms are mild and infrequent, a quick reliever may be the only medication you will need to control your illness.

BETA-AGONIST BRONCHODILATORS

Of all the quick relievers, the most effective and most widely used are the beta-agonist bronchodilators, taken by inhalation. The full name of this medication is *beta-adrenergic agonist*.

ADRENALINE (EPINEPHRINE)

The very first bronchodilator with beta-agonist properties was purified from the adrenal glands of animals and was called adrenaline. You may recall having been treated as a child in your doctor's office or hospital emergency department with adrenaline shots for severe bouts of asthma. These injections provided rapid and powerful relief by causing the bronchial muscles to relax, but, as you may also recall, they had numerous unpleasant side effects. They made your heart race and pound in your chest, they made you feel shaky and jittery inside, and perhaps they gave you a headache or made your blood pressure rise. Epinephrine is another name, more commonly used in the United States, for adrenaline. You may also have heard it referred to simply as epi.

ISOPROTERENOL

As you might imagine, considerable progress has been made in the development of beta-agonists since epinephrine was first purified and chemically synthesized for medical use in 1901. The first major advance was the modification of epinephrine to eliminate the undesirable effect of constricting blood vessels throughout the body, causing high blood pressure. In 1948 a derivative of epinephrine called isoproterenol, which achieved this goal, was introduced. It was given the brand name Isuprel, and if you are old enough and have had asthma long enough, you may remember using an Isuprel Mistometer for quick relief of asthma symptoms.

The Isuprel Mistometer incorporated a second major improvement—a convenient and highly accurate method of delivering an exact dose of medication each time: the multidose metered-dose inhaler (MDI). This device fits in your pocket or purse and delivers a spray of medication that you breathe into your bronchial tubes. It is hard for most people with asthma to imagine life before metered-dose inhalers, when inhaled medications were administered in forms that now seem quaint and old-fashioned, such as bulb nebulizers, cigarettes, water pipes, and steaming pots of boiling liquid.

Believe it or not, epinephrine is still available today for inhalation. It is the active ingredient in Primatene Mist, a perhaps familiar bronchodilator sold over the counter (no prescription needed). We discourage our patients from using over-the-counter bronchodilators because they are less effective, shorter lasting, and have more side effects than prescription bronchodilators. Overusing these bronchodilators to treat asthma attacks, while neglecting to treat the swelling and mucus plugging of the bronchial tubes, can result in disaster. Better to get your medicines, and complete medical care of your asthma, under the supervision of a physician.

BETA-2 AGONISTS

Fortunately, the third major advance in the development of modern-day beta-agonist bronchodilators was the further modification of epinephrine and related chemicals to minimize their cardiac effects while maintaining their bronchodilating effects. In technical terms, this development is spoken of as the minimizing of the beta-1 (heart) effects while maintaining the beta-2 (bronchial) effects. This brings us to our modern-day beta-agonist bronchodilators, such as albuterol. They are described as selective beta-2 adrenergic agonists—and now you know why!

Bronchial-selective beta-adrenergic agonists like albuterol are available as tablets or liquid formulations as well as by inhaler. We focus in this chapter on the inhaled form—even though manipulating inhalers can be difficult and frustrating—for the following reasons: when inhaled, beta-agonists begin to work faster, dilate the bronchial tubes more effectively, and have fewer unpleasant side effects. In a very young child who has difficulty inhaling the medicine, a liquid preparation may at times be your only option—but we only rarely find this necessary.

Modern beta-agonists exert most of their effects on the bronchial tubes, which is to say that they are relatively selective for the bronchial tubes, but they are not perfectly selective. When inhaled, the side effects are few, if any, but can include heart pounding, a jittery feeling, and shakiness. The standard dose in adults is two inhalations, or puffs. Fortunately for those adults and children who are particularly sensitive to these unpleasant effects of the beta-agonists, one inhalation—with consequently fewer side effects—may suffice to open the breathing tubes.

As we noted above, most of the quick-acting bronchodilators, whether inhaled or swallowed, help keep the breathing tubes open for about four hours. When they wear off, if you are still having asthma symptoms, you can take another dose (one to two puffs). In an asthma flare-up, when the bronchial tubes are severely narrowed, you can use your bronchodilator more often to get through a difficult period—even as frequently as every 20 minutes. We discuss treatment of asthma attacks elsewhere (Chapters 10, 11, 12, 16, and 17). Here we simply emphasize that these modern beta-agonists are very safe to use if you need them. Serious heart complications are very rare, even at ten or more times the standard dose.

The selective beta-2 agonists are available by prescription only. The most widely used quick reliever is albuterol, available as a generic albuterol inhaler and also sold under the brand names Ventolin and Proventil. Other commonly prescribed beta-2 agonists include metaproterenol (Alupent, Metaprel) and pirbuterol (Maxair). These medications all come in inhaler devices small enough to fit in your purse or pocket, so they can be within easy reach whenever you need a puff or two to quiet your coughing or wheezing and restore your breathing to normal.

Facts and Fictions About the Beta-agonist Bronchodilators

If you have had asthma for some time, not only have you almost surely been given a bronchodilator inhaler, you also have experience using it and have opinions about the right way to use it. In speaking with our patients, we find that certain myths have grown up about these bronchodilator inhalers, sometimes based on outdated practices, sometimes based on false information. Here are four common misconceptions about the inhaled beta-agonist bronchodilators.

Fiction 1: Because the benefit from most of the quick-acting inhaled bronchodilators lasts for only approximately four hours, you should use quick relievers four times daily to keep the bronchial tubes open throughout the day.
Fact: This is not necessary. In experiments conducted at several academic research centers, it was found that regular use of quick-relief bronchodilators did not improve well-being or prevent asthma flare-ups. The current recommendation is that you use your quick-relief bronchodilator only when needed to quiet your asthma. When you are feeling well, there is no need to use it on any regular schedule.

Fiction 2: You need to take two puffs from your bronchodilator inhaler before using your anti-inflammatory (controller) inhaler, for maximal delivery of the anti-inflammatory medication to your bronchial tubes.

Fact: Not so. The idea was that the bronchodilator would open your bronchial tubes, allowing the inhaled anti-inflammatory medication to penetrate deeper into the system of bronchial tubes. However, most of the time your bronchial tubes are sufficiently wide open to permit delivery of the anti-inflammatory medication without any need for pretreatment with a bronchodilator. Having to wait five to ten minutes or more for the bronchodilator to work is likely only to make you skip use of the important, preventive anti-inflammatory medicine.

Fiction 3: When using any of your inhalers, you should wait one minute between each inhalation.

Fact: As long as you use your inhaler correctly—shaking it first, then slowly breathing in after releasing the medication from the inhaler, and holding your breath for about five to ten seconds after each spray—you don't have to pause before proceeding with the next puff. After you have completed one careful inhalation, you (and your inhaler) are immediately ready for the next puff. We think that waiting a minute or more between puffs unnecessarily slows you down and makes it more likely that you will forget to take some of your medication.

Fiction 4: You need to wait at least four hours between doses of your quick-acting bronchodilator.

Fact: This is not true during an acute attack of asthma. If you use your bronchodilator inhaler and are still having difficulty breathing due to your asthma, you don't need to wait several hours before using it again. If you are having worsened asthma symptoms and need quick relief, you can safely use your inhaler as often as every 20 to 30 minutes for two to three hours without significant risk of harmful side effects. When using bronchodilator inhalers this often for a short period of time, you may experience jitteriness and racing heart. Even so, unless you have a serious heart condition, there is no danger to your heart.

However, if you do need your bronchodilators this often, you are having a serious flare-up and should take immediate action to prevent breathing difficulty that can be potentially dangerous. Keep in mind that while you may be getting short-term relief from your bronchodilator inhaler, your asthma may be worsening as the breathing tubes become more swollen and filled with

Usual Dosages of the Inhaled Beta-2 Agonist Medicines

Medication	Dosage for Adults	Dosage for Children	Comments
METERED-DOSE INHALERS (MDI)			
Albuterol, pirbuterol, metapro-terenol	2 puffs 3 or 4 times a day as needed, 2 puffs 5 minutes before exercise	2 puffs 3 or 4 times a day as needed, 1–2 puffs 5–15 minutes before exercise	If you need increasing amounts to control your asthma, you may need additional treatments: Talk to your doctor. If you need to use every day, talk to your doctor. You may double your usual dose if your asthma suddenly becomes worse, but also call your doctor.
NEBULIZER SOLUTION			
Albuterol	2.5 mg every 4–8 hours as needed	1.25–2.5 mg every 4–8 hours as needed	Can mix with cromolyn or ipratropium nebulizer solutions. You may double your usual dose if your asthma suddenly becomes worse, but also call your doctor.

Source: National Heart, Lung, and Blood Institute, Bethesda, MD

mucus. You are overusing bronchodilators if you are delaying other, crucial treatments, usually in the form of anti-inflammatory medications. If you find that you are not improving after two treatments with your quick-relief bronchodilator spaced 20 to 30 minutes apart, give your health care provider a call to discuss further steps to take.

Medications That Can Have Bad Interactions with Beta-agonists

- Antidepressants known as monoamine oxidase (MAO) inhibitors
- Beta-blockers, medications used (in tablet form) to treat various heart conditions and high blood pressure (see Chapters 13 and 14) and (as eye drops) to treat glaucoma

MEDICATION DELIVERY DEVICES: THE CHALLENGE OF GETTING INHALED MEDICATIONS INTO THE BREATHING TUBES

THE METERED-DOSE INHALER

When they were first introduced in 1956, the metered-dose inhalers revolutionized asthma treatment. Here was a device that administered the same amount of medication (a "metered dose") each time you used it. All you had to do was squeeze the pump and breathe in the medication. Not only that, you could carry your metered-dose inhaler in your purse or slip it into your pocket and have it handy whenever you needed it.

However, many people find these standard inhalers, developed to deliver quick-acting bronchodilators (and many other asthma medications), difficult to use. If you are one of these people, it may be that no one ever showed you how to use a metered-dose inhaler properly. We would like to take this opportunity to instruct you in the proper use of the metered-dose inhaler. No matter how long you have been using one, there is no harm in reviewing proper technique. We often find that inhaled medicines that have not been helping our patients suddenly begin to work well when they are actually breathed in correctly for the first time. Remember these two points: 1) you are not alone in the struggle to master this technique, and 2) a variety of inhalational aids and alternative devices have been developed to help you get the medicine you need to go where you need it to go!

Many people have been told first to breathe out all of the air from their lungs before releasing the medication from the inhaler and breathing in. We suggest that you skip this step because it unnecessarily complicates the process and it sometimes triggers spasm of the bronchial tubes.

Asthma specialists debate whether it is better to close your mouth around

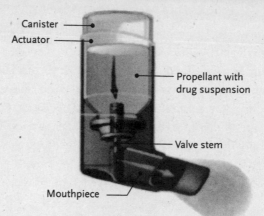

Canister

Actuator

Propellant with
drug suspension

Valve stem

Mouthpiece

FIGURE 8: HOW TO USE YOUR METERED-DOSE INHALER (MDI) EFFECTIVELY

- First, shake the inhaler a few times to make sure the medication is evenly mixed.

- Close your lips tightly around the mouthpiece of the inhaler. Alternatively, you can hold the mouthpiece an inch or two from your mouth.

- Press down on the canister to release the medication.

- Start breathing in as soon as you press down on the canister or even just before (if you delay taking a breath too long, a lot of the medication will settle in your mouth). Breathe in through your mouth, not your nose.

- Take about three to five seconds to pull in a slow, full breath.

- Hold your breath for about five to ten seconds so the medication can settle onto the breathing tubes. If you breathe out immediately, you lose some of the medication in your exhalation.

- Remember that two puffs (the usual dose) doesn't mean two squirts and one breath. It means one squirt and one slow breath in (and breath out), followed by a second squirt and a second slow breath in. It does not work to spray two puffs into your mouth and then breathe both in at once. In the same way, if you use a spacer chamber with your inhaler, take one breath in for each spray delivered into the chamber. Do not "load up" the chamber with multiple doses. If you do, much of the medication will be left behind in the chamber.

- Young children can use metered-dose inhalers with the help of attached inhalational aids or spacers (see Chapter 12).

Number of Puffs Per Canister for Several Common Beta-agonist Drugs

MEDICINE	NUMBER OF PUFFS PER CANISTER
Ventolin, Alupent, Metaprel	200
Maxair Autohaler	400

the mouthpiece of the inhaler or hold the device an inch or so from your mouth, held wide open. Either method is fine. The latter ("open-mouth technique") allows the spray, which exits the canister at a speed of approximately 60 miles an hour, to slow down somewhat before you inhale it. For reasons having to do with evaporation of moisture and the distribution of the sizes of particles within the spray, somewhat more medicine can get into the bronchial tubes using this method. The advantage of putting the mouthpiece of the inhaler directly into your mouth ("closed-mouth technique") is that the medicine at least starts out in the right place, and no special aim is required. In our experience, most people find the closed-mouth method easier.

Do's and Don'ts of the Metered-Dose Inhalers

DO:

1. Shake the device before inhaling, to thoroughly mix its contents. Two or three quick shakes will suffice.

2. If using a new inhaler for the first time, "waste" one spray into the air. Priming the inhaler in this way ensures that the next spray will contain a full dose of the medication. Similarly, if your inhaler has not been used for two weeks or longer, release one spray into the air before using.

3. You can wash your inhaler by pulling the metal canister out of its plastic holder, then running water over and through the plastic holder. Allow it to dry thoroughly before reassembling. It is best is to allow it to air-dry overnight. Then carefully reseat the nozzle of the metal canister in its receptacle at the base of the plastic holder.

4. Take care that no foreign object gets caught in the mouthpiece of your inhaler. The risk is that you inhale not only medication but also the plastic shoe of a toy doll or some other small intruder!

DON'T:

1. Allow the inside of your inhaler to get wet. Water trapped in the nozzle of the canister will interfere with the release of the correct dose of medication.

2. Hold the device upside down. The mouthpiece needs to be at the bottom; the metal canister sticks out at the top.

INHALATIONAL AIDS: SPACERS

A simple device called a spacer can make the use of a metered-dose inhaler a lot easier and more effective. We recommend spacers for people who have difficulty coordinating the hand-breath actions that the use of metered-dose inhalers requires, for virtually all children using metered-dose inhalers, and for anyone taking inhaled steroids delivered by metered-dose inhaler (see Chapter 6). If you are good at inhaling your quick-acting bronchodilator from a metered-dose inhaler, there is no need to use a spacer—it provides no added benefit.

A spacer is a hollow chamber that attaches to your metered-dose inhaler. In its simplest form, it is a hollow plastic tube that fits onto the mouthpiece of your MDI; you place your mouth on the mouthpiece of the spacer, and instead of spraying the medication directly into your mouth, you spray it into the chamber, where it remains suspended for a few seconds. You inhale the medication from the other end of the chamber in one or two slow, deep breaths, without any sense of urgency or need for split-second timing.

When you use a spacer, you are less likely to stop inhaling suddenly because a cold blast of medication (released directly from the metered-dose inhaler) hits the back of your throat. The suspension of the medication in the chamber minimizes the "cold blast" effect.

Another feature of many spacers is a built-in whistle that sounds when you breathe in too rapidly. The whistle helps train you to inhale slowly, which in turn helps distribute the medication throughout the system of bronchial tubes. A spacer that we recommend for children in particular is called InspirEase. It uses a collapsible, accordionlike plastic bag instead of a solid plastic tube. You

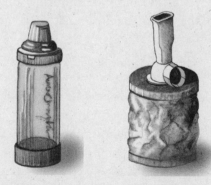

FIGURE 9: TWO COMMONLY USED TYPES OF SPACERS, AEROCHAMBER (LEFT) AND INSPIREASE
Spacers can make the use of a metered-dose inhaler a lot easier and more effective.

can watch the bag collapse and expand with each breath in and out, which lets you know that your child is actually getting the medication. Disadvantages of this device are: 1) to deliver medication into the plastic-bag holding chamber, you need to remove the metal canister of medication from its plastic holder in the metered-dose inhaler and place it in the pipe-stem-like attachment that connects to the plastic bag; 2) over time the plastic bag tends to crack and needs replacement; and 3) it is difficult to clean.

We almost always recommend spacers for children who are old enough to use metered-dose inhalers. Children are usually ready to use an inhaler when they are able to hold their breath underwater, since these activities involve an equivalent amount of breath control. Most children can reliably manage this task at about age 7. In very young children, we like to use spacers that come with attachable face masks, such as the Aerochamber and OptiChamber devices. One such spacer, made by Pari, has a removable mask that can also be used with a nebulizer (see below).

It is safe to say that spacers introduce no risk or side effects. Spacers can be washed in soap and lukewarm water, rinsed, and allowed to drip-dry. The only downsides to spacers are their size—they don't fit into your purse or pocket as easily as your inhaler does—and the added cost (approximately $20 to $30).

ALTERNATIVE METHODS FOR INHALING BETA-AGONIST BRONCHODILATORS

A crucial step in inhaling medication from your metered-dose inhaler is timing the puff just as you are beginning to breathe in. Spray too early, and much of the medication settles on your tongue and throat before the flow of air into your lungs can pull the medication with it. Spray too late, and you have no breath left to pull the medication deep into your lungs. Spray way too late, and the medication is blown away from your bronchial tubes while you exhale. Wouldn't it be good if there were an inhaler that would not release medication until it sensed that you were breathing in?

One such device is available with one of the beta-agonist bronchodilators. The medication is pirbuterol (Maxair) and the device is called an Autohaler. It is described as a breath-actuated inhaler, and it looks similar to an MDI. You prepare the inhaler to release medication by lifting up a lever at the top of the device, thereby spring-loading the metal canister inside. You then put your lips tightly around the mouthpiece of the inhaler and simply breathe in. As you start to breathe in, your effort is detected and the medication spray is released (you hear a click confirming its release). Your job is to keep pulling in the slow, steady breath needed to distribute medication along the many bronchial tubes, then hold your breath for five to ten seconds to allow the medication to settle from the air onto the walls of the tubes. Once you reset the lever on top, you are ready for a second release of medication.

For the Autohaler to work, you need to pull air in with sufficient force for the device to detect your inhalation. You need to hold the device upright while setting the lever on top; and when you grip the device, you must be careful that your fingers aren't blocking the air entry ports at its bottom. You cannot use the Autohaler with any medication canisters other than Maxair; they won't fit. Nor can the Autohaler be used with a spacer.

NEBULIZERS

A nebulizer uses a jet of air (or oxygen) to convert a liquid form of medication into a fine mist that is delivered by routine, quiet breathing to your bronchial tubes. The mist is not irritating, and no special coordination is needed to inhale the medication effectively. You simply breathe in and out from the nebulizer mouthpiece (or mask), and as you breathe, the medication is delivered throughout the lungs.

Quick-acting bronchodilators such as albuterol and metaproterenol are available in liquid form for nebulization. If you or your child has ever needed to go to the emergency department of a hospital for treatment of an asthma

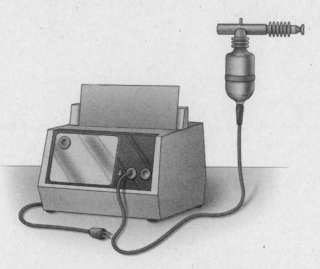

FIGURE 10: ELECTRIC COMPRESSOR AND NEBULIZER
Nebulizers are often the best way to deliver asthma medication to very small children, and to elderly people and others who have difficulty inhaling medicine effectively from a metered-dose inhaler.

attack, it is likely that you received bronchodilator treatments by nebulizer. Even if you are in the midst of a severe flare-up and are struggling to catch your breath, nebulizers are easy to use. The medication is delivered to the airways with each breath, however labored. The usual amount of liquid administered is approximately half a teaspoon, and it takes approximately ten minutes for it to be completely transformed into mist—in other words, it takes about ten minutes to complete a nebulizer treatment.

In the hospital, nebulizers are usually driven by pressurized air or oxygen

Setting Up, Using, and Cleaning the Nebulizer

SETTING UP

1. Plug in the compressor.
2. Insert one end of the tubing into the compressor and the other end into the nebulizer cup.
3. Put the proper amount of medicine in the cup.
4. Attach the cup to the dome.
5. Attach the dome to the T-shaped piece.
6. Attach the T-piece to the mouthpiece.

USING THE NEBULIZER

1. Start the compressor (push the "start" or "on" button).
2. While using the nebulizer you can read, watch TV, listen to music, etc.
3. Hold the mouthpiece in your mouth, keeping the cup level, and take slow, deep breaths.
4. As the medicine in the cup runs out (usually after approximately ten minutes), shake the cup to make sure that all of the medicine is used up. If so, your treatment is done.

CLEANING UP AFTER EACH USE

1. Rinse each piece of the nebulizer with warm running water.
2. Let each piece air-dry, by laying it on a paper towel.
3. When all pieces are dry, put them back together and store them in a clean plastic bag.

CLEANING UP AT THE END OF THE DAY

1. Wash each piece with warm soapy water, and rinse it off with warm running water.

2. Let each piece air-dry.

3. When all pieces are dry, put them back together and store them in a clean plastic bag.

CLEANING ONCE OR TWICE A WEEK

1. Mix 1½ cups of tap water with ½ cup of white vinegar.

2. Soak each piece in this mixture for one hour.

3. Rinse each piece with warm running water.

4. Let each piece air-dry.

5. When all pieces are dry, put them back together and store them in a clean plastic bag.

6. Toss out the water-vinegar mixture—you should only use it once.

available from outlets in the walls of the hospital cubicles or rooms. At home, small electronic air compressors are used for the same purpose. Most compressors are approximately the size of a small toaster; they are attached by tubing to a plastic cup—the nebulizer—which holds the liquid medication. Once medication has been placed in the cup, operation is extremely simple: just push the on-off switch to "on," and the mist begins to form.

You can rent a compressor-and-nebulizer system from a respiratory home-care company, or you can buy one at the pharmacy for about $120 or from a respiratory supply company (including those accessible online via the Internet) for less than $100. Battery-operated systems are also available for use in your car or on a camping trip; they are small and convenient but considerably more expensive.

The great appeal of nebulizer systems is that they are virtually foolproof. Even very small children can receive inhaled medication via nebulizer, using a facemask to make sure the mist gets to their airways. Nebulizers are also often the best way to deliver asthma medication to elderly people and others who, despite repetitive coaching and use of a spacer, have difficulty inhaling medicine effectively from a metered-dose inhaler. Disadvantages of nebulizers are lack of portability (most compressor-nebulizer systems are far too big to fit in your pocket or purse) and amount of time required to administer a full dose (10 to 15 minutes, compared with less than a minute with a metered-dose inhaler).

If your asthma is difficult to control and you have frequent, severe attacks, you might want to have a compressor and nebulizer handy. Anyone who has ever had a life-threatening asthma flare-up that came on quickly should probably have a nebulizer system at home for use while awaiting emergency care.

MDIs AND CHLOROFLUOROCARBONS (CFCs)

Would you ever have imagined that taking care of your asthma is connected to preserving the environment? It is, and here is how. Most inhalers use chemical gases called chlorofluorocarbons (CFCs) to propel the medicine out of the pressurized canister. Developed in the 1930s, CFCs were widely used in pressurized spray cans, refrigeration units, and air conditioners (for example, freon is a CFC). More than a decade ago it was recognized that man-made chemicals—and in particular CFCs—released into the atmosphere were depleting the ozone layer in the upper atmosphere, particularly around the South Pole. (If you are using an inhaler, you are not contributing much to the problem: less than 0.01 percent of all CFCs that entered the atmosphere came from asthma inhalers.)

In response to this environmental problem, more than 130 countries came together in 1987 under the auspices of the United Nations and signed an agreement—known as the Montreal Protocol—to eliminate production and use of CFCs. An exception was made for use of CFCs in medical devices, until suitable alternative delivery systems were developed. Where does this agreement leave people with asthma? The question brings us to the subject of alternatives to CFC-propelled MDIs, and medication delivery systems that do not use chemical propellants at all. However, in the meantime rest assured that CFCs have no effect on your bronchial tubes. Breathed in regularly, day after day, they are totally harmless (as would be many other inhaled gases, such as helium or hydrogen).

OTHER MEDICATION DELIVERY DEVICES

Two alternatives to CFC-propelled MDIs are already available. One involves chemicals called hydrofluoroalkanes (HFAs), instead of chlorofluorocarbons, to deliver the medication. HFAs propel medicines just as effectively as CFCs, but they do not destroy ozone. Two quick-acting bronchodilators, the Proventil and Ventolin brands of albuterol, are available with this ozone-safe propellant and are called Proventil-HFA and Ventolin-HFA. One nice feature of the

HFA-driven inhalers is that the plume of medication that leaves the mouthpiece exits slightly more slowly, and the mist is somewhat finer, so the spray feels softer. As bronchodilators, these HFA formulations act just like traditional, CFC-driven albuterol inhalers, which is to say they are equally effective; however, they cost significantly more.

Incidentally, in our opinion, generic albuterol is equally effective (with the same side-effects profile) as brand-name albuterol (Ventolin and Proventil). Many of our patients feel otherwise, but we have been convinced by carefully done medical experiments demonstrating their equivalence. Only after proving to the Food and Drug Administration that the effects of their generic albuterol were identical to those of brand-name preparations were manufacturers given approval to produce and market their generic equivalents.

The other alternative to CFC inhalers is a whole new type of delivery system, driven by your own inhalation rather than by chemical propellants. The medications contained in these devices come in the form of a very fine, dry powder that can be made into an aerosol by the force of a strong breath in. Besides being ozone-friendly, the so-called dry-powder inhalers are also more user-friendly than metered-dose inhalers. They address the problem of proper timing and coordination, at least in part, by not releasing medication until you breathe in. Some of these new devices also contain a built-in dose counter that lets you know precisely how many doses remain in the inhaler.

For a time, albuterol was available in a dry-powder inhaler called the Ventolin Rotahaler. At present, however, these dry-powder inhalers are only available for administration of controller medications. We will discuss them further in the next chapter. In the future, dry-powder inhalers will likely also be available to deliver quick-acting bronchodilators.

How Do You Know If Your Inhaler Is Empty?

Metered-dose inhalers have no good way for you to tell when they have run out of medication. Ninety-five percent of what is released from the canister with each spray is propellant rather than medication. It is possible that after the medication has run out, some propellant will remain. This remaining propellant will make a sound when you shake the device, and will release a plume when you squeeze down on the canister, causing you to think that you are releasing medication. Eventually, the remaining material is also consumed and nothing comes out of the inhaler, but before this occurs, you may be using a rescue inhaler that has only leftover propellant but no medicine in it—not a good situation. You certainly don't want to rely on an empty canister for relief of your asthma symptoms.

The cost of the inhalers is another reason for wanting to know for sure whether your inhaler is empty. Given that each puff may cost anywhere from 10 to 65 cents, you don't want to discard a partially filled device. At one time we asked our patients to pull the metal canister out of its plastic holder and test whether it would float in a tub of water. If it fell to the bottom or floated with the nozzle up, it was mostly full. If it floated nearly horizontally with the surface, it was empty, or nearly empty. We have stopped recommending this "float test" for the following reasons: first, at best it was a qualitative assessment and didn't distinguish between a device with few puffs of medication left and a totally empty one; second, it turns out that the floatation properties of the different canisters vary considerably; third, the test risks getting moisture into the medication nozzle at the end of the canister, which interferes with its proper functioning.

If you use a medication on a regular basis, as we often recommend for controller medications (see Chapters 6 and 7), then you can simply multiply the number of puffs used each day by the number of days that you have been using a particular inhaler. Subtract this number from the number of puffs in a full inhaler (as determined from the product insert that accompanies each inhaler or from tables provided in this book) and you have the number of puffs left to use. However, for the quick-acting bronchodilators used intermittently for relief of symptoms rather than on a regular schedule for prevention this strategy won't work. It totally fails when you have multiple quick-relief inhalers stationed about your busy life: one at home, one at work, one in your gym bag, one in the car, and so on.

Two "add on" electronic devices can be used to track the number of doses of medication released from an inhaler, but they are pricey and require some degree of technological sophistication. Designed to fit on top of most metered-dose inhalers, the Doser has a computer chip inside that keeps track of how many times it has been pressed. It can only be used with one inhaler at a time and costs approximately $30. Another, more expensive (about $200) unit is called Smart Mist. Your metered-dose inhaler fits inside this device, which can be programmed to track the number of doses left in multiple inhalers placed into the device one at a time. Two additional features of the Smart Mist are that medication is released from the inhaler only when your inhalation is slow and steady, thus training you in proper inhalation technique, and that it can also measure your peak flow and record the trend of your peak flow values over time.

One final, *good* word about metered-dose inhaler technology: these inhalers are manufactured with great accuracy as to their contents (they are highly reliable as to the number of puffs provided in a full canister), and they continue to deliver the exact same amount of medication in each puff, up to the guaranteed number of puffs, even as you get to the last few doses of medicine in the canister.

OTHER QUICK-RELIEF BRONCHODILATORS

NEW FOR THE NEBULIZER: LEVALBUTEROL

Scientists continue to refine the beta-agonist bronchodilators. In Chapter 7 we will discuss the long-acting beta-agonist bronchodilators, which are effective for 12 or more hours. Another refinement was the recent creation of a purified form of albuterol, called levalbuterol (Xopenex). At a dose that causes a similar degree of bronchodilation (0.63 mg), levalbuterol has slightly fewer side effects than albuterol, which can cause jitteriness and heart racing. The decreased side effects have made for its marketing niche. In young children made "hyper" by beta-agonist bronchodilators (with their adrenaline-like side effects), levalbuterol may be less stimulatory. In older people with heart disease such as angina or irregular heart rhythms, levalbuterol may cause less cardiac stimulation. In our opinion, for most patients with asthma the advantages of levalbuterol over albuterol are small and probably not worth the significantly greater cost. Levalbuterol is manufactured only as a liquid for nebulization. So far, no levalbuterol metered-dose inhaler is available.

BRONCHODILATORS BESIDES BETA-AGONISTS

There are quick-relief bronchodilators other than the inhaled beta-agonists that can be used to treat asthma, but they are less satisfactory and not widely used. We have already mentioned beta-agonists in tablet or liquid form, such as albuterol (Ventolin and Proventil), metaproterenol (Alupent), and terbutaline (Brethine). Compared with the same medication inhaled into the breathing tubes, these oral preparations are not as effective in opening the airways, take longer to act (20 to 30 minutes), and cause more side effects—mainly jitteriness and tremor.

THEOPHYLLINE

Another type of bronchodilator, available for swallowing either as an alcohol-based liquid (for rapid absorption) or as a tablet, is theophylline. Twenty years ago, theophylline was the mainstay of bronchodilator therapy. Many people still rely on sustained-release theophylline in capsule or tablet form as a regular controller medication (see Chapter 7). Other formulations once widely used were designed for more rapid absorption and action: immediate-release tablets; an alcohol-based liquid called Elixophyllin; a rectal suppository; and, in the hospital's emergency department, an infusion directly into the veins (aminophylline).

Theophylline is chemically a close relative of caffeine. It shares some of the side effects of caffeine, including a sense of jitteriness and shakiness, and has other potential side effects as well, including nausea, diarrhea, and headache. More troublesome, if you take too large a dose of theophylline, there is a risk for dangerous adverse effects, including seizures and irregular heart rhythms. Because of these potentially very serious outcomes, theophylline has been called the most dangerous of the antiasthmatic medications. Intensive care unit admissions and even deaths have been caused by theophylline overdoses.

Perhaps because of this risk for doing harm, and perhaps because the inhaled beta-agonists act more quickly and strongly to open the breathing tubes, theophylline has fallen from favor among many physicians, especially as a medication for the quick relief of asthma symptoms. Even in our emergency departments, we now almost never use intravenous aminophylline or theophylline, even though it was once a standard treatment for stubborn asthma attacks. However, you may want to remember that caffeine is a weak bronchodilator. If you find yourself in a jam, without access to any bronchodilator medications, you can get a little bit of relief from three cups of coffee—although you will have to say goodbye to a night's sleep.

ANTICHOLINERGICS

Just as the natural body chemical adrenaline stimulates bronchial muscles to relax, opening the breathing tubes wider, there is another natural body chemical, acetylcholine, that stimulates bronchial muscles to tighten or constrict. And just as medicines with adrenaline-like effects have been developed to make bronchial muscles relax, medicines that *block* the constriction of bronchial muscles by acetylcholine have also been developed. These medicines are called anticholinergics.

The first anticholinergic medicine used to treat asthma and other bronchial conditions was atropine, which was extracted from the plant called nightshade or belladonna. This plant is also called deadly nightshade, because excess amounts of atropine can be poisonous.

The next approach was to create anticholinergic medicines that could be inhaled—so that they would go directly to the bronchial tubes and could be used in very small amounts—and that, unlike atropine, would not enter the bloodstream after inhalation. Ipratropium (Atrovent) is just such a medication, available as a metered-dose inhaler and as a liquid for nebulization. It is recommended for treatment of emphysema and chronic bronchitis (see Chapters 2, 14, and 15 for more on these diseases), for which it works well with few side effects, but in general it is not recommended for the treatment of asthma. Why? Because compared with the inhaled beta-agonist bronchodilators, such as albuterol, it is weaker and slower in its onset of action. It takes 10 to 15 minutes to begin working, whereas the relief from the quick-acting beta-agonists starts within one to two minutes. Weaker and slower are not redeeming features when you are trying to catch your breath or get relief from troublesome coughing and wheezing.

If your doctor needs to choose an inhaler for you to keep with you for quick relief of symptoms, he or she will likely choose a beta-agonist bronchodilator rather than an anticholinergic, with the following possible rare exceptions:

- *If you have serious and unstable heart disease.* Under this circumstance, even a little extra stimulation of the heart might cause complications, and ipratropium causes less cardiac stimulation than an inhaled beta-agonist.

- *If you are taking a medication that might adversely interact with beta-agonists.* A rarely used type of antidepressant, called a monoamine oxidase inhibitor (or MAO inhibitor), fits this description. Examples of MAO in-

Usual Dosages of Inhaled Anticholinergic Medicine

MEDICATION	DOSAGE FOR ADULTS	DOSAGE FOR CHILDREN	COMMENTS
METERED-DOSE INHALERS (MDI)			
Ipratropium	2–3 puffs every 6 hours as needed	1–2 puffs every 6 hours as needed	Regular use combined with beta-2 agonists not of proven value
NEBULIZER SOLUTION			
Ipratropium	0.5 mg (2 ml) every 6 hours as needed	0.25–0.5 mg (1–2 ml) every 6 hours as needed	Regular use combined with beta-2 agonists not of proven value

hibitors include phenelzine (Nardil), tranylcypromine (Parnate), and the anti-Parkinsonian medication selegiline (Eldepryl). Ipratropium does not adversely interact with these medications.

The medication Combivent combines ipratropium and albuterol in one metered-dose inhaler. Each spray from a Combivent inhaler releases a standard amount of each of these medicines mixed together. Similarly, the combination of albuterol and ipratropium in a single, pre-mixed solution for nebulization is marketed as Duo-Neb. The two medications together have some additive benefit in treating emphysema and chronic bronchitis. However, there is little if any advantage in asthma, and we do not recommend Combivent or Duo-Neb as part of our routine treatment plan for asthma.

QUICK-ACTING MEDICINES DO NOT PRODUCE LONG-TERM ASTHMA CONTROL

In this chapter we have focused our attention on the medications designed to provide quick relief of asthma symptoms by relaxing tightened bronchial muscles. In Chapters 6 and 7 we discuss the "controller" medications that act to prevent episodes of spasm of the bronchial muscles. In asthma care, one might say a puff of prevention is worth ten puffs of cure.

CHAPTER 6

Controller Medications: The Corticosteroids

WHEN YOUR ASTHMA FLARES UP and the muscles surrounding your breathing tubes contract and cause these tubes to narrow, the quick-relief bronchodilators provide the treatment you need. These medications act quickly and effectively to relax the bronchial muscles, restoring your breathing to normal and making you more comfortable again. And if your symptoms of cough, wheeze, and chest tightness recur, you can simply use your bronchodilator again. So what's wrong with this approach?

There is nothing wrong with it *if:*

• You infrequently experience asthma symptoms (once or twice a week at most)

• You rarely wake up at night due to your asthma (once or twice a month at most)

• You have normal breathing capacity when your lung function is measured

• You never have severe attacks of asthma necessitating emergency care

But if your asthma is troublesome more frequently, or is more severe than this, treating only the bronchial muscle spasm without attending to the underlying inflammation of the bronchial tubes is a mistake.

Here's why. If you rely only on your quick-acting bronchodilator (Primatene Mist, albuterol, or other similar inhaler), you will find yourself bothered by your asthma more than you need to be. Treating only the contractions of the bronchial muscles is a bit like using tissues to stop a bloody nose. If the bleeding is minor and infrequent, this approach works well. But for severe or frequent nosebleeds, inquiring into the underlying cause is necessary: Is there some bleeding disorder or disease of the nasal passageways that can be treated? With asthma, the question is, Why are the bronchial tubes so sensitive to all your asthmatic triggers, and is there anything that you can do to lessen that sensitivity? Rather than reacting to asthmatic symptoms, can you take action to prevent them, or at least to lessen their frequency and severity? Controller medications, especially anti-inflammatory medications, serve this role; they address the underlying problem of inflamed bronchial tubes rather than simply responding to the end product of that inflammation.

Here's another reason not to rely only on your quick-acting bronchodilator: if you do, and find that you need it more and more often, you may also find that it "stops working" for you. As the bronchial tubes swell and fill with mucus during worsening asthma, it becomes increasingly hard to breathe—not so much because the bronchial muscles tighten but because the tubes swell and plug. In this circumstance, causing the bronchial muscles to relax with your bronchodilator inhaler can't be expected to solve the problem. Although it seems that the inhaler is no longer working, in fact the swollen, plugged-up air passageways are the problem, and they require a different treatment. You can protect yourself against asthma attacks and lessen the risk of dangerous ones that don't respond to your bronchodilator inhaler by taking preventive medication (the asthma "controller medications") on a regular basis.

No one likes to take medications every day. We feel as though we are putting foreign chemicals into our bodies; we worry about side effects, both those that are known to occur and those that medical science may not yet know about; and we dislike feeling "dependent" on medicines to maintain our well-being. Particularly if we are young and feeling healthy, why would we take a medicine every day, especially a medicine that may not make us feel better right away?

Controller medications will help you feel better *over time:* usually within two to four weeks you will have fewer asthma symptoms and find yourself less sensitive to asthmatic stimuli and attacks. You will feel as though your asthma is going away, and you will be pleased at how rarely you need your quick-relief bronchodilator.

We all brush our teeth once or twice a day, without a sense of dependence on toothpaste or fear of its side effects. We would suggest that breathing freely and protecting against asthma attacks are every bit as important as keeping teeth white and protecting against cavities. Breathing matters! And fortunately, regular preventive asthma treatments are available that are safe, convenient, and effective.

There are five categories of controller medications:

• Anti-inflammatory steroids

• Long-acting bronchodilators

- Leukotriene blockers

- Mast cell stabilizers

- Anti-IgE therapy

In this chapter, we focus on the anti-inflammatory steroids—the main controller medicines. In the next two chapters, we discuss the other important controller medications.

ANTI-INFLAMMATORY STEROIDS: THE MAIN CONTROLLER MEDICINES

In recent decades our understanding about the importance of inflammation in asthma has grown (see Chapter 1 for a description of what inflammation is). We have learned that people with asthma have airways that are always inflamed to some degree, even when they are feeling totally well. This new understanding has given well-deserved prominence to those medicines that reduce inflammation (called anti-inflammatory medications) for controlling asthma symptoms and preventing asthma attacks. Inhaled anti-inflammatory corticosteroids (called steroids for short) have consistently proved to be the most effective type of controller medication for asthma.

The body makes different kinds of steroids. You have probably heard about the steroids used to build up muscle strength and bulk. In this chapter we are talking about a very different kind of steroids, anti-inflammatory steroids, that we use to treat asthma. These steroids are derived from cortisol, a natural hormone made by our bodies.

Steroids are now a familiar component of modern medical therapies. Steroid injections are used for joints with bursitis. Steroid creams are used for itchy rashes, steroid enemas for colitis (inflammation of the colon), and steroid eyedrops for inflammation of parts of the eye (iritis or uveitis). Steroid tablets or injections are used for severe inflammation, such as the inflammation in rheumatoid arthritis, severe allergic reactions (anaphylaxis), and the rejection of transplanted organs. Cortisone was first used for the treatment of severe asthma attacks in the 1950s, with dramatic, sometimes lifesaving benefit.

Steroid medicines can be inhaled directly into the lungs (inhaled steroids). They can be swallowed or injected by needle into the body, after which they travel through the blood to reach all the body's organ systems (systemic steroids). A great advance in asthma care came in the 1960s, when modification of the structure of cortisol led to the development of new anti-inflammatory steroids, ones that have primarily local effects when applied to a surface such as

Not All Steroids Help Asthma: The Muscle-Building Steroids

If you are young and athletic or if you follow Olympic or professional sports, you may associate *steroids* with illicit drug use for the purpose of muscle building. These other steroid hormones, in particular testosterone and other chemicals derived from it, have muscle-building effects and have been used by athletes to enhance physical performance. Although these hormones and the anti-inflammatory steroids have some chemical similarities—and are therefore both referred to as steroids—they have completely different effects on the body, and on health. The testosterone-derived hormones do not suppress inflammation; the anti-inflammatory steroids do not help build bigger muscles. Because the anti-inflammatory steroids are made by the outer rim of the adrenal glands (called their cortex, or, if referring to more than one, cortices), they are medically referred to as corticosteroids. We will call them steroids for short.

the walls of the bronchial tubes, with minimal effects systemwide. Like a steroid skin cream applied to a red, itchy rash, for the most part they exert their effect where applied and not systemically. Applied directly to the airways, the medication can work to reduce inflammation there without causing the same harmful effects as systemic steroids.

Most patients with asthma who take steroids do so by the inhaled route of administration; inhaled steroids have many fewer side effects than systemic steroids. Systemic steroids are sometimes needed to deal with more severe asthma (often in addition to inhaled steroids), or to help treat asthma flareups. We discuss them later in this chapter.

INHALED STEROIDS

For people who had been dependent on daily use of systemic steroids (often prednisone tablets) to control their asthma, introduction of this new generation of locally active inhaled steroids was nothing short of miraculous. Many people were able to switch from oral steroids to inhaled steroids and maintain good control of their asthma without the many unpleasant and harmful side effects of the oral steroids.

Inhaled steroids have been shown to have the following favorable effects on asthma: they improve the breathing capacity of your lungs, they reduce the frequency and severity of your symptoms, they protect you against asthma attacks, and they improve the overall quality of your life by controlling your asthma. One medical report described a 50 percent lower risk of hospitalization for a severe asthma attack among people using inhaled steroids compared with those not taking these medications.

When you use a quick-acting bronchodilator, your breathing improves and you feel better within just a few minutes. When you use an inhaled steroid, you won't feel any immediate benefit. Steroids reduce the swelling and irritation of the bronchial tubes (the inflammation), but it takes time, typically one to two weeks of regular use. At that point, you will probably experience fewer symptoms and find that you need to use your rescue bronchodilator less frequently.

Unlike your quick-acting bronchodilator, which you carry with you and use when you feel the need, you should take your inhaled steroid *every day*, whether you have symptoms of asthma or not. Leave it at home, but take it every day to prevent your symptoms from occurring. If you develop coughing, chest tightness, or wheezing and need quick relief, don't use your steroid inhaler for that purpose. It won't bring quick relief during an asthma flare-up. It's not a quick reliever (see Chapter 5). But if you take it every day, it will reduce the number of flare-ups you have.

> *"You need to follow your treatments even on the days when you're feeling well. I fell into that trap: once you get over an attack and you're feeling pretty well, you tend to slack off on your medication. I think that it's real important that you keep it up because even though the signs aren't there, you always have asthma."*
> —MARGARET, 60

DIFFERENT INHALED STEROID MEDICINES

For several decades, only three inhaled steroid medications were available to treat asthma: beclomethasone (Beclovent, Vanceril), triamcinolone (Azmacort), and flunisolide (Aerobid). (As noted in Chapter 5, medications have generic and brand names. Throughout this book, we provide brand names in parentheses after the generic name.)

In the last decade, new steroid preparations have been introduced, each with distinctive and potentially advantageous features: these are fluticasone (Flovent), budesonide (Pulmicort), and beclomethasone with a non-CFC propellant (QVAR, pronounced Q-var).

When they were first introduced for the treatment of asthma, inhaled steroids were typically prescribed to be taken four times a day. In truth, few people can remember to take a medicine four times every day, especially if they don't feel immediately better after each inhalation. More recently, it was found that if you take the same amount of medicine divided into two portions each day (for instance, four inhalations twice daily rather than two inhalations four times a day), you get the same benefit without the burden of having to take your medicine so frequently.

Then came the discovery that for milder forms of asthma, using an inhaled steroid once a day works perfectly fine. The Food and Drug Administration has approved once-daily use of budesonide (Pulmicort) for mild asthma, and it is likely that the other inhaled steroids will soon be used in the same way.

FACTS AND FICTIONS ABOUT INHALED STEROIDS

In the previous chapter, we pointed out some of the common misconceptions about quick-acting bronchodilator medications. Several fictions have also grown up about the inhaled steroids.

Fiction 1: If you take inhaled steroids every day, you become dependent on them. You become addicted.

Fact: If you were to stop them suddenly because your asthma went away (when you finally gave away your pet cat or left your job as a welder), your body would not miss them. You would not undergo medication withdrawal, like a smoker withdrawing from nicotine, or even a heavy coffee drinker withdrawing from caffeine. No chemical dependence on inhaled steroids develops, even after years of regular use. (The same does not apply to oral steroids, as we will discuss below.)

Fiction 2: If you take medicines such as inhaled steroids every day, they will lose their effectiveness.

Fact: Although your body can build up a tolerance or resistance to certain medications if you take them for a long time (for example, narcotic painkillers), tolerance does not develop to the anti-inflammatory steroids. They will work just as effectively after months and years of regular use as they did the first few weeks that you took them. And you will not need to take larger and larger doses to achieve the same effect. The same dose has the same effect over time—as long as the stimulus for asthmatic inflammation does not change. (When the stimulus changes, for example during pollen season, if you are sensitive to pollens, you may need to increase your dose of steroids temporarily.)

Fiction 3: Inhaled steroids can cure asthma.

Fact: Inhaled steroids don't cure asthma. They only suppress the asthmatic inflammation of the bronchial tubes for as long as you continue to use them. If you use your inhaled steroids for a few weeks and find yourself feeling better and then stop taking them, it is likely that your symptoms will return. It takes approximately two weeks for the beneficial effects of inhaled steroids to wear off after stopping their use. Asthmatic inflammation will then return, unless something in your environment has changed to prevent its recurrence (such as a reduction in the amount of dust in your bedroom if you are allergic to dust mites and have taken steps to dust-proof your bedroom, or the coming of the first frost if you are sensitive to ragweed pollen). We still lack a one-time cure for asthma. Inhaled steroids are highly effective—as long as you continue to take them.

Fiction 4: You must not suddenly stop taking your inhaled steroids.

Fact: It is true that if you take systemic steroids, such as oral tablets or liquid, for a few weeks or longer, you can become very ill if one day you just stop taking them. However, the same does not apply to inhaled steroids. With regular use of systemic steroids, the adrenal glands stop producing the normal daily amounts of cortisol necessary for routine bodily functioning. The glands shrivel up and are unprepared to resume cortisol production if you stop taking steroid tablets. In routine doses, inhaled steroids have no such effect on the adrenal glands. These glands will function normally, whether or not you continue to take inhaled steroids.

Fiction 5: If you are taking multiple puffs of steroid medicine, you need to wait one minute between puffs.

Fact: Although you will see this recommendation in package inserts, we do not believe that there is any scientific basis for it. As soon as you complete a careful, slow breath in and hold your breath for approximately five seconds, you are ready for your next puff of medication, and your inhaler is ready, too.

DELIVERY DEVICES

Metered-Dose Inhalers

As with quick-reliever medicines (see Chapter 5), metered-dose inhalers (MDIs) are common delivery devices for inhaled steroids. We encourage all patients taking inhaled steroids by metered-dose inhaler to use a spacer with their inhaler. (For more information about spacers, see Chapter 5.) There are two major advantages: first, spacers make it easier to use inhalers effectively, so more medicine gets into the bronchial tubes; second, when you use a spacer, less medicine settles in your mouth. You are less likely to develop an unpleasant side effect of inhaled steroids, a yeast infection in your mouth, if you use a spacer. Also, when less medicine is left in your mouth, less is available to be swallowed and absorbed into the bloodstream, which minimizes the likelihood of side effects elsewhere in the body (such as the eyes, skin, and bones). The Azmacort inhaler, containing the inhaled steroid triamcinolone, has the convenience of being sold with a built-in spacer.

In response to the Montreal Protocol three non-CFC-propelled delivery systems have emerged for the administration of inhaled steroids. One employs an alternative propellant, called hydrofluoroalkane (HFA). Like the inhaled beta-agonist bronchodilators Ventolin-HFA and Proventil-HFA, QVAR utilizes HFA in a pressurized canister to deliver the inhaled steroid beclomethasone. An advantage of this HFA-driven system—having to do with special characteristics of the spray, or plume, of medicine—is that a greater portion of medication can make its way deep into the lungs, where it settles on small bronchial tubes at the lungs' outer edges.

A second option is nebulization of a liquid steroid preparation. The inhaled steroid, budesonide (Pulmicort), is made available as a liquid in prefilled vials called Respules. The liquid medication is converted to a mist for inhalation using a compressor and nebulizer system. We will have more to say about this delivery system for inhaled steroids when speaking about controller medications in young children.

Dry-Powder Inhalers

Dry-powder inhalers (DPIs) are another device for delivering medicines directly into the lungs. DPIs eliminate pressurized canisters altogether. Steroid medication in these devices is available as a very fine powder. Rather than being sprayed out of the inhaler, the medicine is pulled from the inhaler as an aerosolized powder by the force of a breath in. The newer dry-powder inhalers have solved earlier problems: the powders are very fine and nonirritating, with very little, if any, taste. Some of the newer devices are multidose systems, containing as many as 200 doses.

Currently three dry-powder delivery systems are available for use with certain inhaled steroids, and more such devices are likely to be developed and sold in the years ahead. The following features common to all the dry-powder inhalers are worth noting:

1. As previously mentioned, they are free of CFCs and therefore environmentally friendly.

Features and Directions for Use of Specific Dry-Powder Inhaler Devices

Budesonide (Pulmicort) Turbuhaler: Two hundred doses are provided in each container. To prepare the next dose, twist off the plastic cover. Hold the container upright and turn the brown wheel at its base one-quarter turn to the right (clockwise), then back to the left (counterclockwise) until the wheel clicks into position. Then hold the inhaler horizontally up to your mouth, put your lips around the top, and breathe in. The Turbuhaler has a built-in system to indicate when the device is almost empty. A small, clear plastic "window" has been cut into the white plastic side of the container. When only 20 doses remain, a red indicator fills half the window; when the device is empty, the red indicator fills the entire window.

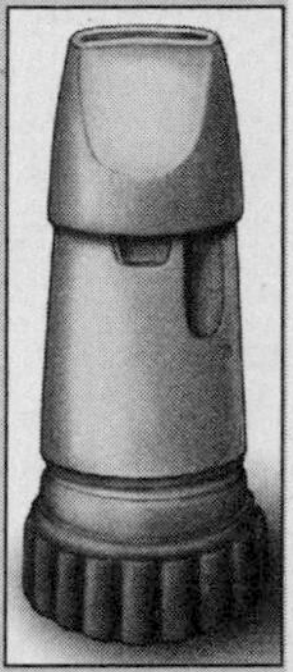

FIGURE 11

Fluticasone (Flovent) Rotadisk: The medication is contained in foil blister packs, each pack containing four doses. To prepare for the first dose, load a blister pack into the tray of the Rotadisk delivery system and slide the tray in and out until the number 4 appears in the window. Next, lift the lid of the device and lower it again to puncture the blister. Now you're all set to inhale the medication, with a rapid, forceful breath in. You can prepare for the next dose by moving the tray in and out until the number 3 appears in the window. The need to reload the Rotadisk after every four doses is a significant disadvantage to this system.

Fluticasone and salmeterol combination (Advair) Diskus: The Diskus device is an excellent delivery system, with 60 doses in each container as well as a built-in counter to indicate precisely how many doses remain. We will discuss the Diskus device further when speaking of the controller medication salmeterol (Serevent) in Chapter 7.

2. They are easier to use than pressurized metered-dose inhalers. The medicine is released by your inhalation rather than by pressing down on the canister, eliminating the coordinated hand-breath action needed with the metered-dose inhaler. To use the dry-powder inhaler properly, after readying the next dose for inhalation, simply place your mouth on the mouthpiece, pull in a strong, steady, full breath, and then hold your breath for approximately five seconds before exhaling. When you are done, rinse your mouth with water and spit out.

3. Dry-powder inhalers are *not* used with spacers. Spacers are meant only for metered-dose inhalers.

4. Compared with metered-dose inhalers, a greater portion of the medicine contained in each dose actually winds up on the walls of the bronchial tubes. The aerosol of dry powder turns out to be more efficient for delivering steroid medicine to the surfaces of the bronchial tubes than the pressurized spray from traditional (CFC-driven) metered-dose inhalers. The greater efficiency of the dry-powder aerosol has to do with the relative size of the microscopic particles generated by the two systems. A greater percentage of the particles released by dry-powder inhalers are of the optimal size for being deposited on the bronchial tubes (rather than settling in the mouth or being breathed back out during exhalation).

5. Some people find that they are unable to get the benefit of steroids from metered-dose inhalers because as soon as they try to breathe in the medication, they cough. Some of the elements of the spray (particularly a chemical called oleic acid) can be irritating. Dry-powder inhalers do not contain these chemicals and are often well tolerated by people who cough using metered-dose inhalers.

Delivery Devices for Inhaled Steroids

MEDICINE	DELIVERY DEVICE
Beclomethasone (QVAR)	Metered-dose inhaler (with HFA propellant)
Triamcinolone (Azmacort)	Metered-dose inhaler (with CFC propellant and built-in spacer)
Flunisolide (Aerobid)	Metered-dose inhaler (with CFC propellant)
Fluticasone (Flovent)	Metered-dose inhaler (with CFC propellant) Dry-powder inhaler (Rotadisk)
Fluticasone with salmeterol (Advair)	Dry-powder inhaler (Diskus)
Budesonide (Pulmicort)	Dry-powder inhaler (Turbuhaler) Liquid for nebulization (Respules)

OTHER ASPECTS OF THE INHALED STEROIDS: DOSE, DOSING SCHEDULE, AND POTENCY

Your doctor will decide how much inhaled steroid to give you, and his or her decision will of course determine how many puffs or inhalations you will be asked to take each day. In choosing the most suitable inhaled steroid preparation for you, your doctor must take into account the differences among the preparations in terms of the amount of medicine contained within a single puff. This amount varies considerably, from 40 micrograms of beclomethasone in QVAR to 500 micrograms of budesonide in Pulmicort Respules. (A microgram is a millionth of a gram, or 1/450,000,000 of a pound.) Some of the pharmaceutical manufacturers have made their inhaled steroid preparations available in more than one amount per puff, providing you and your doctor with additional options.

If your doctor has prescribed your inhaled steroid (or other asthma medication) to be taken twice a day, you may be relieved to learn that you don't need to take the doses exactly 12 hours apart. Twice a day usually means morning and evening (when you get up in the morning and when you go to bed, or even at breakfast and at supper). For most people, it is easier to remember to take medications according to some daily routine (for example, before you brush your teeth in the morning and before bed) rather than by the clock. Doing so is fine, even if it means taking your medications at 8 and 16 hours apart instead of precisely 12 hours apart. No harm is done, and this schedule is preferable to skipping a dose. So, find a convenient schedule that fits with your daily routine and make taking your medication part of the routine. If you miss a dose, just resume your medicine with the next dose. No need to double up on the number of puffs or inhalations to make up for the missed dose.

As noted earlier, all of the inhaled steroids can be taken twice a day rather than the once routine four times a day, and budesonide (Pulmicort) has been approved for once-daily dosing in mild, well-controlled asthma. We anticipate that in the future the same recommendation will be made for the other inhaled steroid preparations as well.

SIDE EFFECTS OF INHALED STEROIDS

Concern about side effects makes many people apprehensive about the idea of taking steroids for their asthma. However, while systemic steroids have many predictable side effects (discussed later in this chapter), there are only infrequent side effects with the use of inhaled steroids. Remember that for steroid

Amount of Medicine in One Puff of Various Inhaled Steroids

STEROID PREPARATION	AMOUNT OF MEDICINE IN ONE PUFF OR INHALATION (IN MICROGRAMS)
BECLOMETHASONE	
Vanceril,* Vanceril DS*	42, 84
Beclovent*	42
QVAR	40, 80
TRIAMCINOLONE	
Azmacort	100
FLUNISOLIDE	
Aerobid	250
BUDESONIDE	
Pulmicort Turbuhaler	200
Pulmicort Respules	250, 500
FLUTICASONE	
Flovent metered-dose inhaler	44, 110, 220
Flovent Rotadisk	50, 100, 250
Advair Diskus	100, 250, 500

*No longer available.

tablets to work, they have to be absorbed from the stomach and carried by the bloodstream to your bronchial tubes. At the same time, the blood carries the medicine to your eyes, bones, muscles, skin, and appetite center, causing havoc. By contrast, steroids delivered directly to the bronchial tubes by inhalation *for the most part* stay right there—on the bronchial tubes. We will come back to what we mean by "for the most part" in a moment.

Local Side Effects

With the inhaled steroids, the most common side effects are local: on the mouth and voice box (larynx). They can cause a dry, irritated throat and can make you susceptible to a yeast infection in your mouth. The yeast is called *Candida,* and the infection is called candidiasis, commonly referred to as thrush. It feels like a sore throat. If you look in a mirror and see white deposits like a superficial white rash at the back of your throat and especially on the roof of your mouth, you may have thrush. You can help prevent it by rinsing your mouth with water after each use of your steroid inhaler, washing away the medication residue in your mouth. Just rinse with water and spit out; or brush your teeth after your dose of inhaled steroid. Thrush is not dangerous. It is easily treated with prescription antifungal medications in the form of a mouthwash (nystatin mouthwash), lozenges (clotrimazole or nystatin lozenges), or tablets to swallow (fluconazole). Over-the-counter mouthwashes like Scope and Listerine are not helpful for thrush.

The other potential local effect of inhaled steroids is a hoarse voice. You may find that you develop a mild hoarseness that comes and goes. It is annoying, but not harmful or dangerous. It reflects the fact that some of the steroid medicine, on its way down into your lungs, passes by (and settles on) your vocal cords. Rinsing your mouth does not help this side effect, because you cannot gargle water as deep as your voice box. If you must, simply stop your inhaled steroids for a day or two and the hoarseness will typically disappear. Then start back on the inhaled steroids.

Systemic Side Effects

Now back to the observation that *for the most part* inhaled steroids remain localized to the bronchial tubes, just as a steroid cream (such as hydrocortisone cream, or Cortaid) applied to the skin acts only on the skin. There are two ways in which steroids taken by inhalation can make their way into the bloodstream. One way is by swallowing the medication residue in your mouth, so it gets into your stomach and is then absorbed into your bloodstream. This possible chain of events is another good reason to rinse your mouth after each use of your steroid inhaler. Also, as we will discuss shortly, using a spacer with your steroid metered-dose inhaler can help minimize the amount of medication that settles in your mouth.

The other route by which some of the medicine can be absorbed into the bloodstream is through the blood vessels in the bronchial tubes. The surface of the bronchial tubes provides only a very thin barrier—thinner than skin—against the absorption of steroids. Fortunately, only very small amounts of the steroid medicine are needed to control the inflammation of the bronchial tubes, so in general only minuscule amounts are available to be carried from the bronchial tubes to other parts of the body—on the order of 1/1,000 of a 10 mg tablet of prednisone.

Nonetheless, if you were to use high doses of inhaled steroids for a long time, after several months you might begin to experience, to a slight degree, some of the typical side effects that we associate with systemic steroids (like prednisone). The eyes are at risk for glaucoma and cataracts, the skin for black-and-blue bruises after only minimal trauma, and the bones for loss of calcium and increased likelihood of osteoporosis.

If you are taking high doses of inhaled steroids (see below for a definition of a high dose), don't despair. For one thing, other controller medicines are now available that will help you and your doctor reduce your dose of inhaled steroids to a lower and safer level. For another, the risk of these serious side effects remains small and is far less than it would be if you needed steroids in tablet form to control your asthma. Finally, you can take action to protect your eyes and your bones. Have periodic eye examinations and have your bone density measured with a specialized but routinely available X-ray test called bone densitometry. Both glaucoma and thinning of the bones are treatable, if they develop. Good general protective strategies for your bones include adequate intake of calcium and vitamin D, weight-bearing exercises, and not smoking cigarettes.

The following guidelines as to what constitutes high doses of inhaled steroids have been suggested by the National Asthma Education and Prevention Program:

What Is Meant by "High Doses" of Inhaled Steroids?

Steroid Inhaler	No. of Inhalations/Day in Adults	No. of Inhalations/Day in Children
BECLOMETHASONE—HFA		
QVAR 40	More than 12	More than 8
QVAR 80	More than 6	More than 4
BUDESONIDE—DRY POWDER		
Pulmicort Turbuhaler	More than 6	More than 4
BUDESONIDE BY NEBULIZER		
Pulmicort Respules 250		More than 4 treatments
Pulmicort Respules 500		More than 2 treatments

FLUNISOLIDE		
Aerobid	More than 8	More than 5
FLUTICASONE—METERED DOSE		
Flovent 44	More than 15	More than 10
Flovent 110	More than 6	More than 4
Flovent 220	More than 3	More than 2
FLUTICASONE—DRY POWDER		
Flovent Rotadisk 50	More than 12	More than 8
Flovent Rotadisk 100	More than 6	More than 4
Flovent Rotadisk 250	More than 2	More than 1
Advair Diskus 100/50	More than 2	More than 2
Advair Diskus 250/50	More than 2	More than 1
Advair Diskus 500/50	More than 1	1 or more
TRIAMCINOLONE		
Azmacort	More than 20	More than 12

Remember that inhaled steroids cut in half your chances of having an attack of asthma severe enough to require hospitalization. Used wisely, and at the lowest effective doses, these medicines are still the best long-term treatment for the majority of people with persistent asthma.

CHILDREN AND INHALED STEROIDS: SPECIAL CONSIDERATIONS

Inhaled Steroids and the Very Young

If your infant or toddler needs inhaled steroids, two methods of delivery are available to you. One utilizes the metered-dose inhaler with spacer chamber and attached face mask. With your child seated comfortably in your lap, hold the face mask to his or her face. Deliver a spray of medication into the spacer chamber and have him or her breathe in and out five to six times to empty the chamber completely and inhale all of the medicine. If your doctor has prescribed two sprays of medicine, you will need to repeat this process. When done, take a damp cloth and wipe the residue of steroid medicine from your child's face and mouth, being careful to gently wipe the surface of the tongue, the inside of the cheeks, and the roof of the mouth.

Face masks attachable to spacer chambers are sold in small, medium, and large sizes. It is likely that you will be able to find a mask just right for your child's face.

The alternative approach, newly available in the last few years, is to deliver the steroid medication via nebulizer. Only one inhaled steroid preparation, budesonide, is currently available in liquid form for administration by nebulizer. A face mask adapter can be attached at the end of the nebulizer, along with devices that swivel conveniently to match the angle at which your child is holding his head. Nebulization continues until all of the medicine has been delivered, usually taking about ten minutes. Again, carefully clean the steroid residue from your child's face and mouth after completion of the treatment. (In our practice, we also make nebulized budesonide an option for adults, especially the elderly, who may not be able to coordinate any of the other delivery systems.)

Infants and babies cannot pull air in forcefully enough to generate an aerosol from dry-powder inhalers. As your child grows older, how can you and your doctor determine whether the child has sufficient inspiratory power to use a dry-powder inhaler? His or her inspiratory flow rate can be measured in a pulmonary function laboratory. Also, for the same purpose, a new, simple handheld device is now available to your doctor, called In-Check Dial (made by Clement Clarke in England). The minimum flow needed for each device is indicated below:

Minimum Flow Rates for Different Dry-Powder Devices

Dry-Powder Inhalation Device	Minimum Inspiratory Flow Rate (liters/minute)
Turbuhaler	30
Aerolizer*	60
Diskus	30

*Discussed in the next chapter.

Possible Effects of Steroids on the Growth of Children

Because the effects of steroid hormones can manifest themselves throughout the body, there has always been special concern about the use of anti-inflammatory steroids in children, because they are still growing and developing. Might the anti-inflammatory steroids, including those administered by the inhaled route, interfere with lung maturation, brain development, or bone growth if given to very young children? Concerns about long-term side effects have made many pediatricians reluctant to prescribe inhaled steroids for children.

In recent years, important research studies about the effectiveness and safety of inhaled steroids in children have added some insight. The first study, called the Childhood Asthma Management Program, was one of the largest long-term studies of pediatric asthma ever conducted in the United States. More than 1,000 children aged 5 to 12 with mild-to-moderate asthma participated in this research project, which extended over four to six years. Some of the children were treated with the anti-inflammatory steroid budesonide (Pulmicort). Others received a controller medication called nedocromil (Tilade), which is a mast cell stabilizer and not a steroid. A third group of children received no controller medication, only placebo inhalers. All of the children had a quick-acting bronchodilator to use as needed and were given extra medicine (steroids in tablet form) if their asthma got worse.

Three important observations came out of this report:

1. Compared with children treated with nedocromil or the placebo, children treated with the inhaled steroid had fewer symptoms of asthma and fewer asthma attacks that required urgent care, hospitalization, or oral prednisone tablets for treatment. The inhaled steroid was a superior controller medicine and was better at preventing asthma flare-ups.

2. As for medication side effects, the inhaled steroid had only a temporary effect on bone growth. After the first year of use, children in all three groups grew at identical rates, and it was predicted that all the children would achieve similar final heights. The conclusion from this large, carefully performed study was that inhaled steroids did not have a harmful effect on growth in children of this age (5–12). Children treated with inhaled steroids did not appear to grow up to be shorter than children with asthma who did not receive inhaled steroids.

3. Inhaled steroids did not affect lung growth and lung function for better or for worse. The lung capacity of these growing children did not differ among the three groups at the start or the end of the study: the inhaled steroid did not stunt lung growth.

We know that inhaled steroids are effective in treating childhood asthma. They lessen symptoms and vulnerability to asthma triggers. Children treated with inhaled steroids have fewer attacks of asthma, and fewer severe attacks.

We now also know that children can use inhaled steroids in low doses without fear of growing up to be shorter than their peers.

What we don't know enough about—and here more scientific study is needed—is the effect of inhaled steroids in very young children, under 5, especially with respect to their developing brains and lungs. No definite harmful effects are known, but we remain cautious because there is enough *theoretical* concern regarding a *possible* effect. For instance, steroids are known to influence the growth of the air sacs of the lungs, the alveoli, which normally continue to mature in the first few years of life. They also might have effects on maturing brain cells and on the density of growing bones.

In our opinion the very real dangers of severe asthma attacks (which are likely to result in the need for steroids in tablet or liquid form) outweigh any theoretical risks of inhaled steroids. As we noted earlier, steroids in tablet or liquid form are fully absorbed into the bloodstream and carried throughout the body; inhaled steroids are primarily deposited onto the bronchial tubes, with only very minute quantities making their way into the bloodstream and thereby to the rest of the body.

The Food and Drug Administration has given approval for the use of inhaled steroids in children, with the following recommendations for starting ages:

Ages at Which Children Can Start Inhaled Steroids

INHALED STEROID	STARTING AGE (IN YEARS) FOR FDA-APPROVED USE
Beclomethasone (QVAR)	6
Triamcinolone (Azmacort)	6
Flunisolide (Aerobid)	6
Budesonide	
Pulmicort Respules	1
Pulmicort Turbuhaler	6
Fluticasone (Flovent)	
Metered-dose inhaler	12
Dry-powder inhaler (Rotadisk)	4

How Can You Tell If You're Nearly Out of Inhaled Medicine?

You should be taking your inhaled steroids on a regular basis, every day. Therefore, you can pretty easily count the number of puffs you have taken since you started to use a new canister of medicine. A useful practice is to write the date that you started using your new inhaler directly onto the device. The total number of puffs in several commonly used steroid inhalers is shown in the table below:

The Number of Puffs in Various Steroid Inhalers

Medication	Number of Puffs in a Full Canister
Beclomethasone (QVAR)	100
Budesonide (Pulmicort Turbuhaler)	200
Flunisolide (Aerobid) MDI	100
Fluticasone (Flovent) 44, 110, 220	120
Fluticasone and salmeterol combination (Advair Diskus)	60
Triamcinolone (Azmacort)	240

SYSTEMIC STEROIDS

Steroid medicines taken by mouth or by injection are carried by the blood to every organ system in the body and are therefore called systemic steroids. Systemic steroids are used when asthma is more severe, or during a bad flare-up. Typically, steroid tablets or liquid to be swallowed (oral steroids) are given for a brief period (a few days, up to two to three weeks) for an asthmatic crisis, when no other medicine or combination of medicines can relieve symptoms or improve breathing capacity.

In very rare instances, *only* steroid tablets or liquid will work to control asthma in a person with severe persistent asthma. We refer to this unusual problem—when oral steroids must be used as a regular controller medication—as steroid-dependent asthma. We will consider this subject further in Chapter 15, "When Asthma Doesn't Get Better." We believe that anyone with steroid-dependent asthma should be referred to an asthma specialist—and if necessary,

Systemic Steroids

Type of Systemic Steroid	Usual Route of Administration
Prednisone (Deltasone)	Tablets
Prednisolone (Prelone)	Liquid
Methylprednisolone (Medrol)	Tablets, injection (including intravenous)
Triamcinolone (Kenalog, Aristocort)	Injection
Dexamethasone (Decadron)	Tablets, injection (including intravenous)

to a specialized center for asthma care—with the goal of finding an alternative and safer means of controlling his or her asthma.

Systemic steroids are often thought of as a double-edged sword—powerful both in their benefits and, over time, in their harmful, undesirable side effects, which are described later in this chapter.

ORAL STEROIDS

Steroids taken as tablets or liquid to be swallowed are the most powerful medicine available to treat asthma. During an asthma attack oral steroids are given in relatively large doses: from 10 to 60 milligrams per day and more (typically one half to 1 milligram per pound of weight in children). (A milligram is a thousandth of a gram; it is 1,000 times more than a microgram.)

For most people who use steroid tablets as a regular controller medicine, once-daily dosing—usually first thing in the morning—suffices. Sometimes the steroid tablets can be taken every *other* day, thereby minimizing side effects. There are three important points to remember if you have taken daily or alternate-day steroid tablets for more than approximately three weeks. It is important to emphasize that these points pertain only to steroid tablets (or syrup) given systemically for several weeks, and *not* to inhaled steroids or a brief—meaning less than three weeks—course of oral steroids.

First, when trying to decrease the dose of oral steroids, you may experience unpleasant side effects. These symptoms of "steroid withdrawal" include generalized aching, depression, and relative lack of energy and appetite.

Second, it is *not* safe to suddenly stop taking your steroid tablets. After several weeks of use, your body may not be able to make the normal amounts of cortisol hormone required for routine functioning. Your adrenal glands may have shrunken (atrophied) and require time to begin normal steroid hormone production again. Without adequate cortisol hormone—a condition called

Common Doses of Oral Corticosteroids

Medicine	Dosage Form	Adult Dose	Child Dose	Comments
Methylprednisolone	2, 4, 8, 16, 32 mg tablets	Short course "burst": 40–60 mg/day as single or 2 divided doses, for 3–10 days	Short course "burst": 1–2 mg/kg/day, maximum 60 mg/day, for 3–10 days	Short courses, or "bursts," are effective for establishing control when initiating therapy, or during a period of gradual deterioration. The burst should be continued until the patient achieves 80% of his or her personal best peak expiratory flow or symptoms disappear. This usually requires 3–10 days but may require longer. There is no evidence that tapering the dose following improvement prevents relapse.
Prednisolone	5 mg tablets Liquid in two strengths: 5 mg/teaspoonful; 15 mg/teaspoonful			
Prednisone	1, 2.5, 5, 10, 20, 25 mg tablets Liquid: 5 mg/teaspoonful			

Source: National Heart, Lung, and Blood Institute

adrenal insufficiency—you may feel weak, light-headed, and nauseated. Your blood pressure and blood sugar may fall dangerously low, and other chemical imbalances may occur in your blood. Adrenal insufficiency is reversed by starting systemic steroids again.

Third, if you undergo severe physical stress—such as a major operation or critical illness—your body may need extra steroid hormone. Normally, your adrenal glands would produce this extra surge of needed hormone, but because of atrophy they cannot. Under these circumstances, you must let any doctor treating you know that you are taking steroid tablets on a regular basis, so that he or she can administer the extra amounts of systemic steroids that you will need. Many people wear a medical alert bracelet with this information (TAKING REGULAR ORAL STEROIDS) in case they are unable to communicate this information in a crisis. We are in favor of these bracelets, for safety's sake.

You can avoid or minimize the side effects of steroid withdrawal by reducing your dose of steroid tablets very gradually, under the guidance of your doctor. Most often (although not 100 percent of the time), the adrenal glands recover normal function again after you have slowly decreased and then stopped your steroid tablets, even after many months and years of regular use. If you have taken oral steroids regularly for more than a year, this process of gradual withdrawal may take as long as several months.

After months of regular use of steroid tablets, side effects inevitably mount up. Some are merely annoying, such as weight gain and bloating, while others are medically quite serious, such as cataracts and thinning of the bones (osteoporosis). Although side effects are not totally preventable, you can take measures to minimize some of them, as outlined in the following table.

Potential Side Effects of Steroid Tablets with Short-Term Use

SIDE EFFECTS	WHAT YOU CAN DO
Greatly increased appetite	If you are overweight, be careful not to overeat.
Retention of fluid and feeling bloated	Be careful to avoid salty foods, and don't add salt to your meals.
Tendency to develop acne	Be more careful about keeping your face clean and dry, using acne soaps and lotions.
Increased blood sugar	Go light on sweets, and call your doctor if you find yourself getting unusually thirsty or passing an unusually large amount of urine.
Increased blood pressure	If you have a tendency to high blood pressure anyway, check with your doctor about how best to monitor your blood pressure while you are taking steroid tablets. Minimize your salt intake.
Increased irritability and mood swings	There is not a lot you can do except just be aware (and warn your friends and family). This side effect will go away as the medicine is tapered. Antianxiety medications (benzodiazepines) are sometimes prescribed for very severe mood swings or agitation.
Menstrual irregularities	There is not much you can do. This side effect will go away as the medicine is tapered. However, if you miss your period completely, let your doctor know.
Vaginal yeast infections	You can take over-the-counter vaginal creams for yeast infection. Yogurt and lactobacillus capsules may help.

Bone and joint damage (called aseptic necrosis)	Avoid more than one alcoholic drink per day. If you feel a new pain in your hips, or in other joints, let your doctor know.

Potential Side Effects of Steroid Tablets with Long-Term Use

SIDE EFFECTS	WHAT YOU CAN DO
Thinning of the skin and a tendency to bruise and experience skin tears	Be more careful of activities that injure your skin.
Cataracts and high pressure in the eyes (glaucoma)	Have your eyes checked every 6–12 months by an eye doctor. Measuring the pressure in your eye (tonometry) is a painless and quick procedure.
Thinning of the bones (osteoporosis)	Calcium and vitamin D supplements plus bone-strengthening medications such as bisphosphonates, estrogen, and calcitonin can help maintain bone mass and protect against osteoporosis. Foods that are rich in calcium include all milk products (milk, cheeses, yogurt, many frozen desserts), nuts and seeds, beans, tofu, orange juice, rhubarb, and saltwater fish.
Possible muscle weakness	If you find yourself having trouble lifting heavy objects or standing up from a sitting position, notify your doctor.
Vulnerability to certain uncommon infections	Preventive antibiotics are sometimes recommended. If you start feeling unusually ill with fever and chills, notify your doctor.

CHAPTER 7

The Other Controllers

IN OUR DISCUSSION OF CONTROLLER MEDICATIONS thus far (see Chapter 6), we have devoted a lot of space to the anti-inflammatory steroids—deservedly so, because they are the cornerstone of preventive asthma management. However, other types of medication offer additional approaches for asthma control. These include long-acting bronchodilators; nonsteroid anti-inflammatory medicines that work by preventing activation of mast cells ("mast cell stabilizers"); and the leukotriene blockers. A novel controller medication just recently approved for treating allergic asthma, called anti-IgE antibody (Xolair), is discussed in the next chapter.

LONG-ACTING BRONCHODILATORS

Like the quick-acting bronchodilators (see Chapter 5), long-acting bronchodilators help keep the muscles around your bronchial tubes relaxed. They generally do not work as fast as the quick-acting bronchodilators, but their effects last longer—bronchodilation lasting 12 hours or more. When taken once or twice daily, the long-acting bronchodilators can provide effective asthma control, especially when used together with anti-inflammatory medications.

Long-Acting Bronchodilators

GENERIC NAME	BRAND NAME
Salmeterol	Serevent
Formoterol	Foradil
Theophylline*	Theolair, Theo-24, Uniphyl
Albuterol tablets	Volmax, VoSpire ER

* Medications available in generic form (that is, manufactured and sold by a company other than the original developer, usually at lower cost).

Examples of long-acting bronchodilators include the inhaled beta-agonist bronchodilators salmeterol (Serevent) and formoterol (Foradil); slow-release theophylline preparations (such as Uniphyl); and slow-release albuterol tablets (Volmax and VoSpire ER).

LONG-ACTING INHALED BETA-AGONISTS

The discovery of salmeterol (Serevent) and formoterol (Foradil) resulted from researchers' efforts to develop bronchodilators that, like albuterol, could keep the muscles around the bronchial tubes relaxed with minimal side effects, but that would work for more than four to six hours. The first of the long-acting inhaled beta-agonist bronchodilators, salmeterol, was introduced in 1995. It achieved these goals and also proved to be a highly successful controller medication. Several studies have shown that when asthma symptoms are poorly controlled, adding a long-acting inhaled beta-agonist to a regimen of inhaled steroids works better than taking higher doses of the inhaled steroids alone. Many people with difficult-to-control asthma find that by combining a long-acting inhaled beta-agonist and an inhaled steroid, they can take lower doses of steroid inhalers or steroid tablets than they would otherwise need, thus avoiding the possible side effects of high-dose steroids.

SALMETEROL (SEREVENT)

It is usually recommended that salmeterol be taken twice daily, although occasionally people who have asthma symptoms only during the daytime may take it once a day in the morning, and people whose asthma bothers them exclusively at night may take it once a day in the evening. It begins to work about 15

Guidelines for the Use of Salmeterol (Serevent)

- Use it no more than twice a day.
- Do not use it for quick relief of asthma symptoms. It is relatively slow to open the airways and is not intended for quick relief.
- If you need quick relief of symptoms, you can use use your quick-acting bronchodilator, such as albuterol, even after you've taken salmeterol that morning or night.
- Keep taking your other medications, such as inhaled steroids, unless your doctor advises you to stop or cut back on them.
- With your doctor, keep track of your breathing and lung function.

to 20 minutes after you inhale it (versus quick-acting bronchodilators, which take effect within 2 to 3 minutes). The morning dose works to prevent asthma symptoms brought on by exercise at any time throughout the day; the evening dose works as a bronchodilator all night long and may help prevent nighttime awakenings due to asthma. The side effects (jitteriness, tremor, racing heart, and muscle cramping) are minimal, and many people do not experience them at all. For additional information on the safety of salmeterol (Serevent) see Chapter 10, page 163.

Until recently, you had two options for delivery devices containing salmeterol: a metered-dose inhaler or a dry-powder inhaler. The usual dose from the metered-dose inhaler was two puffs. As of July 2003, production of the CFC-containing salmeterol MDI stopped, and now the medication is only available as a dry-powder inhaler.

The dry-powder formulation comes in the Diskus device. Meant to last one month, the Diskus contains 60 doses. To prepare to take a dose, open the inhaler by rotating the outer cover to the right (clockwise), using the thumb-hold indentation. Then push the plastic lever to the right as far as it will go; it clicks into position, exposing the opening through which the medication is released. Finally, holding the device horizontally, place your mouth over that opening—your mouth fits over the plastic holder as it does on a harmonica—and pull a breath in forcefully. *One* inhalation from the Diskus is a full dose. The amount of medication released in one inhalation from the salmeterol (Serevent) Diskus is twice the amount that was contained in each spray from the salmeterol (Serevent) metered-dose inhaler. Finally, close the device by pulling the outer cover back into its original position using the thumb-hold indentation. Closing the device will also pull the triggering lever back into position.

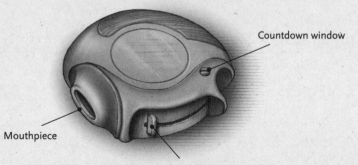

Countdown window

Mouthpiece

Plastic lever

FIGURE 12: THE DISKUS
The Diskus device is a delivery system for dry-powder formulations. It contains 60 doses (meant to last about a month) and has a built-in counter to indicate precisely how many doses remain.

On the outside of the Diskus device you will notice a small opening and a number visible within it, indicating the number of doses of medicine left. With each push of the triggering lever, the number decreases by one. The Diskus is the first device to give a precise indication of the number of doses of medicine remaining in your inhaler.

FORMOTEROL (FORADIL)

Formoterol is another long-acting inhaled beta-agonist bronchodilator. Like salmeterol, it is a beta-2 selective beta-agonist that keeps bronchial muscles relaxed for at least 12 hours with minimal side effects. Like salmeterol, formoterol is meant to be used in combination with an anti-inflammatory medication. Clinical trials have shown that formoterol added to an inhaled steroid is more effective in controlling asthma than using inhaled steroids alone, even at high doses of the inhaled steroids.

Formoterol has two distinctive features that distinguish it from salmeterol. One is that it begins to act very rapidly. Like the quick-acting inhaled bronchodilators, it starts working within two to three minutes. Note that as a controller medicine, formoterol is meant to be taken regularly, usually twice daily, and not carried with you for quick relief of symptoms. Because of its long duration of effect (at least 12 hours), it should *not* be taken more than twice daily.

The second distinguishing feature of formoterol is the unique dry-powder inhaler device, called an Aerolizer, used to deliver it to your bronchial tubes. Like the Spinhaler device once used to administer cromolyn (Intal) and the Rotohaler previously used to deliver albuterol (Ventolin Rotacaps), the Aerolizer is a single-dose device—each dose of medicine has to be loaded individually. Here is how it is used:

1. The capsule of medicine is removed from its foil container and placed into the base of the Aerolizer.

2. The long neck of the Aerolizer is then swung back into place over the base.

3. When the plastic "wings" on either side of the base are squeezed together, the capsule is broken open and ready for use.

4. To release the medication, you place your mouth around the top of the tube and pull in hard. One inhalation is usually sufficient to empty the contents of the capsule, which constitute one full dose.

5. By rotating the tubelike top of the device and exposing its base, you can view the empty capsule to make sure that you inhaled all of the medicine.

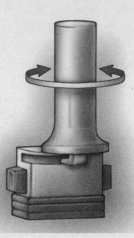

FIGURE 13: THE AEROLIZER
The Aerolizer is a unique inhaler used to deliver the medication formoterol (Foradil). It allows you to check visually to make sure you've inhaled a complete dose of medication.

The obvious disadvantage of this system is the need to load the medicine into it each time you are ready to use it.

As noted, salmeterol (Serevent) and formoterol (Foradil) are highly effective asthma controllers when used in combination with an anti-inflammatory medication, in particular inhaled steroids. They are not recommended for use alone in persistent asthma.

ADVAIR

One pharmaceutical manufacturer has combined its anti-inflammatory steroid, fluticasone (Flovent), with its long-acting inhaled beta-agonist bronchodilator, salmeterol (Serevent), into Advair, a preparation available in a single dry-powder inhaler, the Diskus. Advair makes therapy for even difficult asthma remarkably easy. This combination medicine is prescribed as one inhalation twice daily. With one inhalation, you get a full dose of fluticasone (made available in three different strengths) and a full dose of salmeterol (Serevent). With one medication, you can *simultaneously* treat narrowing of the bronchial tubes due to spasm of the bronchial muscles *and* airway narrowing due to inflammation in the walls of the bronchial tubes. Advair is approved for use in children 12 and older.

We have found Advair both convenient and highly effective as a controller medicine in children and adults. One disadvantage is that the doses of the two

Formulations of the Advair Diskus

ADVAIR DISKUS	FLUTICASONE (FLOVENT)	+	SALMETEROL (SEREVENT)
Advair 100/50	100 micrograms	+	50 micrograms
Advair 250/50	250 micrograms	+	50 micrograms
Advair 500/50	500 micrograms	+	50 micrograms

medicines are linked in "fixed combination" and cannot be adjusted independently. For example, if you want to double your dose of inhaled steroids by taking two inhalations from your Advair Diskus instead of one, you will also get twice as much salmeterol, which is more than the recommended dose.

OTHER LONG-ACTING BRONCHODILATORS

Before long-acting inhaled beta-agonist bronchodilators became available, physicians treating asthma often relied on the long-acting bronchodilator theophylline in tablet or capsule form. (We also discussed theophylline in Chapter 5 under the category of quick-acting bronchodilators.) Throughout the 1970s and 1980s, theophylline played a central role in the treatment of asthma. A variety of different slow-release preparations became available, with brand names such as Theodur, Slophylline, SloBid, Theo-24, Uniphyl, and Uni-Dur. An appealing feature of slow-release theophylline preparations is that they are taken as a tablet or capsule once or twice a day. However, theophylline has important drawbacks. First, side effects are common, including agitation and jitteriness (as you may experience from its chemical relative, caffeine), headache, stomach upset, and diarrhea. Dangerous side effects, including seizures and irregular heart rhythms, can result from excessive amounts of theophylline in the blood.

Second, because the correct dose of theophylline is different for different people and is hard to predict based on your weight alone, it is necessary to measure the amount of theophylline in your blood to make sure that you are receiving the right dose. For this reason, periodic blood tests to check your theophylline blood level are recommended while you are taking it.

A third disadvantage to theophylline is that the amount of medicine that gets absorbed into the blood can increase or decrease while you are taking a stable daily dose because of interactions with other medicines.

None of these three drawbacks to theophylline is shared by the long-acting inhaled bronchodilators salmeterol (Serevent) and formoterol (Foradil). Consequently, the latter have largely replaced theophylline as the current choices for a long-acting bronchodilator to be used along with anti-inflammatory controllers. As a result, several theophylline brands have disappeared from the market. Those still available include Uniphyl, Theo-24, and Theolair, along with generic slow-release theophylline preparations.

A number of our patients with longstanding asthma have used theophylline for many years with good results. Although we generally don't prescribe it for people who haven't used it previously, we don't discourage longtime users who are comfortable with theophylline from continuing to use it. Because of its side effects and because there are better options, we no longer use it for children except on rare occasions.

LONG-ACTING BETA-AGONISTS IN TABLET FORM

Like slow-release theophylline, albuterol has been formulated in special tablets that slowly release medication over a period of several hours. They extend the duration of bronchodilating activity for albuterol to approximately eight hours, and so they are recommended for use three times a day. However, like shorter-acting beta-agonists in tablet form (discussed in Chapter 5), slow-release albuterol (Volmax and VoSpair ER) is not as effective in opening the bronchial tubes as the same medicine delivered by inhalation. Furthermore, if the slow-release mechanism of a tablet is imperfect, you may get a sudden burst of medicine release, with associated adrenaline-like side effects (jitteriness, heart pounding, and so on). We very rarely find occasion to prescribe these tablets.

A LONG-ACTING ANTICHOLINERGIC BRONCHODILATOR

It is likely that a new, ultra-long-acting bronchodilator will become available in the near future. Like its short-acting relative ipratropium (Atrovent), discussed in Chapter 5, this new bronchodilator, called tiotropium (Spiriva), acts by blocking nerve pathways that stimulate constriction of the bronchial muscles. The effects of tiotropium last a remarkable 24 hours, so that once-daily dosing will likely be recommended.

We are hesitant to judge a medicine before its release and before obtaining any firsthand experience with its use. Nonetheless, we anticipate that like ipratropium (Atrovent), tiotropium (Spiriva) will be more appropriate for the treatment of the chronic obstructive pulmonary diseases (for more on these diseases, see Chapters 2, 14, and 15) than for asthma. Our reason is that generally, in people with asthma anticholinergic medications are relatively weak bronchodilators, probably because of the limited contribution made to bronchial tube narrowing by the cholinergic nervous system that anticholinergics are designed to block. Inhaled beta-agonists simply work better.

MAST CELL STABILIZERS

Whereas inhaled steroids have very broad effects on various aspects of inflammation, a mast cell stabilizer has very specific effects. It works to prevent allergy cells called mast cells (see Chapters 1 and 8 for more on mast cells) from breaking open and releasing chemicals like histamine (see Chapters 1 and 8) that contribute to inflammation. Thus this medication, cromolyn (Intal), is referred to as a mast cell stabilizer. When you encounter an allergen to which you are sensitive, a mast cell stabilizer acts to interrupt the allergic response that typically results from that exposure. It is purely preventive: if you have already developed coughing and wheezing after an allergic (or other) exposure, it will not relieve your symptoms.

When cromolyn was first introduced in the 1970s, it came only in the form of a dry-powder inhaler, administered via a Spinhaler. Cromolyn (Intal) powder was relatively coarse. It could be irritating to the throat and could worsen an asthmatic cough. The Spinhaler and cromolyn capsules are no longer made in the United States, but cromolyn is now available as a liquid for nebulization and in a traditional metered-dose inhaler. Another mast cell stabilizer, nedocromil (Tilade), is no longer being produced.

The great appeal of cromolyn, especially for the treatment of asthma in children, is that it is virtually free of side effects. It is not a steroid, so it evokes none of the concerns associated with steroid use. However, as a long-term controller medication, it has a number of shortcomings that have prompted an ongoing search for alternative preventive treatments for childhood asthma. These shortcomings include the following:

1. Cromolyn (Intal) has to be administered four times daily to be effective as a controller medicine. Most generally healthy people find it difficult to take a medication four times a day over an extended period. Imagine the difficulty in getting a young, active child to sit quietly for 10 to 15 minutes four times a day while inhaling cromolyn nebulizer solution.

2. Cromolyn is only modestly effective, especially when compared with inhaled steroids. It does not provide protection against severe asthma flare-ups as reliably as the inhaled steroids do.

3. Increasing the dose of cromolyn does not increase its protective effect. Unlike inhaled steroids, upping the dose does not help during asthma flare-ups.

One particular use of cromolyn is worth mentioning: it effectively blocks exercise-induced bronchial narrowing when taken as a single dose 15 to 20 minutes before exercise. (For more on this use of cromolyn, see Chapter 11.) The quick-acting inhaled beta-agonist bronchodilators, such as albuterol, are usually used for this purpose, but cromolyn offers an alternative for people who are especially susceptible to the jittery side effects of albuterol. It can also be taken in addition to albuterol (or other quick-acting bronchodilators) if albuterol alone does not prevent exercise-induced symptoms of asthma. Cromolyn does not help reverse exercise-induced bronchoconstriction once it has occurred. Turn to your quick-relief bronchodilator for that purpose.

Many pediatricians who remain concerned about possible long-term side effects of inhaled steroids continue to prescribe cromolyn. As we learn more about the safety of inhaled steroids in children, asthma specialists and other physicians are recommending the mast cell stabilizer less and inhaled steroids more, especially for children with more severe asthma.

The Mast Cell Stabilizers

MAST CELL STABILIZING DRUG	DOSE (IN MILLIGRAMS)
Cromolyn (Intal)	
by Spinhaler (no longer available in U.S.)	20 per capsule
by metered-dose inhaler	0.8 per puff
by nebulizer	20 per nebulizer treatment

LEUKOTRIENE BLOCKERS

Years of careful scientific research successfully pinpointed an important group of inflammatory chemicals, called leukotrienes, that are produced by mast cells and other allergy cells called eosinophils (see Chapters 1 and 8). Leukotrienes can cause many of the effects we associate with asthma. They stimulate bronchial muscles to contract. They cause excess mucus to form in the bronchial tubes and promote leakage of fluid into the walls of the bronchial tubes. They attract additional allergy cells into the airways. Collaborative research among scientists at Harvard Medical School in Boston and the Karolinska Institute in Sweden led to the identification of the leukotrienes in 1978. In 1982 the discovery was honored with the Nobel Prize in Physiology or Medicine.

One of the observations that led to the identification of the leukotrienes was the finding that antihistamines—which block the action of the inflammatory chemical histamine and are effective in treating allergies in the nose and elsewhere—do not prevent or relieve asthma. The failure of antihistamines to affect asthma made it clear that inflammatory chemicals besides histamine must be contributing to asthmatic reactions in the bronchial tubes. Some of those chemicals turned out to be leukotrienes.

In 1996 the first medication to block the activity of leukotrienes, zafirlukast (Accolate), became available. Because of the many effects of leukotrienes, this leukotriene blocker was difficult to categorize as a bronchodilator or an antiinflammatory medication. By stopping the activity of leukotrienes, it had both effects. Since then, two additional leukotriene blockers have become available: montelukast (Singulair) and zileuton (Zyflo). As a group, the leukotriene blockers represented the first new type of antiasthmatic medication developed in more than 20 years.

The three currently available leukotriene blockers are all taken by mouth (swallowed):

- Zafirlukast (Accolate) is taken twice daily on an empty stomach.

- Montelukast (Singulair) is taken once daily. A chewable tablet is approved for use in children as young as 2. A granular sprinkle that can be used to treat asthma in infants as young as 12 months has recently become available.

- Zileuton (Zyflo) has to be taken four times daily for maximal effectiveness, although it has some benefit when the dose is reduced to two to three times a day. The manufacturer of zileuton has announced that it will cease production of this medication at the end of 2003.

Zafirlukast (Accolate) and montelukast (Singulair) block the action of leukotrienes after the body makes leukotrienes, just as antihistamines block

Leukotriene Blockers

GENERIC NAME	BRAND NAME	DOSE
Montelukast	Singulair	10 mg once daily in adults; 5 mg chewable tablet once daily in children age 6 to 14; 4 mg chewable tablet once daily in children age 1 to 5; 4 mg oral granules in children age 6 to 24 months
Zafirlukast	Accolate	20 mg twice daily
Zileuton	Zyflo	600 mg four times daily

the action of histamine. Zileuton (Zyflo) inhibits the formation of the leuko-trienes in the first place. For some people, leukotriene blockers work very well—lessening symptoms, improving breathing capacity, and reducing the frequency of asthma attacks. For mild asthma they may be the only preventive medication needed. Leukotriene blockers offer additional advantages: they come in tablet form, so no coordination of inhaler devices is needed; and because they are not corticosteroids, they have none of the potentially harmful effects of steroid tablets.

Not everyone with asthma benefits from leukotriene-blocking medications, however. As many as 40 percent of adults with asthma experience no improvement when taking them. For the most part, we can't predict who will (or won't) respond well to these drugs, with one exception. Individuals with aspirin-sensitive asthma make relatively large amounts of leukotrienes and are particularly likely to improve on leukotriene blockers (see Chapter 11 for more on this subject).

SIDE EFFECTS OF LEUKOTRIENE BLOCKERS

People who take leukotriene blockers rarely experience side effects. Two to four percent of people taking zileuton (Zyflo) develop liver inflammation. Although this is an unusual side effect, doctors order periodic blood tests to monitor liver function as a precaution when a person starts taking zileuton. If liver inflammation does occur, it is generally mild and goes away when the medication is stopped.

A very rare complication of zafirlukast (Accolate) and montelukast (Singulair) is a generalized outpouring of the allergy cells called eosinophils into blood vessels throughout the body, called eosinophilic vasculitis, or Churg-

Strauss syndrome. This reaction can involve allergic inflammation at multiple sites, including the lungs (in a pneumonia-like reaction), heart, nerves, and skin. It happens once in approximately 60 million patient-years of treatment with these medications. (One patient taking the medication for one year = 1 patient-year. Two patients taking the medication for one year, or one patient taking the medication for two years = 2 patient-years.) It has occurred almost exclusively in people with severe asthma who were taking regular steroids in tablet form but in whom the oral steroids were withdrawn after they were started on the leukotriene blocker. This complication, though serious, is so rare that it does not influence our use of these medicines. However, when using leukotriene blockers in people with severe asthma who are attempting to withdraw from daily oral steroids, we recommend particularly careful monitoring for adverse effects.

In this and the two preceding chapters, we have covered a lot of territory, touching on nearly all the medications currently available to treat asthma. The one exception is a novel, "biotech" therapy just recently approved for use in the treatment of asthma, called omalizumab (Xolair). In the next chapter, we will discuss this new therapy and explore additional asthma treatments still under development and potentially available in the years ahead. In the third part of this book, devoted to the management of asthma, we will revisit all of these medications and examine how they are best used.

CHAPTER 8

New Asthma Therapies

ASTHMA THERAPY HAS ADVANCED remarkably in just a generation or two. If you are a middle-aged reader, you may have heard of asthma sufferers in your grandparents' generation who sought relief from their symptoms by smoking cigarettes filled with dried leaves of the stramonium plant, also called thorn apple, jimsonweed, or, more formally, *Datura stramonium.* The active ingredient of stramonium is atropine, an anticholinergic bronchodilator like ipratropium (Atrovent)—but with many more side effects. (See Chapter 5 for more on ipratropium.) Both the bronchodilators and the medication delivery systems used to treat asthma have come a long way since then.

Still, as good as asthma treatment has become, it is not perfect. Many people dislike having to inhale medicines, and even the newer generation of dry-powder inhalers are not foolproof in delivering medication to the bronchial tubes. In addition, concerns linger about the long-term safety of some of the medications, particularly the inhaled steroids, although it should be at least somewhat reassuring to know that after approximately 30 years of availability, and after use by many millions of people with asthma, no epidemic of harmful effects from inhaled steroids has occurred.

We eagerly await advances in asthma therapy for two other reasons. First, despite taking several of the current antiasthmatic medications, a small minority of people with severe asthma continues to be troubled by asthma symptoms and recurrent asthma attacks. Their asthma fails to respond to any treatment except relatively high doses of steroid tablets (such as prednisone). They are caught between a rock and a hard place: suffering from frequent coughing, wheezing, and nights of disturbed sleep, or from steroid-induced symptoms such as weight gain, mood swings, high blood sugar, and high blood pressure. This small subgroup of people with "steroid-dependent asthma" is in need of new approaches to treatment.

The second aspect of asthma that calls out for advances in treatment (and is described in Chapters 3 and 15) is "airway remodeling"—the permanent scarring that some people with asthma, perhaps 10 percent or so, eventually develop in their bronchial tubes. Even when at their best, they have limited lung capacity. Unlike most people with asthma, their breathing is impaired even when they are feeling well. We have yet to identify the causes of the irreversible changes in the structure of their bronchial tubes or find treatments that can prevent or possibly reverse these changes.

Based on past developments in asthma therapies, new asthma treatments are likely to emerge from three general sources: 1) refinements of current treatments; 2) precisely targeted treatments that grow out of detailed understanding of the specific steps and interactions involved in the inflammatory process of asthma; and 3) serendipity—unexpected treatments found when looking elsewhere. Examples of new medicines from these sources exist now. The long-acting inhaled beta-agonists salmeterol (Serevent) and formoterol (Foradil) are refinements of older, shorter-acting beta-agonists. The leukotriene blockers emerged from the discovery of previously unknown inflammatory chemicals, the leukotrienes, and their important role in asthma. (See Chapter 7 for a discussion of these medications.) The just-released immune-modifying drug omalizumab (Xolair), discussed later in this chapter, grew out of a refined understanding of the role of the key allergy protein in asthma, IgE.

A fourth avenue of discovery is just around the corner: treatments based on analysis of our genes. Around the world, researchers are making intensive efforts to determine which genes—and which of the proteins made by these genes—are linked with asthma. Armed with this information, scientists will be able to study how these specific gene products either cause asthma or affect its severity and to figure out how to interfere with these processes.

REFINING ANTIASTHMATIC MEDICATIONS: NEW MEDICINES FROM OLD

NEW INHALED STEROIDS

An ideal inhaled steroid would have potent local effects on the bronchial tubes with no generalized harmful effects beyond them. It would be a very powerful agent for suppressing asthma but would not raise any concerns about damage to the eyes, bones, skin, and other parts of the body.

This holy grail of the inhaled steroids does not appear to be just around the corner. However, promising new inhaled steroids to watch for will continue a positive trend in the development of these medicines: they will be strong in suppressing asthma, *relatively* free of side effects at usual doses, and convenient to use. One agent, already available in Canada and several other countries around the world, is mometasone (Asmanex). This steroid formulation is already approved for use in this country as a nasal steroid spray (Nasonex). Experiments have shown it to be an effective asthma controller medication when given only once daily, whether taken in the morning or the evening. It is delivered by dry-powder inhaler in Canada; the dry-powder device, called Twisthaler, looks similar to the Pulmicort Turbuhaler (see Chapter 6). A non-CFC metered-dose inhaler containing mometasone is also expected. (For a discussion of CFC-free inhalers, see Chapter 5.)

Another steroid compound under development has a unique feature—it is activated by enzymes along the bronchial tube walls. The medication, called ciclesonide (brand name not yet given), has shown promise in clinical trials, causing very few effects beyond the lungs. It, too, will probably become available as a dry-powder inhaler (Cyclohaler) and as a CFC-free metered-dose inhaler to be taken once daily.

New Bronchodilators

Theophylline (see Chapters 5 and 7 for more on theophylline preparations) works as a bronchodilator by boosting the amount of a specific chemical signal—cyclic adenosine monophosphate (cyclic AMP)—within bronchial muscle cells. It does so by inhibiting the enzyme called phosphodiesterase, or PDE. In brief, theophylline blocks the action of PDE and thus acts to relax the bronchial muscles.

It turns out that there are different forms of PDE and that it is possible to block one or more of these forms without blocking them all. This scientific observation has spurred efforts to find chemical compounds that, by blocking unique forms of PDE, might act as bronchodilators but not cause the nausea or heart stimulation associated with theophylline. Theophylline is a blunt instrument, blocking multiple forms of PDE. Selective PDE inhibitors are under development—in particular, inhibitors that block PDE type 4 (one of at least seven different subtypes of PDE so far identified). The hope is that blocking this specific subtype of PDE that is related to bronchial constriction will maximize the benefit of treatment while minimizing some of the unwanted side effects that result from blocking other subtypes.

Several pharmaceutical companies are testing their PDE_4 inhibitor drugs on people with asthma and chronic obstructive pulmonary diseases, or COPD. (For more on COPD, see Chapters 2, 14, and 15.) Drugs in this category share the suffix "-milast." One PDE_4 inhibitor drug currently undergoing testing is called cilomilast (Ariflo). It can be taken as a tablet twice daily, with seemingly few side effects or interactions with other drugs. Preliminary observations suggest that cilomilast (Ariflo) may be more effective for the treatment of COPD than of asthma. Nonetheless, having a theophylline-like bronchodilator that is safe, relatively free of side effects, and easy to use would seem desirable, if only for the convenience of asthma treatments in tablet form.

Another medication refinement in the works involves purification of the long-acting inhaled beta-agonist bronchodilator formoterol (Foradil). Like albuterol, formoterol (and all the beta-agonist bronchodilators) exists as a 50:50 mixture of identical molecules with mirror-image shapes, the "left-handed" and "right-handed" formoterol molecules. These differently shaped molecules do not act the same way. One shape (designated R,R) acts as a powerful bronchodilator; the other shape (S,S) does not, and may even lessen the bronchodilating effects. By developing a purified preparation of only (R,R)-formoterol, one pharmaceutical company hopes to create a stronger and longer-lasting bronchodilator. (R,R)-formoterol offers the prospect of an inhaled bronchodilator that acts immediately upon use and continues to work for 24 hours—a once-daily inhaled bronchodilator.

NEW MEDICATION COMBINATIONS

New therapies for asthma can involve a simple repackaging of a combination of already existing medications. The Combivent metered-dose inhaler (albuterol plus ipratropium) and Advair Diskus (fluticasone [Flovent] plus salmeterol [Serevent]) are prime examples. (See Chapters 5 and 7, respectively, for a discussion of these medications.) The former combines two quick-reliever medications. Because ipratropium (Atrovent) is primarily used to treat chronic bronchitis and emphysema rather than asthma, we have not encouraged the use of Combivent for our patients with asthma. On the other hand, the combination of an inhaled steroid and a long-acting inhaled bronchodilator in Advair Diskus has proved highly convenient and effective for people with moderate and severe asthma. As discussed in Chapter 7, this combination inhaler is formulated so that with one inhalation morning and night, you receive both a powerful anti-inflammatory medication and around-the-clock bronchodilation.

Another pharmaceutical company is preparing a similar combination. It will mix the inhaled steroid budesonide (Pulmicort) with the long-acting inhaled bronchodilator formoterol (Foradil) in a combination metered-dose inhaler called Symbicort. Treating the dual aspects of asthma, bronchial inflammation and bronchial muscle constriction, with a single inhaler holds great appeal. In addition, because of the quick onset of effect of formoterol (Foradil), Symbicort will provide immediate symptomatic improvement. It will also overcome the disadvantage of the current formoterol delivery system;

as we noted in Chapter 7, a single capsule of formoterol has to be added to the dry-powder delivery system (the Aerolizer) with each use. Like all other metered-dose inhalers, Symbicort will contain multiple doses ready to go.

NEW INHALATIONAL DELIVERY DEVICES

It is a sure bet that as traditional CFC-driven metered-dose inhalers are gradually phased out of production, new devices will be created to deliver both traditional and newer inhaled asthma medications. The technical challenge is to create devices that are simple to use, economical to make, sturdy, and portable. The best of these devices will contain multiple doses of medication and have numerical dose indicators so you can tell exactly how many doses you have used and how many remain. They will also disperse the medicine in a way that ensures that as much as possible gets deposited on the walls of the bronchial tubes, and as little as possible winds up in the mouth and throat. Medical requirements dictate that the exact same amount of medication is released with each inhalation. Other desirable features are that even during an asthma attack, when your breathing power is limited, your weaker breath is sufficient to pull in a full dose of medicine; and that variations in heat and humidity have little effect on the dispersal of powdered medications.

Three other developments are worth mentioning. One involves the purified form of albuterol, levalbuterol (Xopenex; see Chapter 5 for more on levalbuterol). Until now, this bronchodilator has been available only as a liquid for nebulization. In the near future, a pocket-sized formulation will probably be marketed: a metered-dose inhaler with an ozone-friendly propellant (hydrofluoroalkane, or HFA—see Chapter 5 for more on these propellants). Once levalbuterol becomes available in a metered-dose inhaler, direct comparison can be made with the old standby albuterol metered-dose inhalers. We can then learn for certain whether at conventional doses the purified form of albuterol really is stronger, besides being more expensive, and whether it truly has fewer side effects.

Another noteworthy development involves a new device to be used with dry-powder inhalers. As noted in Chapter 6, we encourage all our patients to use a spacer with their steroid metered-dose inhalers, to minimize the amount of medication that settles in the mouth and throat. So far, no similar device is available for steroid medicines delivered by dry-powder inhaler. The Aero filter proposes to remedy this situation. This simple plastic device can be attached to dry-powder inhalers and is meant to trap the larger particles that would otherwise tend to be deposited in the mouth and throat, while allowing the smaller particles, destined to settle on the breathing tubes, to pass through.

A third interesting development to watch relates to novel techniques in particle engineering. Dry-powder inhalers of the future may contain carefully engineered particles that help in settling the medicine on the bronchial tubes, leaving less medicine behind in the throat. One such proprietary manufacturing process, PulmoSphere technology, creates hollow and porous particles with favorable aerodynamic properties. Both bronchodilators and anti-inflammatory inhalers may take advantage of this sort of technology in the future.

All of this technological development is likely to mean more choices for you in the future. Do you prefer to take your inhaled medicines from a CFC-free pressurized spray or from a dry-powder inhaler? Do you prefer the flexibility of using individual medicines in separate inhalers, or the convenience of combining them in a single device? Do you want to be able to see medicine in a capsule before you take the drug, and an empty capsule after taking it? These are among the options that are likely to become available to you in the years ahead.

ASTHMA DESIGNER DRUGS: THE AGE OF BIOTHERAPEUTICS

A revolution in the treatment of asthma and other allergic diseases looms just around the corner. Our understanding of the molecular biology of asthma has advanced at a great pace. We know in detail about the molecules (immunoglobulin E, or IgE for short) that recognize the allergens we breathe in. We have discovered the so-called IgE receptors that help IgE molecules stick to the surface of inflammatory cells. We have identified the molecules that act as signals to instruct other cells to make IgE molecules (interleukin-4), and other signals that attract allergy cells such as eosinophils to the bronchial tubes (interleukin-5). We have discovered molecules that help the allergy cells stick to blood vessel walls so that they can make their way from the blood to the bronchial tubes (ICAM-1, VCAM-1, VLA-4). Finally, we have identified other molecules (called lipoxins) that seem to put a brake on this inflammatory reaction.

A very much abbreviated "scorecard," listing only a few of the many "players" in allergic inflammation as well as some of their actions, appears in the following table. (For an overview of the allergic reaction, and what allergies have to do with asthma, see Chapter 1.) In fact, the cast of characters is enormous, and each is a potential target for a drug that might interfere with allergic inflammation, whether in the form of asthma, hay fever, eczema, hives, food allergy, or anaphylaxis (a severe allergic reaction throughout the body leading to dangerously low blood pressure).

Molecules That Affect Inflammation

BIOLOGICAL MOLECULES (ABBREVIATION)	THEIR ROLE IN ALLERGIC INFLAMMATION
Immunoglobulin E (IgE)	One end of the molecules sticks to, or binds to, mast cells; the other end recognizes and binds to specific allergens
Interleukin-4 (IL-4)	Stimulates production of IgE; recruits eosinophils to the bronchial tubes
Interleukin-5 (IL-5)	Attracts eosinophils to the bronchial tubes and helps sustain them there
Adhesion molecules: intercellular cell adhesion molecule (ICAM), vascular cell adhesion molecule (VCAM), very late (activation) antigen (VLA)	Molecules on the surface of eosinophils that help eosinophils traveling in the blood stick to blood vessel walls before they exit the blood for the bronchial tubes
Lipoxins	Recently discovered molecules that dampen the inflammatory response

ANTI-IgE THERAPY

As of July 2003, an exciting new biotherapeutic drug has been approved for use in allergic asthma by the Food and Drug Administration. Called omalizumab (Xolair, pronounced zo-lair, with emphasis on the first syllable), it is an injected medicine designed to remove IgE antibodies from the blood. It is recommended for people with moderate or severe persistent asthma, particularly those who have not achieved good asthma control with conventional asthma medications or have had unacceptable side effects from them.

Its creation was a scientific tour de force. Scientists stimulated mice to make antibodies that would recognize and bind to, or stick to, human IgE molecules. They used a special technique to isolate mouse cells that would produce only this one type of antibody, a pure preparation of anti-IgE antibodies. These antibodies, all of exactly the same structure, are called monoclonal antibodies. They come from a single clone (that is, a genetically identical type) of antibody-producing cells.

It was not enough that these antibodies could recognize and bind to IgE as it circulated in the blood. They needed to bind to IgE at a specific point. If they stuck to the IgE molecules at any other point, they would act like an allergen and set off the whole cascade of allergic responses. The scientists managed to develop monoclonal antibodies that stuck to IgE exactly at the point where it would otherwise bind to the surface of a mast cell. As a result, the IgE molecule could no longer stick to a mast cell, and the monoclonal antibody did not trigger an allergic reaction.

But the scientists were not done yet. If an antibody made by a mouse is injected into a human being, the body's immune system will recognize the antibody as a foreign substance and work to get rid of it. So the scientists engineered a solution: 95 percent of the structure of the anti-IgE antibody would be composed of a human antibody molecule with identical structure, and only 5 percent—the critical IgE-binding part—would be composed of mouse components. The result is described as a humanized monoclonal anti-IgE antibody.

Why would anyone go to the trouble and massive expense of creating a humanized monoclonal anti-IgE antibody? The answer is based on our belief that IgE is central to asthma and many other allergic processes. People with asthma tend to have increased levels of IgE molecules in their blood. As noted in Chapter 1, the IgE molecules stand as sentinels, prepared to recognize allergens and to signal mast cells to release histamine, leukotrienes, and other inflammation-causing chemicals. In people with allergies, mast cells whose surfaces are loaded with IgE molecules lie in wait in the bronchial tubes, the skin, the lining of the eyes, the nose, or the intestinal tract. What if enough IgE molecules could be removed from the surface of these mast cells so that they would no longer burst open when people with allergic sensitivities were exposed to allergens? What if it were possible to protect against these allergic responses regardless of the specific allergen, whether cat or dog, pollen or dust mite, cockroach or peanut? Anti-IgE antibody therapy appears to have just such a protective effect.

More than 800 people with allergic asthma participated in two experimental studies to test the effect of treatment with anti-IgE therapy. People recruited for these studies had moderate or severe persistent asthma. They were taking regular inhaled steroids, and some needed daily steroids in tablet form to control their asthma. In one study omalizumab (Xolair) was administered by intravenous infusion every two weeks; in the other it was given as injections into the skin every two or four weeks. Both studies included a group of people with asthma who were assigned at random to receive infusions or injections of a placebo (an inactive treatment). For several weeks, all participants in the studies continued their usual medicines in addition to anti-IgE treatments (or placebo). In the final weeks of these studies, the subjects attempted to reduce the dose of their steroids (inhaled or oral) and, if possible, to stop them altogether.

What were the results? For one thing, the anti-IgE treatments dramatically reduced the amount of "free" IgE molecules—that is, IgE molecules circulating in the blood. Measured in nanograms (one billionth of a gram) of IgE in each milliliter of blood, the average level of free IgE fell from approximately 1,000 to approximately 10. The consequence: subjects receiving anti-IgE therapy felt better. Their symptoms were somewhat fewer, their peak flows higher, and their response to questions about their quality of life more favorable than those of subjects randomly assigned to received placebo. When it came time to try to reduce their anti-inflammatory steroids, more subjects receiving anti-IgE therapy were able to reduce or discontinue steroids than were subjects in the placebo group. For instance, in one of the two studies (the one in which omalizumab was given as injections in the skin), 40 percent of the subjects given anti-IgE treatment could stop using their inhaled steroids altogether, versus 19 percent in the placebo-treated group. Subjects treated with omalizumab also had fewer serious flare-ups of their asthma.

Among the findings made in these studies was that anti-IgE therapy is well tolerated. Side effects were few: an occasional subject developed hives at the site of medication injection. In sum, it can be said that anti-IgE therapy proved helpful to a group of people whose asthma was very active. It is a well-tolerated, targeted therapy without any of the side effects associated with steroids. It offers new hope for people with severe, steroid-dependent asthma that they will find an alternative to oral steroids for daily control of their asthma. For people with asthma and other allergies, this medication may alleviate not only their asthma but also their other IgE-medicated allergic diseases (like allergic rhinitis and conjunctivitis). In the future, it may also be used to treat food allergies. Preliminary studies using a very similar anti-IgE monoclonal antibody have showed great promise in treating peanut allergy. At the same time, omalizumab (Xolair) is not curative of asthma or so dramatically effective that all other medications for asthma can routinely be stopped. Treatment needs to be continued for as long as you have asthma (that is, indefinitely).

Omalizumab dosing is based on your blood IgE level and your weight. Depending on the dose of anti-IgE antibody that you require, it is administered once or twice monthly by injection under the skin. It is approved for use in adults and in children 12 and older. Its cost depends on dose, but can amount to tens of thousands of dollars per year. Whether removing IgE antibodies from their blood will leave people less well able to fight parasitic infections—

the presumed beneficial function of IgE antibodies—has yet to be demonstrated.

The approach that led to the development of omalizumab represents the dawning of a bright new era of biotherapeutics in the treatment of asthma. Other molecules are being created and tested for their effects on the vast variety of individual steps in the allergic process: blocking interleukin-4, blocking interleukin-5, blocking adhesion molecules, mimicking the action of lipoxin, and many others. Some of these treatments can be given by inhalation rather than injection. All are being carefully monitored for potential harmful effects as well as for desired therapeutic outcomes. Judging from the success of this approach in another chronic inflammatory disease, rheumatoid arthritis, there is every reason to believe that in the next several years additional new treatment options will become available to people with asthma and allergies. At least initially, because of their expense, these biotherapeutic agents will probably be most appropriate for those in whom current therapy has either been ineffective or caused harmful side effects.

GENE-BASED ASTHMA RESEARCH

The decoding of the human genome has provided scientists with another powerful approach to deciphering the mysteries of allergy and asthma. Around the world, researchers are focusing intensive efforts on determining which genes, and which of the chemicals whose production they direct, are linked with asthma. We'll probably have at least some of the answers within the next several years. Armed with this information, we can then study how these proteins and other chemicals contribute to asthma and allergies.

Some genes probably make proteins that influence our tendency to recognize foreign allergens when they enter our bodies. These are the genes that make us atopic, or sensitized to common allergens. Others probably contribute to the abnormal twitchiness of the bronchial tubes that is characteristic of asthma. Identifying the specific genes may point the way to new treatments that we can now only begin to imagine.

Asthma will almost certainly be found to result from the inheritance of many variant genes, some essential in causing the disease, some responsible for the variation in asthma in different people (some who have allergic asthma, others who don't; some who have mild disease, others who have severe disease that resists the usual therapies). This complexity makes the treatment of asthma with gene therapy a very distant prospect.

Although gene-based asthma research hasn't yet produced new therapies, it has led to important insights that may help explain why individuals react differently to the same medications. Genetic differences among us may explain, for instance, why some people with asthma respond well to treatment with leukotriene blockers, whereas others derive no benefit. In the future, we may be able to do something quite extraordinary: we may be able to figure out, at the very beginning of your treatment, the best medicines for you. That would be a big step forward compared with the trial-and-error method doctors must sometimes use today to find what works best for you. The day may come when analysis of your "asthma genes" can predict how you will react to certain medications, thereby making it possible to match you with a "personalized" asthma medication regimen that fits you like a custom-made suit.

For instance, recent studies have pointed to a genetic explanation for why a small subgroup of people with asthma react differently to inhaled beta-agonist bronchodilators. Some people actually do worse when they use the short-acting beta-agonist bronchodilators (such as albuterol) four times a day, every day. Researchers found that these people have tiny variations in the structure of their genes that govern production of receptor molecules for the beta-agonist drugs. As a result, their so-called beta-agonist receptors—to which the beta-agonist bronchodilators attach themselves—differ slightly from the usual beta-agonist receptors. This variant form of the beta-agonist receptor seems to account for the unique response to regular use of short-acting beta-agonists in this particular group. In the future we can expect more such revelations about genetic variations that will explain why medications affect people differently.

Modern asthma research advances on many fronts. Basic research attempts to identify the causes and mechanisms of asthma at the level of individual cells and molecules. Epidemiological research examines the course of the disease over time and seeks patterns in its frequency and severity. Clinical research explores how people experience asthma and how asthma treatments can help make living with asthma easier. Collectively, these efforts have already led to new asthma and allergy medications, new types of treatments, and whole new treatment strategies, some of which we've glanced at here. Some readers may have had the opportunity to participate in asthma research, contributing in their own way to this progress. Given how far we have come since the days of extracting adrenaline from the adrenal glands of cows, the prospect of dramatic new approaches, and perhaps even the development of an asthma cure, may well become a reality in the not too distant future.

CHAPTER 9

Complementary and Alternative Therapies

MANY PEOPLE WITH ASTHMA consider and sometimes try nontraditional therapies, those not routinely recommended by Western-trained doctors, nurses, and pharmacists. Like others with asthma, you may have turned to complementary and alternative medical therapies in the hope that one or more of these might make you better. ("Complementary and Alternative Medicine," or "CAM," is the language used by the National Institutes of Health to describe therapies considered unconventional by most Western medical practitioners, and thought by some to "complement" more conventional Western therapies.) Overall, the percentage of adults in the United States using CAM therapies rose to 42.1 percent in 1997—up from 25 percent in 1990—according to a study conducted by Dr. David Eisenberg, who heads the Division of Research for Complementary and Integrative Medical Therapies at Harvard Medical School.

WHY PEOPLE TURN TO ALTERNATIVE THERAPIES

People use CAM therapies for many reasons. For one thing, medical treatment for asthma can be frustrating. Inhaled medications can be tricky to use properly, and daily medications can feel burdensome and can occasionally cause unpleasant side effects. For another thing, many people worry about potential harmful side effects from long-term medication use, especially use of steroids. Some people feel uncomfortable about putting any "foreign chemicals" into their bodies and are most comfortable taking no medicines at all, even aspirin. Moreover, faithful adherence to treatment programs does not guarantee freedom from asthmatic symptoms or from frightening asthma flare-ups. Some people turn to CAM therapies to get better control of their asthma.

In our own approach to CAM therapies, we seek to keep an open mind. We acknowledge that some wonderful medicines have come from natural sources. No doubt others will follow. At the same time, we have a healthy skepticism about the value of many CAM therapies. Some have not been sufficiently tested and remain unproven in terms of both their efficacy and their safety. Others are just plain useless, the product of hucksterism, false hope, and greed. Too often in our practice, patients come to us with glossy advertisements that they have received in the mail, promoting remedies too good to be true. These advertisements promise, it sometimes seems to us, comfortable breathing, perfect respiratory health, and long life, all from some magical "natural remedy." The claims are usually based on the testimonials of a few individuals and are without even a shred of scientific evidence. In addition, *natural* does not necessarily mean "harmless." Some "natural" therapies have proven to be very dangerous. Some herbal therapies, for example, have been found to cause serious organ damage and even death. For instance, the dietary supplement ephedra, used for weight loss and bodybuilding, has been associated with high blood pressure and strokes.

Where does that leave us, as Western-trained physicians, and you, as an informed consumer? We wish to learn from other cultures and other systems of belief, yet we do not want to be the suckered victims of schemes based on "smoke and mirrors." We want to think creatively about novel approaches while not slipping into wishful thinking.

In our opinion, there is a way to make thoughtful and reasoned decisions about CAM therapies. The solution is based on the scientific method. Put the proposed CAM therapy, as you would any therapy, to a test. Compare it with a placebo in an experiment in which one group of people receives the CAM therapy and another group receives the placebo, or inactive treatment, with neither group knowing in advance whether they are getting the CAM therapy or the placebo. Does it work better than a sugar pill, or sham treatment, or worse? If it is safe and effective, we are eager to incorporate it into our practice. If it is no better or worse than a placebo, it should be dismissed as quackery.

The promising news in this regard is that more and more such experiments are being conducted. Many are being performed under the auspices of the National Center for Complementary and Alternative Medicine, established in 1998 as a branch of the National Institutes of Health. The center is dedicated to supporting scientific research on CAM and to evaluating alternative medical treatments for their efficacy and safety. Some of its studies will undoubtedly focus on CAM for asthma.

Let's examine some of the more popular CAM therapies for asthma and what we have learned about them using modern techniques of analysis.

ACUPUNCTURE FOR ASTHMA

Traditional Chinese acupuncture is perhaps a good starting point, because its use is so widespread for many health conditions, not just asthma.

According to Chinese medical theory, energy, or "qi," flows through the body along pathways called meridians. Along the meridians are "points," where acupuncture needles can be inserted to restore the balance of energy flow thought to be disrupted by disease. As the popularity of acupuncture has increased, researchers have been devoting more attention to understanding how it might work in Western medical terms, and to determining what conditions it might alleviate.

The National Institutes of Health convened a panel in 1997 to look at existing research studies on acupuncture and see what conclusions could be drawn from them. The panel concluded that acupuncture has been shown to be effective for postoperative dental pain, the nausea of pregnancy, and nausea following surgery or chemotherapy. The panelists listed asthma in a group of conditions for which acupuncture was of uncertain benefit. They felt that it *might be* a potentially useful adjunctive treatment, and noted that more high-quality studies were needed.

What sort of study is needed? Ideally, in a large group of patients with asthma of similar severity, one group of people is given real acupuncture and the other group "pretend" acupuncture. "Pretend acupuncture" involves placing needles at sites in the body that are thought to have nothing to do with the meridians relating to asthma. One group receives real acupuncture twice a week for several weeks, the other group "pretend acupuncture" for the same frequency and duration. During and after this period, patients and doctors evaluate how the asthma is doing. Neither the patients (who have never had acupuncture before) nor the doctors are told which treatment they are receiving.

This type of experiment has been performed—although only on a small scale—on at least four occasions, by researchers in the United States, Canada, Australia, and Sri Lanka. In each case, the results were the same: no difference could be found between real and pretend acupuncture. The real acupuncture did not help the patients feel better, improve their lung function, or reduce their need for traditional asthma medications.

Nor is it safe to assume that acupuncture "can't hurt." Acupuncture needles, if not sterilized and disposable, as required by the Food and Drug Administration, can transmit blood-borne infections. The needles can cause local burns and carry a very small risk of puncturing the lung.

Nonetheless, some of our patients tell us that acupuncture helps them. If you decide to try acupuncture, make sure you see a licensed practitioner who uses sterilized, disposable needles. Ask about insurance coverage. Some health insurance plans offer partial coverage for acupuncture. And as with any CAM therapy, talk with your physician about it.

STUDIES DON'T SUPPORT CHIROPRACTIC CARE FOR ASTHMA

You may be one of many people who have sought chiropractic treatment for a musculoskeletal problem—perhaps for low back pain or for a stiff neck that bothers you from time to time. Roughly speaking, chiropractic theory is based on the assumption that your back or neck pain are related to misaligned vertebrae, and that realigning the vertebrae through spinal manipulation may relieve these problems.

The idea that chiropractic treatment can make your asthma better derives from the view that nerve irritation caused by misalignment of the vertebrae adversely affects the chest wall and airways, and that correcting the misalignments can reverse these effects. However, in one carefully done study published in the *New England Journal of Medicine,* the addition of chiropractic spinal manipulations to usual medical care for a period of four months had no effect on the control of childhood asthma. The children who got real chiropractic treatment did not do significantly better than those who got simulated treatment. They did not feel better, have better lung function, or have less need for their quick-acting bronchodilator. Similarly, in an earlier study of chiropractic treatment for adults with asthma, there was no significant improvement in the group who received real chiropractic treatment compared to the group who received simulated treatment.

In our opinion, chiropractic treatments, if they have value at all, are best left for problems of the muscles, bones, and joints. They do not play a role in the management of disorders of the bronchial tubes.

IS THERE A ROLE FOR HOMEOPATHY?

Another widely used CAM therapy, homeopathy is based on the principle that "like cures like"—in other words, that small doses of certain drugs can alleviate the very symptoms that they themselves cause when given in large doses. Superficially, homeopathy would seem to resemble immunotherapy, or allergy shots (see Chapter 4), which you may have considered or tried for your asthma-related allergies. With allergen desensitization, you receive incremental concentrations of an allergen injected into the skin, with the goal of eliciting a different, nonallergic immune response. In homeopathy it is thought that the much-diluted formula of a homeopathic remedy might make your body tolerant of that chemical and thereby make your asthma better. There are big differences, of course: 1) injections stimulate an immune reaction, but ingestion by mouth may not, and 2) immunotherapy uses allergens to which you have been proven to be allergic, whereas the chemicals used in homeopathy are not clearly related to asthma in any way.

Studies of homeopathic treatments for asthma have given mixed results: some showed modest improvements among patients treated with homeopathy; others found no difference between homeopathy and placebo treatment. However, it is difficult to draw clear conclusions from these studies because of their short duration and small number of participants. In addition, these few studies used different homeopathic remedies, making it impossible to draw broadly applicable conclusions from the results. In general, studying homeopathic remedies poses a special challenge because in regular practice the treatments are individualized. The remedy chosen for you is likely to differ somewhat from the one selected for someone else, making comparisons more complicated. To date, using scientific methods, it has not been possible to show a clear-cut beneficial effect on asthma from any homeopathic treatments.

WHAT ABOUT HERBS?

Between 1990 and 1997, the use of herbal remedies in the United States rose by a whopping 380 percent, according to a study on CAM usage conducted by Dr. David Eisenberg. Some herb watchers report that as many as 40 percent of Americans currently use some type of herbal remedy.

Herbs as asthma treatments are by no means a new phenomenon. Various kinds of herbs have been used around the world for thousands of years to treat asthma. Ephedrine is derived from ma huang, the ancient Chinese herbal remedy for asthma. Theophylline is closely related to caffeine and was first isolated from tea leaves. People of your grandparents' generation may have tried to smoke away their asthma with cigarettes filled with the leaves of the stramonium plant. In the early 1800s, a daily spoonful of mustard seed was reportedly recommended for asthma. Among the more dubious treatments we've heard about, camel and crocodile droppings (although these can't accurately be termed "herbal"!) are said to have been used in ancient Egypt. In more recent days, people in this country have tried herbs traditionally used by other cultures, including licorice root, slippery elm bark, and ginkgo biloba. However, despite their widespread use, convincing evidence is lacking that herbal remedies are effective for asthma, or even that they are entirely safe.

THE PRODUCTION AND SALE OF HERBS ARE NOT REGULATED

In the United States no conventional medicine can be released for use by the public until approved by an agency of the federal government—the Food and Drug Administration. The FDA also monitors the production process for each conventional medicine, to make sure no impurities are introduced into the tablet or spray. There is no such agency to evaluate the benefits and risks of herbal therapies, or to monitor their production. Herbal remedies are not classified as drugs, so they are not subject to FDA standards.

For our part, we would like to see more scientific studies of the safety and efficacy of herbs, including studies focusing on their interactions with pharmaceutical medicines. For example, a new dietary supplement is being developed to reduce the production of leukotrienes in people with asthma. Derived from the borage plant, it contains a combination of two fatty acids: gamma-linolenic acid (GLA) and eicosapentaenoic acid (EPA). It has been heralded by its manufacturers as a "medical food product" that, when included in the diet, reduced leukotriene production in 78 percent of people with asthma. But is it helpful in the treatment of asthma? The only way we will ever know is if an unbiased group of investigators performs an experiment in which one group of asthmatic subjects receives the dietary supplement and another group does not, and asthma control among the two groups is compared. This study has not yet been performed.

IS THERE AN ASTHMA DIET?

Several theories maintain that changes in the Western diet over the past 20 years may have contributed to making asthma more common in this country. There is some evidence in support of this, but it is far from proven.

One theory argues that our diets contain too much salt and too much of certain fatty acids (the omega-6 fatty acids, such as linoleic acid). Another theory holds that we lack sufficient magnesium, antioxidants (for example, vitamins C and E), and certain other fatty acids (the omega-3 fatty acids, such as eicosapentaenoic acid [EPA], found, for instance, in dark-meat fish).

However, in the Nurses' Health Study, conducted by investigators affiliated with Brigham and Women's Hospital and Harvard Medical School, more than 75,000 adult women completed dietary questionnaires and were evaluated for their risk of developing asthma over ten years. No food group or vitamin was found to have a definite relationship with their likelihood of developing asthma.

Ask patients with asthma about their own experiences (as was done in a questionnaire distributed in Melbourne, Australia), and you find that most patients have tried to change their diets in one way or another to make their asthma better. Common preparations added to the diet (reported in this study) included calcium supplements, vitamin C, multivitamins, fish oil supplements, primrose oil, and herbal remedies. Commonly avoided foods included nuts, dairy products like milk and chocolate, sausages and frankfurters, pickled onions and gherkins, and fruitcake. Also reported to cause asthmatic symptoms were red wine, flavored toothpaste, and food additives (for example, monosodium glutamate and sulfites).

Among these dietary substances, only sulfites—preservatives commonly found in processed potatoes, shrimp, and dried fruit, as well as in wine and beer—are in fact known to cause asthma attacks, and they cause such attacks only in certain sensitive individuals.

So, except for sulfites, there is no proven link between your diet and your asthma. Certainly, if you believe that something you are eating is making your asthma worse, by all means eliminate it from your diet. It is often said that drinking too much milk or eating too many dairy products causes you to make excess mucus in your bronchial tubes. If you find this to be true for you, avoid these dairy products. However, in general, we do not have enough information to recommend any special, asthma-reducing diet applicable to people with asthma or allergies. You need not restrict your diet in any special way, and you need not supplement it in any special way. As Maimonides said approximately 800 years ago, "Moderation in food type is the key to keeping the bronchioles open."

REDUCING STRESS MAY HELP YOUR ASTHMA

Whether or not you choose to try a special diet or any of the CAM therapies discussed above, you may find that your sense of control over your asthma—and perhaps even your symptoms—improves with certain lifestyle practices that you can cultivate on your own. One of these is stress reduction.

If you have asthma and hypersensitive airways, it is possible that moments of great excitement or stress cause some narrowing of the bronchial tubes and more than the usual sense of breathlessness. As anyone with poorly controlled asthma knows, just having the disease, and not knowing when or where you might have an asthma attack, can be a source of stress. In the event of an asthma attack, when your breathing becomes rapid and shallow, anxiety about your breathing can only make things worse. And while asthma medications are necessary to reduce the likelihood of asthma attacks and to quiet asthma when it flares up, some of them can also make you jittery.

A point that we emphasized in Chapter 4, on asthma triggers, bears repeating here: while asthma was once thought to be a psychological condition, it isn't. It is most definitely a disease of the bronchial tubes of the lungs. Stress may worsen asthma, or it may make you feel worse when you have symptoms of asthma, but it does not cause you to have asthma in the first place. Stress relaxation and psychological counseling cannot be expected to make your asthma go away.

Still, our patients often report that they feel better, and their asthma becomes less bothersome, when the stressors in their lives have been eliminated or reduced. The difficult divorce has been finalized, the financial crisis has passed, the child's illness has been cured—and now the patient can breathe more easily. Sometimes we can't eliminate major stresses from our lives, but we can learn to cope with them more effectively. Here is where stress reduction techniques come into play.

A wonderful thing about stress reduction practices is that while they are likely to help reduce your overall stress, in the event of an asthma attack they also provide a resource that you can draw on to help you stay calm, or to calm down. For example, if you have been practicing some form of breath awareness, you can turn to your practice to help you slow down and deepen your breathing when your asthma is acting up. (Remember, however, that breathing

Research on Asthma and Stress

A team of researchers led by one of our colleagues, Dr. Rosalind Wright of the Beth Israel Deaconess Hospital in Boston, conducted an intriguing study recently on the relationship between stress levels in new mothers and wheezing in their babies. The researchers telephoned the mothers once every two months, until the babies were 14 months old, and asked them to rate their levels of stress in the past month. They found more wheezing among babies whose mothers reported higher levels of stress. The researchers are continuing to follow the children to see whether those with stressed mothers are more likely to develop asthma or not. This study is yet another approach to trying to understand the complex relationship between stress and asthma.

practices are not a substitute for your quick-reliever medication and perhaps other needed medical attention.)

ASTHMA SUPPORT GROUPS

Support groups for people with various illnesses are another tried-and-true complement to medical treatments. Our support group meetings at the Partners Asthma Center begin with a physician discussing a topic of general interest to people with asthma, such as making your home safe for asthma, new medicines, or exercise and asthma. Then a social worker takes over and facilitates a group discussion. People talk about all kinds of things, from the techniques they use to warm the air they breathe on cold winter days, to their embarrassment about using their inhalers in public, to how their family members react to their asthma.

> *"I was in an eight-week asthma support group with people of very different ages and from diverse walks of life. I think we all came away feeling less alone and more secure. We talked about our most frightening asthma attacks. And we learned tips from each other about how to prevent an asthma attack, and if we couldn't prevent it, how to deal with it, and steps we could take to keep ourselves calm in the process."*
> —MARGARET, 60

Our patients sometimes tell us that they experience "support burnout" at home. They feel that they are overburdening family members with concerns they have about their asthma. A support group gives them the opportunity to talk about their experiences of asthma in a new and welcoming venue. People also sometimes share experiences of frightening asthma attacks that they haven't ever spoken about before. One of the most important outcomes of these groups is that people help each other feel less alone with their asthma and more empowered about how to deal with it.

PART III

Caring for Your Asthma

CHAPTER 10

Finding the Treatment That's Right for You

Over the past decade we have witnessed two dramatic shifts in the way medical doctors and scientists view asthma. The first change relates to how serious this disease is considered. For a long time, asthma was considered to be a mild and harmless illness. It was quipped that people with asthma could be expected to wheeze right into old age. Although this assessment is reasonable and realistic in many cases of asthma, perhaps even in most cases, it is not true in all instances, especially among people who are untreated or inadequately treated. Asthma can be a cause of frightening shortness of breath, of life-threatening low blood oxygen, and even of death.

Fortunately, death from asthma remains rare. Of the estimated 15 to 17 million people with asthma in the United States, only approximately 5,000 (approximately 1 in 3,000 people at risk) die each year. However, virtually all of these deaths are preventable with good medical care.

The risk of death is of course only one measure of the importance of a medical condition to our society. The burden of illness can be measured in other ways too: days lost from work and school, urgent medical visits and hospitalizations, and medical costs.

Throughout the 1980s and early 1990s, the number of people in the United States dying of asthma *increased* each year, as did the frequency of emergency room visits and hospitalizations for asthma and the amount of health care dollars spent on the disease. It became clear that asthma is not always mild and innocuous. With the help of the National Institutes of Health, and under the auspices of its National Asthma Education and Prevention Program, the nation's medical community focused its attention on this disorder as a common, important, potentially serious, and treatable condition.

A CHRONIC CONDITION

The other major "sea change" in our view of asthma was based on improved medical understanding about the disease. We have come to perceive asthma not as an occasional or intermittent illness that goes away between attacks. We recognize now that asthma does not "go away" when you feel well and then return when you begin to cough or wheeze or feel short of breath. Your asthma is always there, sometimes symptomatic, sometimes not. Asthma now is understood to be a chronic condition, present day in and day out, even when you feel entirely well and do not have any signs of a breathing disorder.

As discussed in Chapter 1, the tendency of asthmatic bronchial tubes to narrow excessively does not disappear even when asthma symptoms do. Some people experience the symptoms of their asthma infrequently, others repeatedly, still others on a daily basis. Asthma symptoms, when they come, may be mild, or they may be severe and even life-threatening. Regardless of the severity of symptoms, the susceptibility of the bronchial tubes to narrowing is always present. Under the "right" set of circumstances, with exposure to the "right" stimuli, anyone with asthma can develop symptoms and is at risk for an asthma attack.

GOALS OF MODERN ASTHMA CARE

Before discussing the use of medications in the day-to-day management of asthma, it is worth specifying what the goals are for these therapies. Most important, our goals have changed from simply relieving asthma symptoms when they occur to preventing them in the first place. We are using regular (daily) medications to make the asthmatic airways less asthmatic—which is to say, less vulnerable to being sent into spasm by stimuli in our environment. Prevention means not only fewer symptoms but also a reduced risk of asthma attacks, fewer emergency room visits, and fewer overnight hospitalizations.

The goals of good asthma care, as identified by members of the National Asthma Education and Prevention Program, are as follows:

- Prevent persistent and troublesome symptoms (for example, coughing or breathlessness in the night, in the early morning, or after exertion)

- Maintain normal or near-normal lung function

- Maintain normal activity levels (including exercise and other physical activity)

- Prevent recurrent exacerbations of asthma and minimize the need for emergency department visits or hospitalizations

- Provide optimal pharmacotherapy with minimal or no adverse effects

- Satisfy patients' and families' expectations of asthma care

This is not to say that we expect you never to experience symptoms of your asthma. Medical science has not come that far yet. It does mean, however, that our goal is to ensure that most of the time asthma does not interfere with your feeling well and doing whatever you would like to do.

BEING "ASTHMA SMART"

To accomplish the goals listed above, you need to become a partner in your own care. Some things you, the patient, need to do are:

- Make good decisions about avoiding stimuli in your environment to which you may be allergic or otherwise sensitive.

- On occasion, measure your lung function.

- Adjust your medications when your lung function deteriorates.

- Recognize warning signs of a severe asthma attack, and react to these signs quickly.

By no means do you have to manage your asthma alone. You can always call your doctor, arrange an urgent medical visit, or dial 911 in an emergency. But if you are well informed and skilled in caring for your own asthma, crises can be avoided. You will develop self-confidence in your ability to make good decisions about asthma management and develop the sense that you are in control of your asthma and not at its mercy.

We propose five steps to becoming "asthma smart."

STEP ONE: LEARN ALL THAT YOU CAN ABOUT ASTHMA

As one of our patients once said, "You need to get a degree in asthma." By reading this book, you are well on your way to learning about how your lungs work and what goes wrong in your lungs when you have asthma.

Before this, you may have been like most people and taken your breathing for granted. We are generally not called upon to visualize the system of breathing tubes that carry air in and out of our lungs or to consider what happens when these air passageways narrow.

But if you have asthma, you need to understand why these tubes are vulnerable to narrowing, and that there are different causes of narrowing that require different types of treatment. You need to know what the causes, or "triggers," of airway narrowing are for you and how to avoid them. And you need to know the names of your different medications, how to use them, and what they are meant to do.

The Five Steps to Becoming "Asthma Smart"

1. Learn all that you can about asthma.
2. Get the most out of your visit to the doctor.
3. Prevent asthma problems before they occur.
4. Know when you are getting into trouble with your asthma.
5. Be ready to respond to worsening of your asthma.

Additional learning resources are suggested at the end of this book (see page 309), and you may find additional useful information at your doctor's office and online via the Internet. Don't forget to be a critical reader: not every promotional brochure advertising one product or another will give you accurate and unbiased information. If you are uncertain about the accuracy of what you have read, discuss the information with your health care provider.

STEP TWO: GET THE MOST OUT OF YOUR VISIT TO THE DOCTOR

If your asthma care rests in the hands of your primary care physician, as it does for most people, you may have to use your visits to discuss things other than your asthma. Your doctor may need to address other medical problems and perform routine health maintenance—for example, scheduling a cholesterol test or a mammogram. We encourage you to find the time at least once a year (and more often if your asthma is bothering you) to focus your attention, and your doctor's, on your asthma. Here are some of the things that we routinely ask our patients, and that your health care provider will probably want to find out from you:

- Are you having coughing, wheezing, shortness of breath, or chest tightness?

- Do you wake from your sleep because of your asthma?

- Can we review your asthma medications? What are you taking for your asthma? What are the doses? How many puffs of your inhaler are you taking, and how often?

- How often do you need to use your rescue inhaler (for example, albuterol)?

- Have you had any serious attacks of your asthma?

- Have you had any new exposures at home or at work or school?

- How physically active have you been? Do you exercise regularly? Does your asthma limit your ability to exercise?

- Have you experienced any side effects from your medications?

Just as important as the questions your doctor asks you are the things you need to ask your doctor. Here are some sample questions you may want to ask your health care provider:

- Are these still the best medications for me to be taking?

- Should I consider increasing or decreasing the dose or frequency of use of any of my medications?

- Am I using my inhaler properly? Is there someone in your office who can go over the proper use of the inhaler with me?

- Can we measure my breathing today with a peak flow meter or spirometer?

- What should I do if my asthma gets worse? Can you recommend an asthma "action plan" for me? How would I contact you or someone in your office in an emergency?

You can probably add a dozen of your own special questions and concerns. It is a good idea to write down your questions in advance and to bring your list, with your list of asthma and other medications, to your office visit.

STEP THREE: PREVENT ASTHMA PROBLEMS BEFORE THEY OCCUR

As emphasized throughout this book, you can prevent flare-ups of your asthma in two ways: by avoiding the things that set off your asthma, and by taking preventive medications before an anticipated exposure. Sounds simple, but of course it is not.

Some triggers of your asthma are everywhere and cannot be totally avoided, such as dust, springtime pollens, and air pollution. Often you can't anticipate when you will come in contact with your asthma triggers, such as your neighbors' couch, the favorite lounging area for their new pet cat. And who among us can predict when our next viral respiratory tract infection will occur?

Still, prevention is often possible and certainly worth the effort. For instance, if you smoke cigarettes and your child has asthma, you can reduce his or her symptoms to a large extent simply by no longer smoking inside your home. No medications required; no cost involved! If you have asthma and are allergic to cats, finding another home for your pet cat can improve your asthma health dramatically and may prevent the next trip to the emergency department or travel plans canceled because of an asthma attack. (See Chapter 4 for more information on avoiding asthma triggers.)

Sometimes you can minimize the effects of a onetime exposure to one of your asthma triggers by taking medication before the exposure. Very effective, for example, is the use of your quick-acting bronchodilator (such as albuterol) before exercising or walking outside in very cold air. Taken five to ten minutes before the exertion, it can successfully prevent asthma symptoms that would otherwise be stimulated. Use your inhaled bronchodilator before entering a smoky nightclub, and you may find that you can tolerate the secondhand smoke without coughing and chest tightness.

For people whose asthmatic symptoms are generally mild and occur infrequently (no more than once or twice a week), carrying a quick-acting bronchodilator and using it when symptoms occur often proves satisfactory. However, for anyone who experiences severe symptoms or whose symptoms occur quite regularly, daily preventive medicine is recommended. Taking anti-asthmatic medications (also called controller medicines) every day once or twice daily can reduce the frequency of your symptoms dramatically and can protect you from flare-ups of asthma (see Chapters 6 and 7).

STEP FOUR: KNOW WHEN YOU ARE GETTING INTO TROUBLE WITH YOUR ASTHMA

Sometimes asthma attacks are surprisingly easy to ignore. They may come on gradually. As your breathing worsens, you reduce your activities so that physical exertion won't make you short of breath. You may blame your persistent cough on a head cold or "allergies," not associating it with worsening of your asthma. Or perhaps your wheezing goes away after you use your bronchodilator medication, only to recur a few hours later. You find yourself using the bronchodilator inhaler more and more frequently, grateful for the relief that it provides and not noticing how often you have come to use it.

The danger is that all this happens while your air passageways are narrowing, and it is becoming progressively more difficult to move air in and out of your lungs. Even though you don't realize it, the narrowing is proceeding to the danger point. It becomes difficult to draw a breath in even while you are sitting at rest. You feel as though an elephant is sitting on top of your chest. The oxygen in your blood falls dangerously low, and you feel that you may not be able to draw in another breath.

If you are not attentive to early signs of worsening asthma, it may seem as though severe breathing difficulty had come on "suddenly." "Suddenly" your quick-relief bronchodilator is no longer working.

If you're not sure that your symptoms are due to your asthma and not some other cause, like a bad head cold, you have a great resource available to you to answer this question: your peak flow meter. Take five seconds, blow forcefully into the peak flow meter, and you will instantly know whether your asthma is getting worse, and by how much. The value of measuring your peak flow to alert yourself to worsening asthma is emphasized in Chapters 2, 3, and 16.

Being "asthma smart" also means being alert to deterioration in your child's asthma. Here are some warning signs to watch for in a young child:

- Rapid breathing

- Nasal flaring (that is, the sides of the nose pulling wide open with each breath)

- Persistent coughing

- Eating poorly and not wanting to participate in usual activities

- Bluish discoloration of lips and fingers

STEP FIVE: BE READY TO RESPOND TO WORSENING OF YOUR ASTHMA

Recognizing that your asthma has gotten worse is half the battle; the other half is being prepared to take action to get it back under control. Have a plan. Know that in a crisis you can use your quick-acting bronchodilator more often than four times a day. In fact, if you are having severe difficulty with your asthma, you can use your rescue bronchodilator as often as every 20 to 30 minutes if necessary. And you can take as many as four puffs at a time.

Know that for a mild deterioration of your asthma, beginning inhaled steroids (or doubling your usual dose of inhaled steroids) can often restore your breathing to usual. You can double your dose of inhaled steroids by taking twice as many puffs, by taking the medication twice as often each day, or by switching to a preparation that is twice as strong.

Know that for a severe attack of asthma—when you have become short of breath with minimal exertion, or when your peak flow is less than half your normal value—steroids in tablet form are the most effective remedy to relieve your symptoms and increase your peak flow. Because steroid tablets take several hours to exert their anti-inflammatory effect, you will need to take it easy and rely on your bronchodilator inhaler while waiting for the steroids to begin working.

An essential strategy for dealing with an asthma attack is to know how and where to get help. (See Chapter 16 for more strategies.) Family, friends, medical providers, telephone advice, and emergency help can be called on in a crisis, especially if you have made them part of your asthma plan in advance.

MATCHING YOUR TREATMENT TO YOUR ASTHMA

Imagine that you have asthma and only a quick-relief bronchodilator such as albuterol to treat your symptoms when they occur. How do you know if carrying your inhaler with you and using it when you experience chest symptoms is sufficient treatment for your asthma? Are there other treatments that you should be taking? Our recommendation will depend on the severity of your asthma.

MILD INTERMITTENT ASTHMA

Many people with asthma have very mild disease. If you are among these relatively fortunate people, your symptoms are both mild and infrequent: perhaps a tickle in the throat and upper chest with coughing and a bit of chest tightness when you're around furry animals. Perhaps only when running on a cold winter's day do you develop wheezing and labored breathing that disappears within an hour or so after you come back inside. Most of the time you feel well, and if you check your peak flow, it always seems to be normal (see the chart in Chapter 2, page 30, for the normal range of peak flow for a person of your sex, age, and height).

For mild intermittent asthma it is appropriate to use only the quick-relief bronchodilator as needed. If you have asthmatic symptoms, you can use your inhaler to make these symptoms go away quickly. There is no need, and no benefit, to using the bronchodilator inhaler every day on a regular schedule.

Although it is true that what causes your asthma is thought to be a lingering inflammatory reaction in your bronchial tubes, in your case this inflammation is so minimal that it does not interfere with your breathing and makes your bronchial tubes only slightly more twitchy or reactive than normal.

It isn't likely that your asthma will become worse or that you'll develop permanent scarring in and around your breathing tubes if you don't take an anti-inflammatory medication. Only if you acquire a new pet cat, move into a moldy basement apartment, or take up smoking—that is, come in contact with new stimuli that may worsen airway inflammation—is your asthma at risk to worsen dramatically. You and your doctor can periodically measure your breathing capacity. As long as it remains normal, no daily preventive medication is necessary.

For asthma of any severity, a good strategy is to use your quick-relief bronchodilator *before* an anticipated exposure to one of your asthma triggers. The most common example would be exercise, and we will discuss this subject (treatment of exercise-induced airway narrowing) in the next chapter. If you have read the previous chapters in this book, you now understand enough about asthma to know that exposure to allergens like a pet cat will trigger more than just spasm of the bronchial muscles. The allergic swelling and mucus production brought on by exposure to the allergen will *not* be prevented by using a bronchodilator beforehand. In this instance, using your bronchodilator preventively only buys you a little time . . . and in fact you probably don't want to spend too much time around the cat even if you can prevent immediate symptoms.

Antiallergic treatments can be tried preventively before an anticipated exposure to the cat. The mast cell stabilizing medicine cromolyn (Intal) is useful in this way, as are leukotriene-blocker tablets such as montelukast (Singulair) and zafirlukast (Accolade). However, these antiallergic treatments tend to be only partially effective. They should not be relied on to prevent all symptoms related to an intense allergic exposure. Whenever possible, avoidance remains the best and most reliable strategy.

MILD PERSISTENT ASTHMA

Some people have generally mild asthma symptoms, but they suffer these symptoms frequently. If you're in this category, you are not disabled by severe shortness of breath or continuous wheezing, but you notice that you are often aware of your asthma. You often need to use your bronchodilator inhaler to feel fully comfortable in your chest.

Perhaps you wake up during the night, use your inhaler, and quickly go back to sleep, thinking that mild nighttime asthma symptoms are not out of the ordinary. Perhaps you need to use your inhaler repeatedly at work, at school, when you first wake in the morning, or when you first lie down at night. You have become accustomed to getting asthma symptoms and making them go away quickly with your inhaler. Experiencing some asthma has just become a part of your life. If you check your breathing when you feel well, you are reassured to find it normal. These are the signs of mild persistent asthma, which is best treated with regular preventive medicine.

In recent years medical thinking has changed about how best to manage asthma of this severity. A strong consensus has emerged that this burden of asthma symptoms is unacceptable and that daily preventive medication should be taken to reduce the frequency of symptoms. What is more, this preventive medication should be one that has anti-inflammatory properties, not just another bronchodilator (which targets only the bronchial muscles). A leukotriene blocker or an inhaled steroid would be our first choice. Pediatricians still sometimes prescribe cromolyn (Intal) for asthma of this severity, but the four-times-a-day dosing needed for maximal benefit from cromolyn seems an unnecessary imposition.

Some physicians will recommend a leukotriene blocker to treat mild persistent asthma; others prefer an inhaled steroid. The choice is debated in medical literature, without a clear winner. On the one hand, leukotriene blockers are easy to take. You can swallow a tablet once or twice daily. For children as young as 2, a leukotriene blocker is available as a chewable tablet taken once daily (montelukast [Singulair]). The leukotriene blockers are virtually free of undesirable side effects.

On the other hand, inhaled steroids are the stronger medication, more often and more thoroughly preventing asthmatic symptoms and protecting against asthma attacks. Most of the large-scale medical studies showing the benefits of anti-inflammatory treatment in preventing severe asthma attacks, and even protecting against death from asthma, are based on the use of inhaled steroids, not leukotriene blockers.

Mastering the use of the inhaler devices used to administer many of the inhaled steroids can be tricky, and side effects do occasionally occur, including sore throat, hoarse voice, and yeast infections in the mouth (oral candidiasis, or thrush).

However, at the low doses needed to control mild asthma, the risk of long-term adverse side effects, even in children, is thought to be negligible. (See Chapter 6 for more information on potential long-term side effects.) Recent studies have shown that the inhaled steroids can be taken effectively once daily in mild asthma; schedules that call for administration more than twice a day are old-fashioned and unnecessarily burdensome.

So what is our preference for treating mild persistent asthma—a leukotriene blocker or an inhaled steroid? In children less than about 5, we find ourselves trying the leukotriene modifier first. If symptoms of asthma persist, we switch to an inhaled steroid. In older children and adults, we often recommend once-daily inhaled steroids first. They are well-tolerated and more frequently effective.

Remember that having the option of more than one effective treatment is a good thing. Treatment can be tailored to individual needs and preferences, then changed if that approach is not working well either because of lack of benefit or because of unpleasant side effects.

You may wonder why you need to take regular preventive asthma medications for mild persistent asthma at all. Why not just continue to use your bronchodilator as often as necessary as long as it isn't causing any harmful symptoms? The best argument in favor of preventive therapy is that you will feel better. Take medicine as little as once or twice a day, and you will find that you rarely have asthma symptoms. You almost never have your sleep disturbed by your asthma, you haven't needed to use your bronchodilator inhaler in days or weeks, and you feel as if your asthma is going away. The small amount of medication needed to achieve this goal is generally free of any unpleasant side effects, and is also free of any long-term harmful effects.

The other major benefit from beginning preventive therapy is protection from severe asthma attacks. People taking regular preventive medications have fewer attacks of difficult breathing, fewer vacation plans canceled because of asthma, and fewer emergency room visits and hospitalizations for severe asthma.

MODERATE PERSISTENT ASTHMA

Now imagine that you have symptoms of asthma every day. Or that once or more every week you wake from your sleep coughing and wheezing (some people describe dreaming of difficulty breathing, then waking to find that they are really having asthma symptoms). You use your bronchodilator with good relief of symptoms, but find that each inhaler lasts barely one month, or less. Despite your best efforts, you cannot get the peak flow meter to register much more than half to three quarters of the target value anticipated for a person of your age and height. Asthma attacks that send you rushing to the doctor's office or the local hospital are all too frequent. In other words, imagine that you have moderate persistent asthma.

Here's another scenario: imagine that your doctor has already prescribed an inhaled steroid for your asthma. You have used it twice daily faithfully for more than two weeks, and yet you are still regularly experiencing asthma symptoms. Our treatment goals of infrequent use of your rescue bronchodilator (no more than once or twice a week), sleeping through the night, and being able to exercise without limitation seem a far-off pipe dream. Your asthma remains troublesome despite recommended treatment for mild asthma: you have moderate persistent asthma.

Switching to a high-dose, high-potency steroid inhaler is one strategy that may bring moderate persistent asthma under control. For example, your doctor might ask you to switch from QVAR 40 (40 micrograms of the steroid beclomethasone in each puff) to QVAR 80 (80 micrograms of beclomethasone in each puff). Or you might change from Azmacort (100 micrograms of the steroid triamcinolone in each puff) to the Pulmicort Turbuhaler (which contains 200 micrograms of budesonide in each inhalation). Or your doctor might change your Flovent inhaler from Flovent 44 (with 44 micrograms of the steroid fluticasone in each puff) to Flovent 110 or even Flovent 220, which contain 110 micrograms and 220 micrograms of fluticasone per puff, respectively.

Another effective strategy is the addition of a long-acting inhaled beta-agonist bronchodilator such as salmeterol (Serevent) or formoterol (Foradil) to the steroid inhaler, so that you are taking two inhaled medications twice daily. The appeal of this approach is that it allows you to minimize the amount of steroid medication inhaled, thereby avoiding its potential long-term side effects. (For more on these medications, see Chapters 6 and 7.)

In recent years these two strategies for treating moderate persistent asthma (higher doses of an inhaled steroid versus the addition of a long-acting bronchodilator to a low dose of an inhaled steroid) have been compared in carefully controlled medical studies. In these studies, one group of patients was randomly assigned to receive inhaled steroids at high doses. The other group was instructed to maintain use of their inhaled steroid at the original low dose and to add a long-acting inhaled bronchodilator.

A consistent finding in these studies was that the latter strategy was more effective. People had fewer symptoms and achieved better lung function if they took low doses of inhaled steroids in combination with a long-acting bronchodilator. Those who received treatment for both bronchial muscle contraction *and* airway inflammation felt better and experienced fewer asthma attacks. These studies, ushering in the modern approach of using multiple controller medications in preference to one controller medication prescribed at the largest tolerable dose, have had a major impact on how we now treat asthma.

Taking two different inhaler medications twice daily may seem like a bit of a chore. As noted in Chapter 7, one pharmaceutical company has created an appealing solution to this drawback: one dry-powder inhaler (Advair) that contains both a powerful steroid medication and a long-acting bronchodilator. It has been designed so that one inhalation delivers the equivalent of *two* puffs of steroid medication (fluticasone) and *two* puffs of the long-acting bronchodilator salmeterol. An added advantage of the Advair delivery device, called a Diskus, is a built-in counter that indicates the number of doses remaining in the inhaler.

Assessing the Safety of Salmeterol

In February 2003 the pharmaceutical company that manufactures salmeterol (Serevent), GlaxoSmithKline, notified the Food and Drug Administration that it was terminating a large-scale experiment on the safety of salmeterol. At the time that the experiment was stopped, researchers had enrolled nearly 26,000 people with asthma in an observational study in which one group was assigned at random to receive salmeterol and the other group, a placebo inhaler, in addition to whatever other medications they were taking for their asthma. The results were inconclusive at the time that the study was stopped, but a trend was emerging that indicated the occurrence of more severe asthma episodes and more deaths from asthma attacks in the group that had been assigned to receive salmeterol. In particular, it was found that African Americans and people who used salmeterol as their only controller medication were at increased risk of life-threatening exacerbations.

One explanation may be that in many of the problem cases salmeterol was used as a sole controller medication in asthma without any accompanying anti-inflammatory medication. We would discourage this approach. Asthma represents an allergic-type inflammation of the bronchial tubes. In anyone with more than very mild asthma, that inflammation should be treated with anti-inflammatory medication: an inhaled steroid, a leukotriene modifier (such as Singulair or Accolate), or a mast cell stabilizer (Intal). Taking only a powerful bronchodilator like salmeterol might lead to a scenario similar to the following: You feel well—so well that you spend the day playing with the new kitten or mowing and raking the tall grass. Although salmeterol keeps the bronchial muscles relaxed, it does not address the swelling of the bronchial tubes and excess mucus formation resulting from your allergies. You might be falsely lulled into a sense of well-being while your asthma rapidly deteriorates into a full-blown attack of difficult breathing. Salmeterol might do its job (bronchodilation) while masking the effects of inflammatory swelling and plugging of the breathing tubes.

Other possibilities exist to explain the bad outcomes in a few people taking salmeterol. Perhaps because of genetic variations in some people, salmeterol's long-acting, constant signaling that the bronchial muscles should relax paradoxically causes those muscles to relax less. Or perhaps in some people salmeterol interferes with the relaxing effects of quick-relief bronchodilators such as albuterol. In the months and years ahead these and other possible explanations will be carefully explored and analyzed until we understand the exact mechanism that accounts for these findings.

From what we know now our conclusions are: Don't stop your long-acting inhaled bronchodilator (salmeterol or formoterol) based on this preliminary report; don't take regular salmeterol in the absence an anti-inflammatory medicine such as an inhaled steroid; and with your doctor keep track of your breathing and lung function. As long as you maintain good breathing, you can rest assured that your long-acting inhaled bronchodilator is helping, not hurting.

If you are someone who prefers to keep the amount of medication you take to a minimum, you may wonder: If you have added a long-acting inhaled bronchodilator to your inhaled steroid and find yourself doing exceedingly well, can you now stop the inhaled steroid altogether? Theory would suggest not, since asthma involves persistent bronchial inflammation that needs to be treated with anti-inflammatory therapy, not just bronchodilators, even if they are highly effective, twice-daily bronchodilators.

In this case the outcome of medical studies supports the theory: although it may be possible to reduce the dose of inhaled steroids (as we will discuss in more detail below), stopping the inhaled steroid altogether leads to worse asthma control and greater risk of asthma attacks.

You may also wonder about using other combinations of controller medications. What about a combination of inhaled steroid in low doses and a leukotriene modifier for moderate persistent asthma (for example, fluticasone [Flovent] plus montelukast [Singulair])? Or how about combining a leukotriene modifier with a long-acting inhaled bronchodilator (for example, zafirlukast [Accolate] plus salmeterol [Serevent])?

We currently know about the first combination: an inhaled steroid plus a leukotriene modifier. This combination works well, improving the control of asthma over that achieved with the inhaled steroid alone. In direct comparisons, it does not appear to be as effective a combination as an inhaled steroid plus a long-acting inhaled bronchodilator, but it does offer yet another effective alternative to increasing the dose of inhaled steroids to very high levels.

The second combination—a leukotriene blocker and a long-acting inhaled bronchodilator—has not yet been tested in a large group of people with moderate persistent asthma. This experiment is being conducted, but the answer is still a few years away. In the meantime, if for some reason it is desirable to try this combination, you and your physician should carefully monitor your asthma (including with peak flow measurements) to find out whether or not it provides good asthma control and freedom from asthma attacks.

SEVERE PERSISTENT ASTHMA

Fortunately, the smallest group of people with asthma find themselves in our last category of disease severity: severe persistent asthma. If you are in this group, you need your quick-acting bronchodilator several times a day and often during the night when awakened by asthma symptoms. You often have attacks of difficulty breathing that keep you out of work or school and in your doctor's office or the emergency room of your local hospital. Your breathing capacity may be reduced, less than half the normal value, even on a good day.

You are all too familiar with prednisone, the powerful steroid medication in tablet form. It works to control your asthma but causes innumerable side effects. In these circumstances you often develop a love-hate relationship with it. It rescues you from having to gasp for breath, and you feel that you can breathe normally again. But at high doses, prednisone causes you to gain weight, changes the contours of your face, raises your blood pressure and possibly your blood sugar, causes insomnia, and makes you short-tempered. So you and your doctor are eager to reduce the dose of prednisone and possibly stop it altogether. But as you do, your breathing worsens and the coughing, breathlessness, and wheezing return.

Sounds pretty desperate, but even severe persistent asthma can often be brought under good control with modern asthma medications. Here we might combine all three types of controller medications: an inhaled steroid, a long-acting inhaled bronchodilator, and a leukotriene modifier. Sound overwhelming? It isn't, because we have available the combination inhaler (Advair) that delivers both steroid and long-acting bronchodilator in one inhalation morning and night, and the leukotriene blocker is a tablet taken once or twice daily.

Beginning in the summer of 2003, yet another option has become available for treating moderate and severe persistent asthma: omalizumab (Xolair). For people with allergic asthma (by skin test or blood test), this anti-IgE monoclonal antibody can improve symptoms and allow the reduction of the dose of steroids (inhaled and/or oral). Symptoms lessen and the frequency and duration of severe asthma attacks decreases. Treatments are administered as an injection into the skin once or twice a month. Because of the expense of this therapy and its novelty, referral to an asthma specialist for consideration of its use is probably appropriate.

In the past decade we have come a long way, such that even the worst asthma can generally be tamed with appropriate therapy. We say "can *generally* be tamed" in acknowledgment of the fact that some people with asthma continue to struggle with active symptoms even when faithfully taking our most powerful preventive medications. Some people with asthma cannot function without prednisone tablets taken daily (or every other day). Severe, "steroid-dependent asthma" is a special challenge, one that calls for the help of an asthma specialist and possibly a specialized center for asthma care. We address some of the relevant issues in the care of steroid-dependent asthma in Chapter 15, "When Asthma Doesn't Get Better."

"STEPPING DOWN" YOUR MEDICATION

At times when you are free of asthma symptoms, you would probably be tempted to start skipping some of your doses of asthma medications. Naturally, if you feel well, you are less inclined to take medications on a regular basis, especially if you perceive that you no longer need them. Evening doses of your twice-daily medications get skipped; some days you "forget" to take your medicines altogether. What is wrong with that, as long as you are feeling well?

Well, *maybe* nothing is wrong with cutting back on your medications when you are doing well. It makes sense for you (and your health care provider) to reduce the intensity of your medical therapy when you are doing well and when circumstances have changed so that it is reasonable to think that less medication might continue to provide good control of less severe asthma.

In fact, we encourage this "step down" phase of your treatment: finding the lowest dose of medication(s) that will keep you breathing well. We particularly encourage finding the lowest appropriate dose of inhaled steroids. These medications have the greatest potential for some harmful effects *when used in high doses* for many months and years (such as glaucoma, cataracts, thinning of the bones, and easy bruising of the skin).

Now that your asthma is under good control, it is appropriate to try to find, in collaboration with your doctor, the lowest dose of inhaled steroids that will maintain that good control. In mild asthma, once-daily dosing with the inhaled steroid may prove sufficient (any less than once a day has not been proven to work).

TRIAL AND ERROR IN STEPPING DOWN ASTHMA THERAPY

There are some caveats to consider when "stepping down" your asthma therapy. The obvious one is that your asthma control could get worse. You may start experiencing the same asthma symptoms to which you had happily said goodbye. You may begin to rely again on your quick-acting bronchodilator inhaler, whereas before you had come to enjoy rarely, if ever, needing it. No harm done, however. You can simply "step back up" to the treatment program you were using before. We would expect you to regain good asthma control promptly once you have returned to the more intensive regimen.

This trial-and-error approach assumes that when your breathing worsens you begin to experience asthma symptoms and you pay attention to those symptoms. For some people, these assumptions are not valid. You may be someone who doesn't cough and wheeze until your bronchial tubes narrow quite severely. Or you may ignore warning signs of deteriorating breathing capacity as "a little tickle in my throat." In any case, it is wise to check your breathing regularly with your peak flow meter when reducing your medications. A decreasing peak flow number will be a good indicator that your asthma is worsening. A stable peak flow number is reassurance that your bronchial tubes are wide open.

COMBATING THE RISKS OF STEPPING DOWN TREATMENT

More troublesome is the possibility that stepping down the intensity of your asthma treatment will put you at increased risk for an asthma attack. Might you reduce your medications to the point where you become vulnerable to a severe flare-up of asthma, even though you feel good and your peak flow remains normal? This is a real possibility, as found in a medical study in which people with good control of their asthma continued their long-acting inhaled bronchodilator but stopped their inhaled steroid. After stopping their inhaled steroid, people treated with only the inhaled bronchodilator experienced preserved breathing capacity but more often developed exacerbations of their asthma, sometimes needing steroid tablets to treat asthma attacks.

As this study showed, without any treatment of asthmatic inflammation, your bronchial tubes remain twitchy and you are at risk for asthma attacks. Continuing some anti-inflammatory therapy every day is a good idea for all but the mildest form of asthma (mild intermittent asthma).

Ways to Measure Inflammation—Future and Present

But how small a dose keeps you protected? How low a dose of inhaled steroids will maintain protection against serious asthma attacks? Would it be safe to switch off inhaled steroids altogether and take only a leukotriene blocker as your preventive medication?

We are not yet in a good position to answer these questions. We don't have a way of measuring asthmatic inflammation of the bronchial tubes that tells us whether or not the inflammation is being adequately suppressed. Researchers are testing some potential indicators. It is possible that measuring the concentration of certain gases in the air that we exhale may reflect asthmatic inflammation along the surface of the bronchial tubes.

Nitric oxide, one of the candidate gases being studied, is exhaled in higher concentrations in people with asthma than in people without asthma, and treatment with inhaled steroids reduces the amount of exhaled nitric oxide.

Another potential measure, not as easily obtained, would be the amount of inflammatory material in sputum that is coughed up. Finding many allergy-type cells (eosinophils) in expectorated sputum might indicate inadequate suppression of inflammation and high risk for asthma attacks. Neither these

Tips for How Best to Reduce Your Controller Medicine

There is no one correct method, but we have the following suggestions for you to consider, in collaboration with your doctor.

- You may not experience the full impact of reducing your inhaled steroid dose for approximately two weeks after the change. It is a good idea to wait at least two weeks before proceeding with any further changes in your medications.

- If you choose to reduce your inhaled steroid to once-daily dosing, it matters little whether you take it in the morning or in the evening. The best time of day to take it is at a time that you will most likely remember every day.

- The long-acting inhaled bronchodilators exert their effect for approximately 12 hours after each dose. If you are eager to reduce all of your controller medications to once-daily dosing, you can try taking the long-acting bronchodilator only once a day. Use it in the morning if your asthma symptoms occur exclusively during the day; use it in the evening if your asthma symptoms occur exclusively at night.

- Stopping any of your controller medications suddenly may not be the best approach, but it will not cause medication withdrawal symptoms. A possible exception is very high doses of inhaled steroids—more than 2,000 micrograms per day—in which case a gradual reduction is safest.

nor other experimental approaches have yet proved both useful and practical in routine clinical practice.

One tool at your disposal to help you keep an eye on possible deterioration of asthma and risk of an asthma attack is the variability of your peak flow. As an example, imagine that when your asthma is under good control, your peak flow is consistently 350 to 400 liters per minute. When you reduce your medications, you may start noticing greater fluctuations in your peak flow readings: some mornings you hit 400, other mornings only 280, but when you check your peak flow later, it is back up to 400. This variability of peak flow is a warning that an asthma flare-up may be coming. It would be best to increase your medications again, until the peak flow readings are once again steadily in the 350-to-400 range.

WHY NOT STAY ON MEDICATION?

You may have a very different view of managing your asthma. Once good control has been achieved, you may have no desire to reduce your medications to the absolute minimum. You may wish simply to continue a good thing, as long as you can be reassured that there is nothing harmful about using these medications for the long term. And with the exception of high-dose steroids, there are no known long-term side effects of asthma medications. With inhaled steroids, at doses of more than 1,000 micrograms per day, you run a small risk of developing some of the same side effects as with steroid tablets, such as prednisone or Medrol.

We conclude this chapter on managing your asthma with the stories of three patients who experience and manage their asthma quite differently. You may find that one of their stories bears resemblance to your own experience.

"I was diagnosed when I was little," says Laurie, age 15. "I started wheezing around age 5. I was coughing and couldn't breathe. They said it was the cold air."

Soccer was one of the first sports Laurie played, at the age of 11. She would often be short of breath after running and would need her inhaler. Now in high school, she plays soccer in the fall, basketball in the winter, and runs track in spring.

Laurie has no allergies and gets short of breath only when she is "overactive" in sports or is outside in cold air. She has never required a controller medication.

"I haven't had any problems with asthma for a good while, at least six months," she says. "When my asthma does bother me, my chest hurts, and I get a feeling in my throat like an itch that I can't reach, and a dry cough and maybe a little wheeze, but mostly it's a dry cough. It gets annoying if I try to clear my throat and it doesn't go away. It usually goes away if I take two puffs of my inhaler. It has never been that bad where I feel like I can't breathe. It's just there. The worst is after I run up and down the field or the court a lot, and I'm gasping and it takes five or ten minutes to go away.

"I don't worry about every little thing I do," she says. "I keep it in my mind. Having asthma makes me different, but you can talk about it. Talking about it opens up people's eyes to the differences between people."

Laurie, who participated in the Partners Asthma Center Swimming Program, says the program "helped me talk to other kids who have asthma. I met kids who lived one street away from me and found out they had asthma. You find out you're not alone, that there are other people you can talk to who you thought didn't have problems like this and you find out they do."

Richard, age 36, thought he had outgrown his childhood asthma and allergies. But when he was in his twenties and undergoing intense physical training in the Boston Police Academy, a severe asthma attack proved him wrong. "We had to run down to a field and do push-ups and sit-ups in the grass," he says. "I started getting hives, and then wheezing, and having more and more of a feeling of weight on my chest. It was hard to get that breath. When we were standing at attention, they would say, 'Breathe through your nose, not your mouth.' I couldn't get enough air. They told me to sit down in the grass, and that's when the attack came on."

Richard was taken by ambulance to the hospital. Thereafter, he sought out a specialist who "started me on lots of meds and then gradually weaned me down." Although he could have gone back to the police academy once his asthma was under control, Richard took a civilian job in the firearms section of the police department, where he still works today.

"Hopefully we've got it licked," he says. "I haven't had an asthma attack except occasionally when I get a cold that settles in my chest. Then I get a little tightness in my chest and occasional wheezing.

"I haven't used Ventolin in a long time. I use Advair twice a day. I do well on breathing tests. I still run some, play golf, and swim. My asthma doesn't limit me in any way, but I always keep my inhaler with me and know not to put my face in the grass!

"If you think you have asthma, see someone who specializes in breathing problems," Richard advises. "When I did, that's when everything started to come under control. You work out a course of action with your doctor and then you stick to it."

"I'm surprised I wasn't diagnosed sooner," says Margaret, 60, who learned she had asthma at age 24, when a bad cold accompanied by wheezing and difficulty breathing prompted her to see her doctor.

Margaret is the youngest of ten children, six of whom have been diagnosed with asthma as adults. She was "always bronchial" as a child, she says, noting that the colds that settled in her chest and kept her home from school abated when she was a teenager but started up again when she was a young adult.

When she was first diagnosed, Margaret took a long-acting bronchodilator tablet, theophylline, and albuterol as needed. "My asthma was sporadic," she says, "but it wasn't controlled. As I got older, it seemed to get worse, perhaps because there were more smokers around and because I got a lot more colds that exacerbated it. There was a period of time when I was on prednisone a lot and when family plans were often disrupted." Margaret recalls having to come in from sledding with her children because the cold air set off her asthma. On several Thanksgivings, her mother had to take over the cooking because an asthma attack landed Margaret in the hospital.

Some of her asthma episodes have been particularly frightening, says Margaret. "I can remember one night coming downstairs to use my nebulizer. I couldn't set it up because I didn't have enough breath, and I didn't have enough breath to call my husband for help."

With the help of her physician, Margaret has gotten her asthma under control. She now takes a leukotriene blocker and a combination inhaler with both steroid and long-acting bronchodilator in it. When she gets a cold or feels uncomfortable in her chest, she takes additional inhaled steroid medication. She used to take her albuterol frequently but rarely needs it now. She has only had to resort to prednisone, which was once a fairly routine part of her treatment regimen, three times in the last two years.

"Besides faithfully taking my medications, I try to exercise and eat well," she says. "I think this helps." She is also careful to avoid her triggers. "I am very sensitive to smoke, and if I go somewhere where there is smoke, I try to leave, or if I have to be there, I try not to stay long."

All three of Margaret's children—a son and two daughters—have asthma, as do two of her five grandchildren.

"I subscribe to two asthma magazines to try to keep on top of new medications that might be out there," she says, "and to let my children know about them."

CHAPTER 11

The Many Faces of Asthma

ASTHMA, IN DIFFERENT PEOPLE and in different situations, shares the common property of intermittent airway narrowing due to a persistent, underlying "twitchiness" of the bronchial tubes. Yet asthma has many different facets. In subsequent chapters we will talk about special issues regarding asthma in children, in women, and in older people. Here we discuss the unique features of several other "faces" of asthma.

EXERCISE-INDUCED ASTHMA

High school senior and athlete Tania, age 17, was diagnosed with asthma when she was 5 years old. "I remember having allergy skin tests and being allergic to everything," she says. "I was sick a lot growing up. I was the skinny little girl who couldn't do anything."

She considers herself lucky to have gotten good medical care for her asthma, which she takes "seriously," she says. "I have to use multiple inhalers, but it has been worth it. I do kickboxing, spring track, and in my freshman year I was on the high school gymnastics team. I run two to five miles a day."

Tania always takes her bronchodilator inhaler with her on a run. "Even if I have to shove it down into my Spandex shorts, it's always there," she says. "Anyone with asthma who does sports and doesn't have an inhaler handy is a fool. Coaches now know more about asthma, and they trust me to take care of myself. When my father was growing up with his asthma, he was basically told to sit on the couch and not to move!"

Sometimes a coach who is ignorant about asthma will accuse an athlete of being "hysterical," she says, and not acknowledge that the athlete has real physical limitations. But, notes Tania, "asthma is not a lack of mental toughness—it's a breathing problem. For me, it feels as though a heavy weight has been placed on my chest. I can't pull in a deep enough breath, and I can't get the weight off. There's just not enough air to breathe."

Her advice to other athletes, or aspiring athletes with asthma? "I don't believe that anyone should say, 'I can't do it because I have asthma.' Sure, if your asthma is acting up, you need to take it easy. That's different. But just the fact that you have asthma shouldn't prevent you from doing any sport or physical activity that you want to do."

—TANIA, 17

Sometimes exercise can set off your asthma and cause wheezing, chest tightness, coughing, and shortness of breath. That being the case, is it good for people with asthma to exercise? The answer is a resounding yes. We have even heard from many people that getting into good physical shape seemed to improve their asthma. It can help you lose weight and will certainly improve your exercise capacity, and thus your breathing will be easier.

Your asthma needn't prevent you from maintaining good physical conditioning. With appropriate care to keep your asthma under good control, you should be able to exercise regularly. After all, at the 1996 summer Olympics it was said that as many as 20 percent of the competing athletes had asthma. These athletes won proportionately as many medals as the athletes who did not have asthma. Their asthma didn't stop them, and yours need not stop you.

Some people experience their asthma almost exclusively when they exercise. Only during or after exercising do they develop coughing and chest tightness. A term used to describe their condition is exercise-induced asthma. In fact, although the term is commonly used, it does not accurately describe the relationship between exercise and asthma. The truth is that these individuals have asthma and that their asthma is mainly triggered, or only triggered, by exercise, at least so far.

To take this point one step further, it is worth noting that virtually everyone with asthma will have exercise-induced bronchial constriction. If you have asthma and you exercise vigorously enough, the exercise will cause tightening of the muscles surrounding your bronchial tubes, narrowing the air passageways. As discussed in Chapter 2, in some pulmonary function testing laboratories, exercise on a treadmill or stationary bicycle is used (as part of a bronchial challenge) to test for asthma. If exercise provokes airway narrowing, your bronchial tubes show evidence of the hyperresponsiveness typical of asthma. If intense exercise does not provoke airway narrowing, you probably do not have asthma. Instead, there may be another cause for your exercise-induced shortness of breath, including possibly heart disease, anemia, or a lung disease other than asthma.

WHY DOES EXERCISE TRIGGER ASTHMATIC SYMPTOMS?

It has been recognized for hundreds of years that in people who have asthma, exercise can bring on symptoms. In the past 20 to 30 years, scientific research into exercise and asthma has shed light on how exercise stimulates narrowing of the bronchial tubes.

Subjects participating in experiments on exercise-induced bronchoconstriction provided important clues. They complained of having to come to the pulmonary laboratory on cold winter days, because the cold weather seemed to make their asthma worse. In a key series of experiments, scientists had subjects perform the same exercise under three different conditions. One day the subjects ran on a treadmill while breathing the air at room temperature (approximately 70 degrees Fahrenheit). Another day they ran on the treadmill for the same period of time and at the same level of intensity, but they breathed (through a mouthpiece) air that had been passed through a refrigeration unit so that its temperature was below freezing. On the third test day they performed the same exercise while breathing air that had been warmed to approximately body temperature (98 degrees Fahrenheit) with high water content (high relative humidity). Although the exercise performed on all three test days was the same, the response of the subjects' bronchial tubes was dramatically different. Cold, dry air provoked much greater tightening of the breathing tubes than did room temperature air; the warmed, moist air provoked almost no airway narrowing at all.

The researchers wondered whether exercise itself was even necessary to bring on symptoms, so they extended their experiments in an interesting way. As before, they asked people with asthma to breathe room temperature air, then cooled air, and, finally, air that had been warmed and humidified, but this time the subjects simply sat and breathed just as rapidly and deeply as they would if they were exercising. The subjects were given enough carbon dioxide to breathe to prevent light-headedness from hyperventilation.

Perhaps you can guess the outcome. Rapid, deep breathing caused the same tightening of the bronchial tubes as exercising did. Put another way, rapid, deep breathing caused bronchoconstriction whether the breathing was produced by running on a treadmill or by hyperventilating to the same degree while sitting quietly. Under both conditions, air temperature and humidity are crucial factors, with cold, dry air being the strongest stimulus to bronchial narrowing.

When you breathe heavily—and exercise is the most common reason for doing so—large volumes of air are drawn through the bronchial tubes and deep into the chest. It turns out that for people with asthma, as the bronchial tubes give up heat and moisture to warm and humidify this air, the cooling and drying of the tubes causes the bronchial muscles to contract, narrowing the airways and making it difficult to breathe.

When you are breathing quietly, your nose, mouth, and throat naturally warm and moisten the air that passes through them en route to the bronchial tubes. By the time the air gets to these tubes, it has reached nearly the same temperature and has nearly the same moisture content as the airways themselves. Under these circumstances, little cooling and drying of the airways occurs and all is well.

On the other hand, if you race to catch the bus or run up and down the playing field, you will be taking in several times as much air as usual (as many as five to ten gallons of air per minute versus roughly one gallon per minute when at rest). Then you exceed the ability of the nose and mouth to warm and humidify completely the inspired air. When the cooler, drier air hits the asthmatic bronchial tubes, they predictably contract, and you get short of breath and start coughing.

If you are thinking that running on a hot, muggy summer day seems just as problematic for your asthma as running on some winter mornings, you are probably right—but not because the theory about exercise-induced bronchial constriction is wrong. It is likely that the cause of your symptoms on a steamy summer day has to do with the ozone and smog, and possibly the pollens, in the air that act as bronchial irritants or allergens. In this instance, the temperature and water content of the hot, humid inspired air are not the culprits.

Then there is what *you* bring to the equation—the degree of sensitivity of your breathing tubes. Some people experience a lot of airway constriction with just a little bit of exercise, while others experience only a small amount of constriction even with a lot of exercise. The variation in the twitchiness, or sensitivity, of people's airways (see Chapter 1) accounts for this variation in the severity of exercise-induced symptoms, just as it does for the intensity of symptoms brought on by asthmatic triggers more generally. The more active your asthma is at any given time—in other words, the more twitchy your airways are at any given time—the more susceptible you are to developing symptoms after exercise. For example, people whose asthma is made worse by seasonal pollens often find that they have more exercise-induced symptoms during pollen season.

SYMPTOMS OF EXERCISE-INDUCED BRONCHIAL CONSTRICTION

Although exercise can cause all the usual symptoms of asthma, exercise-induced coughing is particularly common. Symptoms may begin during exercise or may develop a few minutes afterward. Athletes often report three patterns to their symptoms:

- With a short period of exercise (five to ten minutes), symptoms often occur approximately five minutes after stopping exercise.

- With longer periods of exercise—for example, a long run, row, or swim—symptoms may occur while still exercising, about 15 to 20 minutes after the start of exercise.

- In people with poorly controlled asthma, shortness of breath may begin within minutes of starting to exercise and make it necessary to stop.

The asthmatic symptoms brought on by exercise typically subside slowly on their own if you rest. After 30 to 60 minutes you will usually be back to normal. In contrast, a child who needs to catch his or her breath for only a minute or two before continuing to play is probably simply "winded," or out of shape.

Two other aspects of exercise-induced bronchial constriction are worth noting. For a few hours after an episode of exercise-induced bronchospasm, the bronchial tubes develop a resistance to repeated exercise-induced constriction (referred to medically as a refractory period). An exercise period of similar intensity will bring fewer symptoms the second time around during this refractory period. Also, unlike exposure to allergens such as dust mites and cat dander, exercise does not cause the bronchial tubes to become more inflamed and thus more sensitive to other asthmatic triggers. After you have recovered and are back to normal, you won't experience any aftereffects that night or the next day.

A variety of strategies are effective in preventing the symptoms of asthma after exercise. Often on a cold day, you can trap a little bit of warm, moist air in front of your mouth by using a scarf pulled up over your nose and mouth. Cold-weather face masks are also made for this purpose. A warm-up period of light exertion often helps reduce symptoms. Medications taken before exercise are effective in blocking bronchial muscle constriction. Your quick-acting bronchodilator, such as albuterol or pirbuterol (Maxair), taken five to ten minutes before exercise, is particularly effective in preventing exercise from provoking asthmatic symptoms. The mast cell stabilizer, cromolyn (Intal), and the leukotriene blocker, montelukast (Singulair), taken 30 to 60 minutes before exercise can also be used in this way. Remember, the goal of good asthma care is to keep your asthma quiet and to allow you to exercise as fully as you wish. We urge you not to restrict your child (or yourself!) from exercising or participating in competitive sports. Asthma should not be viewed as a handicap to full athletic participation.

WHAT IF NOTHING HELPS EXERCISE-INDUCED ASTHMA?

If, despite these measures, you find that exercise is causing you to have chest tightness, coughing, or wheezing, it is time to rethink your overall asthma control. Any asthma trigger, exercise included, will cause greater airway narrowing in someone whose bronchial tubes are highly twitchy or reactive than in someone whose bronchial tubes are only mildly twitchy.

Your sensitivity to exercise may be a sign of the heightened sensitivity of your airways to any of a variety of asthma triggers. The best approach here is to suppress the underlying reactivity of your bronchial tubes. This goal is generally best achieved by anti-inflammatory therapy, meaning starting an inhaled steroid or increasing your dose. As your overall asthma control improves, you will find that exercise less readily sets off bronchial narrowing.

NOCTURNAL ASTHMA

Christine, 32, learned she had asthma when she was 15 and wound up in the school nurse's office barely able to breathe or even speak. "The nurse said, 'You need to use your inhaler; you're having an asthma attack.' I told her I didn't have an inhaler. I didn't even know what asthma was.

"It's been with me ever since. It's stress-related and allergy-related and exercise-induced, and now it's at night," says Christine, noting that nocturnal asthma only became a problem when she reached her late twenties.

"I will be sleeping, and usually a nightmare that I am choking wakes me up, and I realize I'm having an asthma attack and I reach for my inhaler. Sometimes the wheezing is so loud it wakes me. I don't even leave my inhaler on the nightstand anymore," she says. "I hold it in my hand all night long.

"I use three pillows and pretty much sleep sitting up. I think elevating my chest helps a little bit. Sometimes when the episode is bad and I get really scared, I get up and walk around and wait for it to pass. It's just scary, more scary than the day asthma, because at night you're alone. You don't want to wake your husband, or the baby."

Christine says she thinks her excess weight contributes to night-time asthma episodes. "I've noticed that as my weight has increased, my nocturnal asthma has gotten worse." Acknowledging that she sometimes skips doses of her controller medication, she says that her goal is to stick to her medication schedule and to lose up to 70 pounds. "I think this will help me with the nocturnal asthma and with my asthma overall."

—CHRISTINE, 32

Nocturnal awakening due to asthma is a common event for many asthma sufferers. In one study of more than 1,000 children with mild to moderate asthma, over a one-month period of observation, nighttime awakenings due to asthma occurred at least once in 35 percent of the children (who were being treated with bronchodilator medication only during this period). Nighttime awakenings are even more common in adults and in people with severe asthma. Like exercise-induced asthma, nocturnal asthma is one particular manifestation of asthma, not a separate disease.

In asthma, lung function varies over time. The bronchial tubes may narrow during the day, causing daytime symptoms of asthma. Why shouldn't they narrow at night, causing nocturnal asthma? While it is true that one should not necessarily expect sleep to protect against bronchial tube narrowing, there does seem to be something about the early-morning hours that makes people more susceptible to symptoms. If you could measure your lung function around the clock, you would find that your airways are commonly at their narrowest about 4 A.M. There seems to be a natural daily biorhythm that puts people with asthma at greatest risk for asthmatic symptoms around this early-morning hour. Our cortisol and adrenaline blood levels are at their lowest then; histamine levels tend to be high. In patients prone to develop nocturnal asthma, the movement of inflammatory cells into their airways tends to be greatest around that time.

If you were previously sleeping without disturbances, starting to wake up at night due to asthma is a warning sign that your asthma is becoming less well controlled. It is evidence that the bronchial tubes are becoming more twitchy, that the system of bronchial tubes is becoming more unstable, with a greater tendency to constrict. Nighttime awakenings due to asthma are a useful clue, for you and for your doctor, that it is time to:

1. Do some detective work into the possible causes of your nighttime awakenings, such as allergens in the bedroom, post-nasal drip, or reflex of stomach contents up towards the throat.

2. Intensify your treatment. Highly effective treatments are available, both anti-inflammatory medications that will subdue the twitchiness of the airways and long-acting bronchodilators that will prevent constriction of the bronchial muscles throughout the night.

SPASM OF THE VOCAL CORDS

There is a condition that sounds in many ways like nocturnal asthma but that, in fact, is unrelated. In this condition the blockage to breathing occurs not in the bronchial tubes but in the vocal cords. It occurs in people with or without asthma, and is properly diagnosed as *laryngospasm* (spasm of the larynx, or vocal cords). Nighttime awakenings due to laryngospasm are utterly frightening. Patients report that they wake up unable to breathe at all. It may sound like an exaggeration, but in truth, for a few seconds the vocal cords, at the base of the neck, shut closed, blocking any movement of air in or out of the lungs. For a few seconds there is no air passing in or out, no ability to talk or call out. The best thing to do is not to panic. Within seconds, the vocal cords begin to relax, and a small amount of air can pass between them. At this phase the breathing makes a noise that you might call wheezing, but it is different. It occurs only when you breathe *in*, it has only one note or pitch, and it clearly originates in the throat area. Within seconds, this inspiratory noise (properly referred to as *stridor*) lessens and stops. The whole episode is over in less than a minute, although your heart may keep pounding from the fright!

Spasm of the vocal cords of this sort is probably triggered when some saliva, nasal mucus, or coughed-up liquid hits the densely packed nerve endings that surround this area. It is an uncontrollable reflex, meant to protect your windpipe from the aspiration of foreign material. The vocal cords will always begin to relax on their own. There is no need (or time) to reach for any medication. Continue to try to breathe calmly, and in a few seconds you will find that you can do so again.

ASPIRIN-SENSITIVE ASTHMA

When Sarah, 35, was a law student in her mid-twenties, the Advil she had routinely taken for menstrual cramps began to make her asthma flare up. Around the same time, she took Alka Seltzer for an upset stomach and had a bad flare-up. The culprit, she now realizes, was the aspirin in the Alka Seltzer. Now that she is aware of her aspirin sensitivity, Sarah is "on a Tylenol-only diet," she says, for menstrual cramps and other aches and pains.

Sarah also has nasal polyps, which often accompany asthma and as-

pirin sensitivity. Diagnosed with asthma when she was 15 and coughing a lot in gym class, Sarah developed the polyps during her law school years, around the same time that she became aspirin sensitive. Although prednisone tablets have helped shrink the polyps, they haven't helped enough. Like many people with nasal polyps, Sarah has had to have them removed surgically—four times—but typically, they have grown back.

Along with albuterol as needed and a regular inhaled steroid, Sarah takes one of the leukotriene-blocking drugs that are often helpful for people with aspirin sensitivity. Her advice to others with the same condition? "Pay attention to what you put in your body. Get a list of aspirin-based products from your doctor. So many over-the-counter medicines have aspirin in them. You really need to be vigilant."

—SARAH, 35

For the vast majority of people with asthma, taking aspirin has no effect on their asthma, either good or bad. However, for perhaps as many as 5 percent of people with asthma, aspirin can cause their symptoms to worsen, often in the form of a severe and sudden flare-up. If you are a member of this minority, you are at risk for an asthma attack after taking aspirin. Such attacks can be very severe and sometimes even life threatening. They come on predictably within two hours after swallowing the aspirin tablet or tablets and involve all the usual symptoms of asthma: coughing, wheezing, chest tightness, and difficulty breathing. Asthma attacks in response to aspirin are often accompanied by other symptoms as well, particularly nasal congestion and a runny nose, swelling around the eyes, and sometimes abdominal pain.

Children with asthma rarely have aspirin sensitivity, although it can appear in the teenage years. It does not tend to run in families. Many people with asthma have been advised by their physicians to avoid aspirin because of their asthma. This advice is precautionary, given the possibility that you may have or may develop sensitivity to aspirin. We do not make this blanket recommendation to our patients.

No one knows for sure why a few people with asthma develop this sensitivity in their adulthood. Nor do we know why many people with asthma and aspirin sensitivity also have nasal polyps, an overgrowth of tissue that plugs the nasal passageways. Together, asthma, aspirin sensitivity, and nasal polyps are called Samter's triad (named after the doctor who first described the association, in 1968) or simply triad asthma.

A person who is sensitive to aspirin in this way will also be sensitive to the related medications called nonsteroidal anti-inflammatory drugs (or NSAIDs, for short), even though NSAIDs do not share a common chemical structure with aspirin. The NSAIDs are commonly used to treat the inflammation of arthritis and are routinely taken as painkillers. (Since NSAIDs are anti-inflammatory medications, it might seem logical that they would help reduce the inflammation of the bronchial tubes in asthma, but they don't.) Common NSAIDs available without a prescription include ibuprofen (Advil and Motrin) and naproxen (Aleve).

WHAT WE KNOW ABOUT THE WORKINGS OF ASPIRIN SENSITIVITY

Although we can't explain the onset of this unusual sensitivity to aspirin and NSAIDs, we do know something about how it operates. Aspirin and NSAIDs work in a similar way: they relieve pain and reduce inflammation by inhibiting the action of two enzymes in the body called cyclooxygenase enzymes, referred to as COX-1 and COX-2 for short. For reasons we don't fully understand, people with asthma and aspirin sensitivity have an unusual response to the inhibition of the cyclooxygenase enzymes: their bodies react by producing excessive amounts of the inflammatory chemicals with which you are now familiar, the leukotrienes. As you know, these chemicals are released into the airways by allergy cells in the bronchial tubes of people with asthma. They cause spasm of the bronchial tubes and swelling of the walls of these tubes, resulting in wheezing and shortness of breath.

In other words, if you take an aspirin or perhaps an ibuprofen tablet for your headache, the medication will go to work on your headache pain by blocking the action of the COX-1 and COX-2 enzymes in your body. If you have asthma and aspirin sensitivity, the medication will still help your headache, but it will have the added effect of causing your body to produce excess amounts of leukotrienes, which in turn will produce asthma symptoms.

We don't yet know how the medications in the new class of cyclooxygenase inhibitors used to treat arthritis will affect people with aspirin-sensitive asthma. These are rofecoxib (Vioxx), celecoxib (Celebrex), and valdecoxib (Bextra)—you have probably seen them advertised on television. They are called *selective* NSAIDs, or COX-2 inhibitors, because they act selectively, which is to say only on the COX-2 enzyme and not on the COX-1 enzyme. Early evidence suggests that the selective NSAIDs (COX-2 inhibitors) are safe for use by people with aspirin-sensitive asthma, at least in low doses.

HOW DO YOU KNOW IF YOU ARE SENSITIVE TO ASPIRIN?

The only way you can know if you are sensitive to aspirin and related medications is to have experienced an asthma flare-up after taking one of them. There

Medicines That Contain Aspirin or NSAIDs

OVER-THE-COUNTER MEDICATIONS	PRESCRIPTION MEDICATIONS
Aspirin	**Aspirin-containing medicines**
Ascriptin	Easprin
Bufferin	Fiorinal
Ecotrin	Percodan
Empirin	Zorprin
Halfprin	
Nonsteroidal anti-inflammatory drugs	**Nonsteroidal anti-inflammatory drugs**
Actron	Anaprox
Advil	Ansaid
Aleve	Clinoril
Ibuprohm	Daypro
Ibuprofen	Disalcid
Motrin IB	Feldene
Nuprin	Indocin
Orudis KT	Lodine
	Meclomen
Aspirin-containing medications	Motrin
Alka Seltzer Plus	Nalfon
Anacin	Naprosyn
Aquaprin	Oruvail
Bayer Children's Cold Tablet	Ponstel
BC Powder	Relafen
Cama Arthritis Pain Reliever	Tolectin
Cope	Toradol
Doan's	Voltaren
Excedrin	
Goody's Headache Powders	
Stanback Headache Powders	
St. Joseph's Cold Tablet for Children	
Vanquish	

is no simple blood or breathing test to determine whether you have aspirin sensitivity. If as an adult you have never taken aspirin or NSAIDs, perhaps because your doctor told you to avoid them because of your asthma, then you have two options. One is to continue to avoid aspirin and related medications because of the possibility that your asthma involves aspirin sensitivity. The other is to take a small dose of aspirin in a safe place, preferably your doctor's office, and have your breathing closely observed for several hours thereafter.

If you are among the small minority of people with asthma who have this unusual sensitivity, it is important that you avoid all medications that contain aspirin and nonselective NSAIDs. Many over-the-counter pain relievers, as well as cold, flu, and sinus remedies, contain aspirin. Everyone with aspirin-sensitive asthma needs to become a careful "bottle reader," checking all the medication ingredients before taking anything new. In general, people with aspirin-sensitive asthma can safely take acetaminophen (Tylenol).

TREATING ASPIRIN-SENSITIVE ASTHMA

People with aspirin-sensitive asthma respond normally to all asthma treatments. However, because aspirin-sensitive asthma is characterized by the tendency to make excessive amounts of leukotrienes, we feel that everyone with aspirin-sensitive asthma should try a leukotriene-modifying drug. We begin with the leukotriene blockers montelukast (Singulair) and zafirlukast (Accolate) because they are the easiest to use (once- or twice-daily tablets, with almost no medication interactions).

If there is no benefit from leukotriene blockers, we try the medication designed to stop the production of leukotrienes, the lipoxygenase inhibitor zileuton (Zyflo). However, after the end of 2003, when zileuton is scheduled to be removed from the market, this option will no longer be available. There is currently no alternative medication of this type (a lipoxygenase inhibitor) being made.

Taking a leukotriene-modifying drug does not allow someone with aspirin-sensitive asthma to begin taking aspirin or NSAIDs. The risk of precipitating an asthma attack remains too high, even with regular use of a leukotriene blocker. We use the leukotriene blockers to treat aspirin-sensitive asthma because they are often particularly effective, not because they make taking aspirin products safe. Avoidance remains a crucial part of therapy.

ASPIRIN DESENSITIZATION

Another approach to aspirin-sensitive asthma seems paradoxical: administering very small doses of aspirin until people build up a tolerance to the drug. The risk is considerable, since in some people even a few milligrams of aspirin can trigger a severe asthma attack. The procedure, called aspirin desensitization, is occasionally employed at our Asthma Center. Patients are kept in the hospital overnight under close medical observation.

These patients receive increasing doses of aspirin—and treatment for any asthmatic symptoms that may develop—until they can safely take 325 mg of aspirin. They need to continue to take aspirin on a daily basis indefinitely to maintain their tolerance to it. When successful, this procedure not only makes it possible for patients to take aspirin and NSAIDs safely but also results in an overall improvement in asthma control. Aspirin desensitization is practiced in only a few specialized centers for asthma care.

OCCUPATIONAL ASTHMA

After 22 years as a welder, Freddy, 56, was diagnosed with occupational asthma in 1995. "I started to cough a lot at work, and then I started getting short of breath and having chest pain," he says. "I couldn't figure out what it was." The symptoms continued for about four months, improving at home on the weekends, until one afternoon when Freddy was in such severe respiratory distress that he had to be taken to the hospital. Because of the chest pain, the emergency room physicians thought he might have had a heart attack and admitted him to the hospital. The next day he was told that he hadn't had a heart attack— he had a "breathing problem"—and he was referred to a pulmonologist.

"The lung specialist told me I had occupational asthma and to stop going to work," says Freddy. Though much better now, he remains on permanent disability and gets short of breath especially when exposed to cigarette smoke and other forms of air pollution, and in hot and cold weather. He takes an inhaled steroid regularly and albuterol as needed and requires a short course of prednisone tablets a few times a year.

Freddy's advice to other workers in the welding business? "Stay away as much as you can from those fumes. Eventually, you could get sick, especially if you don't have proper ventilation and a respirator. All my life I worked every day and never got sick before."

—FREDDY, 56

People without preexisting asthma who work in lumber mills and breathe in certain kinds of sawdust on a regular basis sometimes develop asthma as a result. Similarly, bakers may develop asthma because of ongoing exposure to flour dust in the bakery. Recognition of this association has led to the term *baker's asthma* to describe their illness. Among health care workers, exposure to aerosolized protein from latex rubber gloves has produced new cases of asthma in what one would imagine should be a clean and, in the case of operating rooms, even sterile environment.

Welders, lumber mill workers, bakers, hospital workers, and others who develop asthma for the first time after inhaling workplace substances known to cause bronchial sensitization have occupational asthma. The term *occupational asthma* is sometimes mistakenly used to describe preexisting asthma that is made worse by the work environment. If you have had asthma for some time and you work in a library, you may find that your asthma gets worse if you are around dusty old books. But this circumstance is not what is meant by *occupational asthma*. Workplace environments may aggravate your asthma, and you may need to seek alternative arrangements to prevent worsening symptoms every day at work. *Occupational asthma* refers specifically to the *new onset* of asthma in a previously healthy worker, whose asthma is *caused* by repetitive inhalation of chemical stimuli in the workplace.

Substances in the Workplace That Can Cause Asthma

AGENTS	OCCUPATIONS
Animal Products: Dander, excreta, serum, secretions	Animal handlers Laboratory workers Veterinarians
Plants: Grain, tea, flour, tobacco, hops, dust	Grain handlers Tea workers Bakers Natural oil manufacturing workers Tobacco and food processing workers Health care workers
Enzymes: *Bacillus subtilis,* pancreatic extracts, papain, trypsin, fungal amylase	Bakers Detergent, pharmaceutical, and plastics workers
Vegetable: Gum acacia, gum tragacanth	Printers Gum manufacturing workers
Other: Crab, prawn	Crab and prawn processors

(continued on next page)

Agents	Occupations
Chemicals: **Diisocyanates**—toluene diisocyanate (TDI), methylene diphenyl diissocyanate (MDI)	Polyurethane industry workers Plastics workers Workers using varnish Foundry workers
Anhydrides—phthalic anhydrates, trimellitic anhydrates	Epoxy resin and plastics workers
Wood dust—oak, mahogany, California redwood, western red cedar	Carpenters Sawmill workers Furniture makers
Metals—platinum, nickel, chromium, cobalt, vanadium, tungsten carbide	Platinum- and nickel-refining workers Hard-metal workers
Soldering fluxes	Solderers
Drugs—penicillin, methyldopa, tetracyclines, cephalosporins, psyllium	Pharmaceutical and health care industry workers
Other organic chemicals—urea formaldehyde, dyes, formalin, azodicarbonamide, hexachlorethylene diamine, dimethyl ethanolamine, polyvinyl chloride pyrolysates	Hospital workers Chemical, plastics, and rubber industry workers Laboratory workers Foam insulation manufacturing workers Food wrapping workers Spray painters

Adapted from M. Chan-Yeung and S. Lam, "Occupational Asthma," *American Review of Respiratory Disease* 1986; 133:686–703.

Woodworkers and bakers are among those prone to developing occupational asthma. Auto body shop workers and others who use spray paints containing chemicals known as isocyanates are also particularly susceptible; so are people in the plastics industries who are exposed to chemicals called epoxies and anhydrides. Animal care workers—people who work with laboratory animals, in veterinary offices, or with farm animals, for example—are another group prone to occupational asthma. Exposure to high concentrations of formaldehyde—an occupational hazard among textile workers, insulators, and embalmers, among others—can also lead to this form of asthma.

These are just some examples of occupations with disproportionately high rates of occupational asthma. Over 250 airborne substances found in the workplace, including animal- and plant-derived proteins, metals, and organic chemicals, have been identified as potential causes of asthma.

Some people have developed asthma immediately after a single, high-dose exposure (rather than multiple exposures over time) to chemicals such as ammonia, chlorine, or hydrochloric acid. An intense, usually accidental exposure to noxious fumes can lead to persistent coughing, wheezing, and breathlessness. People with this form of occupational asthma, often referred to as reactive airways dysfunction syndrome, frequently recover gradually over time. Occupational asthma of this type, which is much less common, is thought by some experts to be an airway injury rather than typical asthma.

How Occupational Asthma Develops

Sensitization to an inhaled stimulus such as flour dust or wood dust at work can develop over weeks or months, and can even take years to cause asthmatic symptoms. Once the bronchial tubes have developed sensitivity to the substances, usually an allergic-type sensitivity, further exposure causes the bronchial tubes to narrow and swell. When symptoms develop, they usually follow a fairly predictable pattern: at first they occur only during exposures at work, or hours afterward. Perhaps the worker first notices a nagging cough at the end of the workweek. The cough noticeably lessens during the weekend or other days off from work. With time the allergic sensitivity increases: exposure to lesser amounts of the offending substance brings on asthmatic symptoms. When that happens, coughing and wheezing begin first thing Monday morning and last all week long.

Initially, the lumber mill worker or baker experiences asthmatic symptoms only in response to breathing in the sawdust or the flour dust. Over time, he or she develops wheezing, coughing, and shortness of breath in response to all the usual triggers of asthma (such as exercise, respiratory tract infections, tobacco smoke, and so on). In effect, repetitive workplace exposure to a sensitizing stimulus has created asthmatic airways, with their characteristic property of twitchiness in response to a multitude of typical triggers. You can see that occupational asthma offers an intriguing model for how one might develop asthma outside the workplace. Perhaps if you substitute cockroach or dust mite antigen for isocyanates and flour dust, the same process takes place in the home environment. Repetitive exposures to certain allergens can lead not only to a sensitivity of the airways to those specific allergens, but also to the nonspecific or generalized hypersensitivity of the airways that we recognize as asthma.

For some occupations, the risk of developing occupational asthma is as high as 5 to 10 percent per year. Still, the majority of workers in the same environments do *not* develop asthma. Those who do develop occupational asthma must have a special predisposition. At present we can't identify in advance which workers are vulnerable. Therefore, we can't warn the vulnerable worker to avoid certain occupations. We do know that for some workplace exposures, your risk of developing occupational asthma increases if you have atopy (the genetic tendency to make allergic reactions like hay fever, eczema, and hives) or if you smoke cigarettes. Incidentally, these are also risk factors for developing asthma outside the workplace.

DIAGNOSING OCCUPATIONAL ASTHMA

If you start to develop episodic wheezing, coughing, or shortness of breath at work or after work and if your symptoms get better during the weekend, worsen when you go back to work on Monday, and get progressively worse by Friday, occupational asthma is the likely cause. Occupational asthma is even more probable if a significant number of your coworkers have been diagnosed with asthma.

When symptoms and findings on physical examination (diffuse wheezes heard on examination of the chest) point to a diagnosis of asthma, your doctor can establish the diagnosis of occupational asthma by measuring your lung function before and after work. (See Chapter 2 for details about lung function measurements.) If your lung function is normal before you go to work at the bakery but is below normal after your shift, the evidence is pretty clear that your asthma symptoms are due to flour dust or other allergic stimuli in the bakery.

Your doctor may ask you to gather further evidence on your own by using a peak flow meter to monitor your lung function throughout the day—before, during, and after work. (See Chapter 2 for more on peak flow monitoring for diagnosing asthma.) If your peak flow measurements taken during a period of consecutive days at work (ten days or so) are consistently lower than measurements taken on the same number of days *away* from work (such as during a deliberate work absence pursued for the purposes of diagnosis), that is strong evidence that you have occupational asthma.

CAN OCCUPATIONAL ASTHMA BE CURED?

If occupational asthma is caught early enough and the worker avoids further exposure to the substance that caused it, the asthma may go away. However, over time there comes a point when the inflammation of the airways caused by workplace exposures becomes self-sustaining. In as many as 50 percent of workers who leave the workplace after developing occupational asthma, the asthma persists. The people more likely to recover from occupational asthma are those who are diagnosed earlier, remove themselves from the exposure sooner, and have relatively little reduction in lung function at the time of diagnosis.

If you have been diagnosed with occupational asthma, or suspect that you have occupational asthma, you will want to understand your rights and your employer's responsibilities, and to familiarize yourself with workers' compensation laws and the Americans with Disabilities Act of 1992. You can do so through the Americans with Disabilities Act Web site: www.ada.gov/.

TREATMENT FOR OCCUPATIONAL ASTHMA

The treatment for occupational asthma is the same as for all asthma—quick-reliever bronchodilators and controller medications—but if workplace exposures continue unabated, the worker's asthma is likely to worsen, and he or she may even have life-threatening asthma attacks.

Respirator masks are devices that can filter out impurities in the air, including allergens. They look like the gas masks worn in combat. Occasionally, wearing such a mask makes it possible for someone with occupational asthma to stay in the workplace responsible for his or her asthma. However, in most circumstances, these masks are impractical for routine use: they are heavy, make breathing harder, and look peculiar. (Imagine wearing such a mask for the better part of eight hours a day, five days a week!) Furthermore, they are not always effective in preventing asthmatic symptoms when a person is highly sensitive to an allergen or other workplace stimulus.

As noted above, up to 50 percent of people with occupational asthma continue to have asthma after leaving the workplace that caused it. The Americans with Disabilities Act provides for temporary disability for workers diagnosed with occupational asthma and requires employers to retrain workers if another suitable job is available within the same company. People who remain ill and unable to find employment over two years can apply for permanent disability. Unfortunately, many people continue to work in jobs injurious to their health because they believe they won't be able to get another job with comparable pay.

PREOPERATIVE ASTHMA MANAGEMENT

Most of the special circumstances we describe in this chapter are ongoing, such as aspirin-sensitive asthma or exercise-induced asthma. Preoperative

Things to Remember If You Are Having Surgery

There are several things that you and your doctor need to remember if you are facing surgery:

- **Before surgery, get your asthma under control.** Unless you are undergoing emergency surgery, insist that your asthma be under good control at the time of the operation. If you are in the midst of an asthma flare-up, postpone your elective surgery. If your asthma is "up and down" and you can't predict how you will be on the day of surgery, consult your doctor well in advance of the planned operation to optimize your treatment and ensure well-controlled asthma by the date of your surgery. A peak flow measurement is always useful in judging whether your asthma is well controlled or not.

- **Keep taking your inhaled medications until just before surgery.** Before most operations, you are instructed not to eat or drink anything or to take your usual pills or tablets, so that you arrive for surgery with "an empty stomach." Fortunately, this restriction does not apply to any inhaled medications. You can safely take all of your usual inhaled medications on the morning of your surgery. In addition, bring your quick-relief bronchodilator, such as albuterol, with you to surgery. The surgical team will most likely let you use it immediately before surgery, for protection against spasm of your airways when the breathing tube (endotracheal tube) is placed in your throat. Also, for surgery for which you will be awake, though sedated, using the quick-acting bronchodilator immediately before surgery can minimize coughing or difficulty breathing during the procedure or operation.

- **If you are taking steroid tablets, you will need to get your steroid medicine intravenously during surgery.** People who are taking steroids tablets for their asthma (or have done so for more than two weeks over the preceding six months) cannot do without steroids on the day of surgery. It is not safe to stop your steroid tablets suddenly after your body has adapted to their regular use. Doing so may leave your body without the normal (and necessary) amount of steroid hormone that always circulates through your bloodstream, and without the extra boost of steroid hormone that your body normally produces at times of physical stress, such as surgery. In this circumstance your doctors will give you the steroid medication intravenously at the time of surgery and after surgery, until you can swallow tablets again. You will probably receive an extra amount of steroids on the day of surgery to deal with the added physical stress on the body ("stress-dose steroids"), followed by a rapid dose-reduction back to your usual dose (or to none) over the next few days.

asthma management, on the other hand, poses only an infrequent problem—or so we hope—for any individual with asthma. It is a consideration, however, that should be taken seriously.

Many people with asthma who are facing surgery are appropriately concerned about whether their doctors, including their surgeon and anesthesiologist, will know how to handle their asthma. Poorly controlled asthma increases the risk of complications around the time of surgery, and the intubation performed when general anesthesia is administered (intubation involves passing a tube through your throat into your windpipe) can trigger spasms of the bronchial tubes. The best safeguard against problems at the time of surgery is to remind your doctors, especially your anesthesiologist, that you have asthma. Armed with this knowledge, they can help you take the appropriate precautions to ensure a good outcome.

INNER-CITY ASTHMA

Finally, a few words about inner-city asthma, which is far too prevalent to be appropriately termed a "special" circumstance, except insofar as it often involves inequitable conditions and its treatment poses special challenges.

Imagine bringing up your asthmatic child in an inner-city housing project. Mice and roaches are facts of daily life. City buses park outside your window and idle their engines. Closing your windows in the summer to avoid seasonal pollens means suffocating in the heat. You find yourself having to choose between paying for food and paying for medicines. The emergency department of the local hospital is far more accessible than a medical practitioner in the community. There are many reasons, only a few of which are noted here, that asthma among people living in our inner cities is more severe and potentially dangerous than elsewhere in the country.

Problems Treating Inner-City Asthma

It has been said that treating inner-city asthma is just like treating any asthma—only more so. Environmental control measures to reduce exposure to indoor allergens are just as important, but harder to implement in an aging, multifamily dwelling whose owner has limited commitment to its upkeep. Regular use of preventive medications can reduce the severity of asthma in people living in the inner cities, but lack of access, affordability, and health attitudes grounded in prevention interfere with implementation.

People living in the inner cities face numerous obstacles to effective medical care, including financial, cultural, educational, and language barriers. In addition, lack of transportation and child-care services, depression, and drug or alcohol dependence may all conspire to keep an asthmatic child or adult away from preventive care, perpetuating the cycle of asthmatic crises and emergency interventions.

Effective interventions are possible. Some programs seek to reduce allergen exposures in the home, focusing on cockroach extermination and dust mite control. Others make preventive services available through neighborhood health centers, case managers, and outreach programs. In Los Angeles, a mobile "asthma van" brings asthma care and education to local schools at regular intervals. In Boston, a collaborative advocacy group is working to improve housing and school conditions for people with asthma. In many ways asthma is like infant mortality in the United States. We have the capacity to provide the finest medical care—safe, effective, and well-tolerated—that can be obtained anywhere in the world. The challenge that we face is equitable distribution of that care, including to the poor and disadvantaged.

CHAPTER 12

Special Considerations in Children

KIDS' ADVICE TO OTHER KIDS WITH ASTHMA

"Don't worry about your asthma. Just keep living and take care of your-self. Avoid situations that you think might give you an asthma attack. Just because you have asthma doesn't mean you can't play sports or be an active person. It doesn't mean you have to stop being a regular child just because you are diagnosed with a breathing disorder."
—LAURIE, 15

"It's important that little kids are taught about their disease and severity so that they don't panic. For me, when I was little, not knowing was the worst. When I was little, I used to walk up and down the stairs with my inhaler in my pocket, afraid that I would have an asthma attack. My parents said it wasn't necessary, that I wouldn't have an asthma attack from walking up and down the stairs.

"I know it's kind of embarrassing to take out your inhaler, but you need to in order to survive. I find that teenagers are less likely to take their medications, because there's no one watching over them, or because they're embarrassed. I'm not embarrassed. I carry my inhaler in the front pocket of my bag at all times, and take it out whenever I need it."
—TANIA, 17

"Sometimes if you're around things that make you have asthma attacks, they can really get to your lungs. So kids should try and learn what those things are and stay away from them. If kids don't like taking their in-haler, they should do it anyway, so they don't have to stop doing sports and so they don't get really sick."
—ANDREA, 10

NEARLY 6 MILLION CHILDREN in the United States have asthma, the most common chronic illness of childhood. Asthma is the leading cause of hospital admissions among children and a frequent cause of both emergency room visits and urgent physician visits. Asthma is also the leading cause of school absences. Some children, even those with moderate asthma, may miss a week or more of school each year due to their asthma.

But with careful planning, appropriate medications, and effective communication, your child shouldn't have to miss any more school than other children. Most children with asthma can expect to participate fully in all activities, including sports. Their symptoms can generally be kept under control, and urgent physician visits, emergency department visits, and hospital admissions can be reduced.

For both children with asthma and their parents, everyday situations—school, sports events, play dates, sleepovers, and family vacations—pose special challenges. If you are a parent of a child with asthma, you face important and sometimes pressing questions, such as what to do if your child has an asthma flare-up, when to call the pediatrician, and when to seek emergency care. In this chapter, we try to provide guidance for you and your child. (For simplicity, in the remainder of this chapter we will refer to the child as "she" and "her" rather than "he or she" or "him or her.")

ASTHMA AT SCHOOL

The majority of children with asthma manage fine at school. However, school can be a source of worry and stress. Children with asthma may be more fearful about the possibility of having an asthma flare-up at school than at home, where they are used to turning to a trusted parent for help and reassurance. They may worry—often with good reason—about asthma triggers such as pets in the classroom, dust, cleaning products, chalk dust, and others that you may have eliminated at home. They may feel embarrassed about using their inhalers in front of other children, and may worry that their asthma will prevent them from participating in a much-anticipated sports event or other school activity or might sometimes keep them out of school altogether.

The Asthma Management Conference

The best way to minimize your worries, and those of your child, and to ensure that her asthma is under good control at school is to be certain that the supervising adults know as much as possible about your child's asthma. A good way to communicate this information is to arrange a conference with key people, especially your child's homeroom teacher and the school nurse. It's a good idea to ask your child's pediatrician or asthma specialist to send a letter de-

Topics to Cover at Your Child's Management Conference

- Your child's asthma history
- Medications she is taking and potential side effects
- Medication delivery devices
- Asthma Action Plan
- Her allergies
- How independently your child copes with her asthma, including inhaler use
- How to reach you
- How to reach the health care provider managing your child's asthma
- Plans for treatment when away from school (across the street playing soccer or away from school on field trips)

scribing your child's condition, medications and devices used to deliver them, and her Asthma Action Plan (see Chapter 16 for more on the Asthma Action Plan) to the nurse or other appropriate administrator before the meeting.

Your child will probably not be the first one with asthma at her school, and you may be relieved to discover that the staff is quite knowledgeable about the needs of children with asthma. (Parents often tell us they are reassured when they see the medicine cabinet in the school nurse's office filled with asthma medications and devices.)

At the conference, describe the history of your child's asthma (and any other medical conditions), the things that make it flare up, what medications she is taking, and her particular concerns about her asthma—for example, is she embarrassed about her asthma and reluctant to use her inhaler in front of other children? You may want to note that your child's energy level and ability to concentrate may sometimes be affected if an asthma flare-up has kept her from getting a good night's sleep or if she is experiencing medication side effects, such as a racing heart, jitteriness, headache, or stomachache.

You will also want to communicate how independently your child copes with her asthma. Many children, some as young as 6 or 7, can use inhaler devices effectively and reliably. How well your child takes care of her asthma can be helpful in determining whether it is a good idea for her to carry her own medications with her during the school day, school regulations permitting, or whether they should be kept in the homeroom teacher's desk or in the school health room or nurse's office.

Mention any allergies your child may have, such as to animal dander, dust, seasonal pollens, and other things she is likely to encounter in the indoor and outdoor school environment that may set off her asthma. Emphasize that it is important to keep a close eye on her if she runs outside in the cold air, that she may need treatment before physical activity, and that she will need to be excused from physical activities when her asthma is acting up.

Be sure the school staff knows how to reach you in the event of an emergency and how to contact your child's pediatrician. The school nurse should have a copy of your child's Asthma Action Plan, outlining steps to take in the event of a mild, moderate, or severe asthma flare-up. Communicating your child's needs will help prevent asthma flare-ups, reduce days spent home from school, and lead to a happier and more successful school experience for your child.

INHALERS AT SCHOOL

Some schools allow students of a certain age (usually high school age but sometimes younger) to carry their own inhalers; others do not. Even if you and the school staff agree that your child can be in charge of her asthma medications, it's still a good idea to keep an extra inhaler for her in the health room or teacher's desk, in case she loses her inhaler or it runs out of medication.

Wherever your child's medications are kept at school, and whether your child or an adult is in charge of her inhaler(s), the most important thing is to be sure that she has access to her medications at all times. The supervising adults—homeroom teacher, gym teacher, school nurse, and teacher in charge of a field trip—should always know where the child's asthma medications are and be able to get to them in a hurry. Precious time can be lost if a child is having an asthma flare-up on the playing field across the street and her medications are locked in the homeroom teacher's desk, or if they are in the child's locker and only the child knows the combination. For field trips, be sure to prepare a backpack or waist pouch with any medication equipment your child will need.

HOW ASTHMA-FRIENDLY IS YOUR CHILD'S SCHOOL?

Children with asthma need proper support at school to keep their asthma under control so they can be fully active. You can use the questions below (prepared by the National Asthma Education and Prevention Program) as a measure of how well your school assists students with asthma:

1. Is your child's school free of tobacco smoke all the time, including during school-sponsored events?

2. Does the school maintain good indoor air quality? Does it reduce or eliminate allergens and irritants that can make asthma worse? Allergens and irritants include pets with fur or feathers, mold, dust mites (for example, in carpets and upholstery), cockroaches, and strong odors or fumes from such products as pesticides, paint, perfumes, and cleaning chemicals.

3. Is a school nurse present all day, every day? If not, is a nurse regularly available to the school to help give guidance to students with asthma about medicines, physical education, and field trips?

4. Are children permitted to take medicines at school as recommended by their doctor and parents? May children carry their own asthma medicines?

5. Does the school have an emergency plan for taking care of a child with a severe asthma flare-up? Is the plan clear about what to do? Whom to call? When to call?

6. Does someone teach school staff about asthma, asthma management plans, and asthma medicines? Does someone teach all students about asthma and how to help a classmate who has it?

7. Do students have good options for fully and safely participating in physical education class and recess? (For example, do students have access to their medicine before exercise? Can they choose modified or alternative activities when medically necessary?)

If the answer to any of these questions is no, students face obstacles to optimal asthma control. Asthma that is not well controlled can hinder a student's attendance, participation, and progress in school. School staff, health professionals, and parents can work together to remove obstacles and to promote students' health and education.

The following organizations and publications provide information about asthma and helpful ideas for making school policies and practices more asthma-friendly: the National Asthma Education and Prevention Program (NAEPP) of the National Institutes of Health, whose many printed resources include the "How Asthma-Friendly Is Your School?" questionnaire printed above, and the American Academy of Allergy, Asthma, and Immunology (www.aaaai.org).

Your Child's Rights at School

No matter how good a job you do communicating your child's needs (including the need for quick access to her medication at all times), and no matter how receptive the school staff is, the reality is that there may still be asthma triggers for your child to contend with at school. Carpeting may cause her asthma to flare up. So may chalk dust, cleaning chemicals, the teacher's perfume or cologne, or the classroom rabbit—to name just a few common asthma triggers your child is likely to encounter at school.

You may find it reassuring to learn that if the classroom rabbit's dander makes your child wheeze and cough and have trouble breathing, you are on solid ground in asking to have the animal removed. Two important pieces of legislation protect your child from anything that may interfere with her learning at school or her ability to participate fully in school activities. These are the Americans with Disabilities Act (ADA) of 1992, and Section 504 of the Rehabilitation Act of 1973.

Both statutes entitle people with disabilities to request changes in conditions or policies that exclude them from full participation in public entities and accommodations, including schools. The ADA and Section 504 apply to people with asthma, since asthma is considered a disability when it interferes with "major life activities." Breathing and learning are both specified as major life activities, along with seeing, hearing, speaking, walking, performing manual tasks, caring for oneself, and working. Section 504 applies to all institutions that receive public funding, while the ADA is even more broad-based. Just knowing that your child is legally entitled to a learning environment that is safe and healthy for her can be a comfort.

YOUR CHILD'S ASTHMA AWAY FROM HOME

Birthday parties, play dates, sleepovers, summer camp, and family vacations present another set of challenges for children with asthma. Preparation for these events—including careful communication—is just as important as it is for school.

Visiting Other Children's Homes

Any time your child is visiting another child's home, it is a good idea to call ahead to talk with the supervising adult about your child's asthma, any allergies she may have, what medications she is taking and how they are administered, what to do if her asthma flares up, and how to reach you. Be sure to ask

Talking About Asthma

Making arrangements with other parents for play dates and sleepovers, and having your child's friends visit your home, are natural openings for you and your child to talk with other adults and children about asthma. As with most illnesses, people who don't have asthma or don't have a close friend or family member with asthma may not know much about it. Occasions when children are visiting at your house can also be especially good opportunities for your child to talk about her asthma with her friends.

You and your child may find it useful and fun to watch some of the educational videos about asthma that have been developed for children who have asthma, as well as those who don't. (See the list of videos in the Resources section at the back of this book.) These videos often make use of animated characters (or for adolescent viewers, more age-appropriate characters) to convey the kinds of important messages that you and your child wish to communicate to her friends (and to other adults). One such message is that children with asthma are no different from other children except that they have asthma. Taking the opportunity to be an "asthma ambassador," and encouraging your child to be one too, can help promote understanding about asthma and can also make your child feel good about herself.

about pets. Sometimes pretreating your child with albuterol or cromolyn before a play date at another child's house where there is a cat or dog can spare her an asthma episode. (See Chapters 5 and 7, respectively, for more on these medications.) The pediatrician's or asthma specialist's recommendations about pretreatment should be part of your child's Asthma Action Plan.

Tell your child that you had this conversation. It will not only be reassuring to the two of you, but it will make the supervising adult feel more comfortable. If you are reluctant to share confidential medical history, think about how you would feel if a child visiting your home showed signs of a medical problem that you had not been told about in advance. For example, how would you feel if a child visiting your home started wheezing, had a seizure, or became confused because her blood sugar was low from the insulin shot for her diabetes—and you had not been told about the condition or what to do about it? With proper planning, your child should be able to enjoy play dates and other activities just like any other child.

SUMMER CAMP

Unlike going to school or visiting friends' houses, summer camp means being away from home—and farther away from home—for a week or more. The prospect may make children with asthma and their parents anxious. But your worries, and your child's, can be overcome. If your child wants to go to camp, she doesn't have to miss out because of her asthma. At camp, the camp nurse and your child's counselor are the key people to inform about her medical history, asthma medications, and asthma triggers. While many children with asthma go to camp every summer, some children with severe asthma may require more special attention than most summer camps can provide. But even severe asthma needn't keep your child from enjoying the fun of summer camp. In many areas of the country, the American Lung Association has special asthma camps, staffed by nurses, physicians, and other medical personnel, as well as by camp counselors. At these camps children participate in regular camp activities such as swimming, boating, and arts and crafts. They also learn how to control their asthma better. If you would like to find a nearby asthma camp, contact your local office of the American Lung Association. Some asthma centers may also offer summer programs for children. At Partners Asthma Center, for example, we run a swimming program every summer for children with asthma, where children enjoy swimming and learn how to control their asthma better. They learn that asthma doesn't have to keep them from participating in enjoyable and healthful activities.

TIPS FOR FAMILY VACATIONS

You and your child may naturally feel more relaxed about the prospect of a family vacation together than you do about her first experience of overnight camp. Don't let this make you any less mindful about planning for her asthma care while you are away. Wherever you go, take along a copy of your child's Asthma Action Plan (see Chapter 16) and a copy of her One-Minute Medical History (discussed later in this chapter). It's a good idea to pack more medication than you expect to need, just in case one of her inhalers gets lost, and to take your child's insurance card, in the event that she needs medical attention while you are away from home.

Flying or visiting places at a high altitude is not likely to have an impact on your child's asthma. If you are flying, make sure to have asthma medications in carry-on luggage. Nowadays, we suggest that parents carry a physician's letter detailing their child's diagnosis, medications, and necessary equipment in order to facilitate passage through airport security checks. Your child's asthma doesn't rule out camping, but make sure she doesn't get too close to the campfire, since wood smoke triggers symptoms in virtually everyone with asthma.

Treatment for asthma is similar in developed countries around the world, so you can expect that almost everywhere you go, your child will probably receive good asthma care if she needs it. Your child's asthma needn't keep you from going almost anywhere—you just need to pack a few extra things. Along with your child's medications, be sure to have a list of the generic names and doses. The same asthma medicines used in this country may have different brand names in other countries.

MANAGING ASTHMA IN CHILDREN YOUNGER THAN 5

For younger children who do not have the breath control necessary to perform breathing tests such as spirometry (see Chapter 2 for more on spirometry), we need to rely on medical history and physical examination to make a diagnosis of asthma. In some children, coughing may be the only manifestation of airway obstruction. (Wheezing is most often heard only when listening with a stethoscope.) When we hear that a child coughs for a few weeks with every cold, we begin to think about asthma. Other hints can be shortness of breath

Predictors of Persistent Wheezing (Asthma) in Young Children

Medical studies involving relatively large numbers of children have identified the factors that can best predict whether a child is likely to go on to develop asthma.

Strong predictors of asthma in preschool children with three episodes of wheezing within the past year:

- A parent with a history of allergy or asthma
- Eczema in the first year of life. Eczema, also called atopic dermatitis, is an allergic skin condition, typically causing dry patches of skin behind the ears or in the creases of the elbows and behind the knees.

Weaker predictors:

- Allergy cells (eosinophils) found in increased numbers in the blood
- Wheezing in the absence of a cold
- Allergic rhinitis (allergies of the nose): a persistently runny and/or stuffy nose, with a watery nasal discharge distinct from the thick and discolored secretions of a nasal or sinus infection
- Food allergy

with exercise, or coughing when exposed to cold air. Not surprisingly, many children first come to our attention because of nonstop coughing after a respiratory infection or a day of sledding. Almost every child will have one episode of coughing or wheezing when growing up, but only a minority go on to develop asthma. As we noted in Chapter 2, we start to think about the diagnosis of asthma when a child has had three or more episodes of wheezing or prolonged cough.

Other pieces of medical history increase the likelihood that young children who cough or wheeze will go on to develop asthma. These include eczema within the child's first year of life, and a family history of asthma and allergies. Information about the child's reaction to her environment can also provide important clues. If your child sneezes or rubs her eyes when she is near her pet cat, she is likely to be allergic to cats. If she then begins coughing within a few hours of exposure, or even the next morning, the cat allergy may have triggered an asthma episode.

Even when the history is strongly suggestive of asthma, to be confident about the diagnosis there is still another piece of information that is needed.

Normal Peak Flow Values in Children (in liters/minute)

HEIGHT	PEAK FLOW	HEIGHT	PEAK FLOW
43 inches	147	56 inches	320
44 inches	160	57 inches	334
45 inches	173	58 inches	347
46 inches	187	59 inches	360
47 inches	200	60 inches	373
48 inches	214	61 inches	387
49 inches	227	62 inches	400
50 inches	240	63 inches	413
51 inches	254	64 inches	427
52 inches	267	65 inches	440
53 inches	280	66 inches	454
54 inches	293	67 inches	467
55 inches	307		

Unlike adults, there are no important differences in peak flow rates between male and female children. The range of normal values extends approximately 75 liters/minute above and below the average values shown here.

This confirmatory piece is *time*, since asthma is a chronic condition. We see many children who have an isolated episode of wheezing, and we certainly do not want to tell them or their parents that they have a chronic disease unless we can do so with a great deal of certainty. Often a trial of asthma medication is needed to help make the final determination.

We often ask parents to keep a diary of their child's symptoms: When do they occur, what seems to bring them on, how long do they last, does bronchodilating medication (such as albuterol) make the symptoms better? We explain that bronchodilators such as albuterol begin to work within five to ten minutes and their effect lasts for approximately four hours.

In the office we carefully observe the child's response to a bronchodilator. Do the coughing and wheezing promptly decrease or disappear? Does the child's breathing rate slow? Does the child's blood oxygen level rise (as measured with a medical instrument, called an oximeter, whose sensor is painlessly placed on the skin)?

Once we feel that asthma is the most likely explanation for your child's symptoms, we can select the appropriate medication. The choice of the delivery system is just as important as the choice of medicine. It doesn't help to have the correct diagnosis and the right medicine, if your child cannot take the medicine properly. No doctor's visit is complete without a thorough explanation of how best to give your child the medication, what we anticipate the medication will do for your child, and a discussion of the common side effects. The following vignette illustrates why this communication is so vital:

> John left the office with the diagnosis of asthma and was started on treatment with albuterol. When his mother gave him the first dose at home, he became very shaky. As a result his mother stopped giving him the medication. That night John was unable to sleep because of coughing. His mother brought him to the emergency room, where she reported that her son was allergic to albuterol. The physician in the emergency department explained that shakiness is a common side effect of the medication. When John was treated with albuterol in the emergency room, his coughing stopped and his breathing became more comfortable.

QUICK-RELIEF MEDICATIONS

Albuterol by inhalation is the preferred quick-relief bronchodilator, even in very young children. But how can you get a child less than 5 years old to coordinate the use of a metered-dose inhaler when even adults often struggle to do it correctly? A spacer device with attached face mask allows you to administer medication from metered-dose inhalers to even very young children. Transparent flexible plastic masks in different sizes attach to one end of the spacer; the medication is sprayed into the chamber from the other end. Hold the mask gently to your child's face, covering her nose and mouth. Activate one spray of medicine and watch as she breathes six breaths. With these six breaths, the medication is emptied from the chamber and the treatment is finished. This method is quick and readily portable. Its major disadvantage is the parent's uncertainty about how much medicine the child actually received.

As noted in Chapter 5, an alternative route for inhalation of the quick-relief bronchodilator is the compressor and nebulizer system. A special nebulizer with mask attachment is designed specifically for young children (for example, the Pari nebulizer). Soft, flexible masks of different sizes fit the faces of infants as well as older children. An easily rotated plastic "elbow" allows you to keep the nebulizer cup upright while the mask is positioned at any of a variety of angles. The compressor and nebulizer system can be used to deliver the quick-relief bronchodilators albuterol and levalbuterol (Xopenex). (Xopenex is discussed in Chapter 5. It is similar to albuterol but has slightly fewer side effects and costs more.)

With the nebulizer system, you need not count the number of breaths the child takes; simply continue the treatment until all of the medication has been emptied from the nebulizer compartment. The treatment may last five to ten minutes. It is important to keep the nebulizer and tubing clean. Small amounts of dry medication or saliva from previous treatments can clog the system, including the compressor filter, interfering with its functioning and lengthening treatment times. After each use, simply rinse the nebulizer and tubing with tap water and allow them to air-dry. (For more on nebulizer cleaning, see Chapter 5.)

Although the compressor with nebulizer system is easy to operate, do not underestimate the challenge of using it in a resistant child. Often, it requires considerable patience on your part, as well as some getting used to on the part of your child. We suggest at first letting the child use the mask without medication so that she can become familiar with the equipment. You may find it helpful initially to give treatments with the child sitting in your lap. For the older child, reading a book together or watching a video can help pass the time.

As your child grows older, you may want to move on to a spacer system with a mouthpiece rather than a face mask. When your child has learned to hold her breath underwater, she is ready to make the transition to a simpler inhalational aid: a plastic or metal chamber (examples include Aerochamber, Optichamber, and Vortex). With this system, the metered-dose inhaler (metal

Instructions for Nebulizer Use

- Fill nebulizer with medication as prescribed.
- Have your child seated comfortably.
- Place the face mask over your child's nose and mouth (hold it in place or use an elastic around the head to secure it in position).
- Begin treatment by switching on the compressor.
- Nebulizers need to be kept clean to function properly (follow manufacturer's instructions).
- Compressors need new filters approximately every six months (follow manufacturer's recommendations).

canister and its plastic holder) is fitted snugly into one end of the tube, and the medicine is sprayed into the tube, a hollow chamber. The child puts the mouthpiece at the other end of the tube into her mouth, and inhales the medicine from the chamber. She needs to take a deep breath in and then hold her breath for approximately five to ten seconds. For a second puff of medicine, the same procedure is repeated: shake the inhaler, squirt one puff into the chamber, breathe in slowly, and hold for five to ten seconds. Periodically, the inside of these chambers can be rinsed clean with water and then allowed to air-dry. To be sure that your child is ready to manage one of these inhalational aids, we like to observe her using it properly while still in our medical office. We find that the time we invest during an office visit in explaining the medications and how best to use them is usually time well spent.

For a child who may need some extra time learning to be comfortable with a spacer, we recommend the accordionlike plastic reservoir bag system called Inspirease. The metal canister of the albuterol (or other) metered-dose inhaler is removed from its plastic holder and inserted into the plastic stem of the Inspirease system. The child needs to be able to seal her lips around the plastic mouthpiece. Depressing the metal canister releases one dose of medicine, which is directed into the attached collapsible plastic bag suspended between two plastic disks. When your child breathes in and out, you can watch the bag deflate and reinflate with each breathing cycle. Two or three cycles completely empty the bag of medicine. Using this method, patient, parent, and health care provider can all be confident that the child received the medication. Some of the disadvantages of this device are that it is hard to clean and not very durable. (These spacer devices are illustrated in Figure 9 on page 81.)

205

It is worth emphasizing that children do not become dependent on bronchodilators. Over time they do not need greater amounts of medication to get
the same effects. In fact, unlike other medications, such as antibiotics, the dose
remains the same even as your child grows and gains weight. To some extent,
the dose of medicine reaching the bronchial tubes is automatically adjusted,
because as children get older and breathe more deeply, more of the medicine
released from the inhaler is deposited onto their airways.

LONG-TERM CONTROL MEDICATIONS

Asthma that causes more than occasional symptoms should be treated with a
long-term control medication. Treating it with a bronchodilator only is a little
bit like treating sunburn with a soothing lotion but failing to apply sunscreen
to your child or to take your child out of the sun. The bronchodilator relieves
the immediate problem but fails to address the underlying cause of symptoms
or to prevent the next episode. Don't simply react when your child becomes
sick with asthma; give her medicine that will keep her from getting sick.

The panel of experts assembled by the National Asthma Education and
Prevention Program (see Chapter 3) recently addressed the issue of when to
begin asthma controller medicines in young children. In their *Expert Panel Report: Asthma Update 2002,* these asthma experts concluded that long-term
control therapy should be considered in infants and young children who have
had more than three episodes of wheezing in the previous year and who are at
risk for developing asthma because of their own or their parents' history of allergic diseases. In addition, they recommend long-term control treatments for
children who need bronchodilator treatments more than twice a week or who
have had severe flare-ups of their asthma separated by fewer than six weeks.
These recommendations for beginning regular preventive medicines in young
children with asthma are summarized in the table on page 209.

WHICH LONG-TERM CONTROL THERAPY IS BEST?

There are several options for long-term control therapy (see also Chapters 6, 7,
and 10). In choosing among these options, we consider which is the most appropriate medication as well as which route of delivery will be best. Even the
finest medication will not help the child who cannot or will not take it. Options for the very young child include cromolyn (by metered-dose inhaler or
nebulizer solution), inhaled steroids (by metered-dose inhaler, dry-powder inhaler, or nebulizer solution), and leukotriene blockers (by chewable tablets).
In a large-scale, four-year study of children aged 5 to 12 (at the onset of the

Reasons for Starting Controller Medicines in Infants and Young Children

1. Three or more episodes of wheezing in the previous year that lasted more than one day and affected sleep, and risk factors for developing asthma, namely:

   - A parent with asthma
   - Allergic (atopic) dermatitis diagnosed by a physician
   - Two of the following:
     a. Allergic rhinitis diagnosed by a physician
     b. Wheezing when free of a cold
     c. Excess allergy cells (eosinophils) on a blood test

2. Needing bronchodilator treatments for asthma symptoms more than twice a week

3. Severe asthma flare-ups fewer than six weeks apart

study), treatment with inhaled steroids proved more effective in reducing symptoms and preventing asthma flare-ups (that is, at providing long-term asthma control) than did a cromolyn-like mast cell stabilizer called nedocromil (Tilade). Similar studies done in children younger than 5 are not yet available. In making our recommendations in children this young, we rely on our past experiences, on the conclusions drawn from studies done in older children, and on the recommendations of the expert panel of the National Asthma Education and Prevention Program. Here are the three choices:

- **Mast cell stabilizer:** Cromolyn (Intal) has been available for the treatment of asthma for more than 30 years. To be fully effective, it needs to be taken four times a day (one nebulizer treatment or two inhalations from a metered-dose inhaler with spacer, four times daily). Its great appeal is its complete freedom from side effects and long history of safety, even in very young children.

- **Leukotriene blocker:** Approved for use in children as young as 1, montelukast (Singulair) can be taken once a day as a chewable tablet or sprinkle. It is not a steroid medication. In general, it is not as effective in providing long-term asthma control as an inhaled steroid, but it is easy to give and virtually free of side effects. As a first step for treating mild asthma, montelukast (Singulair) is a suitable alternative to inhaled steroids. Another leukotriene blocker, zafirlukast (Accolate), is approved for children 7 and older.

• **Inhaled steroids:** Inhaled steroids are now recommended as the preferred treatment for young children needing long-term asthma control therapy, just as they are the first-line treatment for adults with persistent asthma. This recommendation is based on the opinion that the inhaled steroids are the most effective control medication and when given in low doses are safe for use even in children younger than 5. Inhaled steroids improve a child's breathing capacity, reduce the frequency of coughing and wheezing, decrease the need for bronchodilator treatments, and decrease the chance of a serious asthma flare-up requiring urgent care, including hospitalization. (For more on steroids and children, see Chapter 6).

One steroid preparation, budesonide (Pulmicort Respules), can be given by nebulization. It is approved by the Food and Drug Administration for use in children as young as 1. Other steroid preparations can be given by metered-dose inhaler with a spacer chamber and attached face mask. There are two precautions to remember when using an inhaled steroid. First, it is important to rinse your child's mouth after each use. An older child can simply rinse with water and then spit out. For a younger child, you will need to take a wet washcloth and wipe the inside of the child's mouth (the top of the tongue and insides of the cheeks). This will protect your child against a painful yeast infection in the mouth called thrush. Second, wipe the skin under the face mask: the nose, cheeks, and chin, where a portion of the steroid medicine is deposited. Over time, steroids applied to the skin can cause it to thin. Again, a simple wipe with a warm, wet facecloth suffices to clean the skin.

In an older child, one who can coordinate a steady inhalation followed by a five- to ten-second holding of the breath, options for steroid delivery include the metered-dose inhaler with spacer (such as Inspirease or the hollow tube chambers discussed above) and a dry-powder inhaler, the fluticasone (Flovent) Rotadisk. For details about dry-powder inhalers in general and the Rotadisk device in particular, see Chapter 6.

We are often asked about the potential for harmful effects from long-term use of inhaled steroids in children. The effects that we watch for include weight gain, mood changes, aggressive behavior, decreased bone growth (short stature), and abnormal functioning of the adrenal glands. The consensus of opinion offered by the expert panel of the National Asthma Education and

Ages at Which Kids Can Start Asthma Medicines

MEDICINES	STARTING AGE (IN YEARS) FOR FDA-APPROVED USE
INHALED STEROIDS	
Beclomethasone (QVAR)	6
Triamcinolone (Azmacort)	6
Flunisolide (Aerobid)	6
Budesonide (Pulmicort)	
Pulmicort Respules (nebulizer)	1
Pulmicort Turbuhaler (DPI)	6
Fluticasone (Flovent)	
Flovent MDI	12
Flovent Diskhaler (DPI)	4
LONG-ACTING BRONCHODILATORS	
Theophylline (Theo-24, Uniphyl, and others)	Less than 1
Salmeterol (Serevent) Diskus (DPI)	4
Formoterol (Foradil) Aerolizer (DPI)	5
LEUKOTRIENE BLOCKERS	
Montelukast	1
Zafirlukast	7
MAST CELLS STABILIZERS	
Cromolyn, by nebulizer	2
Cromolyn, MDI	6

Prevention Program is that when inhaled steroids are used at low doses, these side effects are rare, insignificant, and, if they occur, generally reversible.

Most important is the issue of delayed growth. During the first year of treatment with inhaled steroids, vertical growth tends to slow—on average, by approximately one centimeter, or slightly more than one third of an inch. However, this effect on growth is not sustained in subsequent years of treatment. When children treated with inhaled steroids for more than ten years were followed until they achieved their final height, that height was no different from what was expected in the absence of steroid treatment. In our opinion, the health benefits of inhaled steroids—a wheeze-free child safe from severe asthma attacks—justify the low risk of serious side effects. As with any

Defining Low Doses of Steroids in Children

STEROID PREPARATION	NUMBER OF MICROGRAMS PER PUFF OR TREATMENT	LOW DAILY DOSE (MICROGRAMS)
Beclomethasone (QVAR)	40 or 80	80–160
Budesonide (Dry powder) (Pulmicort Turbuhaler)	200	200–400
Budesonide (Nebulizer) (Pulmicort Respules)	250 or 500	500
Flunisolide (Aerobid)	250	500–750
Fluticasone (Metered dose) (Flovent)	44, 110, or 220	88–176
Fluticasone (Dry powder) (Flovent Rotadisk)	50, 100, or 250	100–250
Triamcinolone (Azmacort)	100	400–800

child, we carefully monitor growth, and we continuously reassess medication risks and benefits over time.

MANAGING YOUR CHILD'S ASTHMA FLARE-UP

Even the best treatment program is not a guarantee against an asthma flare-up. To help your child in the event of an asthma flare-up, you will be best prepared if you have a step-by-step plan of action that you have discussed in advance with your child's pediatrician or asthma specialist. Your child's Asthma Action Plan should be in writing. As you probably know from experience, if your child is in the midst of an asthma flare-up, your best laid plans can be difficult to remember. The action plan will remind you of the first step to take during a flare-up, what to do next if there is no improvement, and when and whom to call if you need more help.

Another important information card to keep handy is your child's one-minute medical history. This is an abbreviated medical history of your child's asthma. Having it in writing ensures that you will be ready to communicate this essential information to any of the health care providers you may encounter when your child is having an asthma flare-up—from your pediatrician or covering doctors to emergency department and inpatient medical personnel.

The One-Minute Medical History

Your child's one-minute medical history should include the following information:

- Diagnosis
- Age of onset of symptoms
- The usual triggers of the child's asthma
- History of asthma or other allergic conditions in family members
- Current status (compared with baseline)
- Current medications, including dosages and times last taken
- History of emergency department visits, hospitalizations in regular pediatric unit or pediatric intensive care unit
- Allergies
- Drug allergies
- Other medical conditions

GUIDELINES FOR RELIEVING AN ASTHMA FLARE-UP

If your child's asthma episodes are mild and infrequent, you may be able to help restore her breathing to normal without even needing to call the doctor. Whether or not you need medical help, the first step to relieve an asthma flare-up is treatment with a quick reliever (see Chapter 5) such as albuterol. The usual dose is two puffs, breathed in slowly and deeply, or one treatment with a nebulized bronchodilator. (See Chapter 5 for more about nebulizers.) If this doesn't work, we recommend that you administer a second treatment 30 minutes later.

If your child is old enough to use a peak flow meter, your health care provider may recommend that you monitor her peak flow (see Chapters 2, 3, 10, 11, 16, and 17 for more on peak flow monitoring) during asthma flare-ups. A peak flow that is greater than 80 percent of your child's personal best indicates a mild flare-up. (Personal best is your child's peak flow on a day when her asthma is under good control.) A peak flow that is 50–80 percent of personal best indicates a moderate flare-up, and a peak flow of less than 50 percent indicates a severe one.

Even without a peak flow meter, you will have a pretty good idea of the severity of your child's asthma flare-up by observing how much difficulty she is having breathing. Look for unusually rapid breathing, wheezing, flaring of the nose, and retraction, or pulling in, of the muscles in the neck and/or between the ribs and pulling in of the skin below the ribs or above the breastbone.

WHEN TO CALL YOUR CHILD'S DOCTOR

We advise parents to call their child's physician if the child does not respond to two treatments (two puffs per treatment) of her quick reliever or to two treatments of her quick-acting bronchodilator delivered by nebulizer 30 minutes apart, or needs quick-relief treatment more than every four hours. However, you should call your child's doctor any time you are uncertain about caring for your child at home. The doctor may advise you to add some more medicine, such as steroid liquid or tablets, or to go to his or her office or to the emergency department.

If your child is having a mild asthma attack, you can drive her to the doctor's office, but it is best for two adults to be in the car: one to attend to the child, and one to drive. If your child is in a lot of distress—for example, if she is unable to speak in complete sentences, is lethargic, confused, or turning blue—it is time to dial 911 and prepare to travel to the hospital by ambulance. In an asthma crisis, do not try to drive your child to the hospital yourself.

CHAPTER 13

Special Considerations in Women

For men and women, maintaining good health, including good asthma control, poses somewhat different challenges. Although one might naturally think that lungs are lungs, and bronchial tubes are bronchial tubes, and that asthma wouldn't be any different in men than in women, in fact there are gender-based differences. Consider the following:

- Before the age of puberty, more boys than girls have asthma, but after puberty asthma is more common among women than men.

- In most studies of severe asthma attacks, women outnumber men in the frequency of emergency department visits and hospitalizations for asthma.

- Pregnancy can have a major influence on the course of asthma.

- For some women, asthma predictably worsens around the time of menstrual periods.

- Birth control pills and hormone replacement therapy may affect asthma in some women.

There are many theories, none proven, about gender differences in asthma. We know that women's lungs are smaller and that their bronchial tubes have a smaller diameter than those of men of the same age and height. This normal anatomic difference may partially explain the tendency toward greater airway narrowing in women with asthma. The situation is the reverse in childhood, when boys' airways are smaller relative to their lung size compared with those of girls. Having relatively smaller airways means being more susceptible to airway narrowing and wheezing, which may explain why more young boys than young girls develop asthma.

Perhaps the differences in asthma between men and women have something to do with the environments in which we tend to spend most of our time. In our culture, as in many others, women tend to spend more time in the home environment than men do. If home is the source of allergens that cause or aggravate asthma—such as dust mites, cockroaches, and furry or feathered animals—women may have greater exposure to these stimuli than men do.

Another reason for the gender difference we see in asthma may have to do with possible differences in the way men and women respond to having asthma. Women may be more aware of their asthma symptoms and more likely to seek medical attention during an asthma attack. This possible difference could contribute in part to observations that emergency department visits and hospitalizations for asthma are more frequent among women than men. In several studies, women were shown to be admitted to the hospital for asthma more often than men and to experience longer hospital stays, suggesting that perhaps women are more severely affected by asthma than men.

We suspect that there are genetic differences between men and women that are relevant to asthma. In the years ahead researchers are likely to identify the genes that make people susceptible to developing asthma, and other genes that influence the severity of asthma. It is possible that some of these genes travel together with the genes that determine gender.

Finally, female reproductive hormones clearly influence asthma, although we don't know exactly how. Estrogen and progesterone may affect how the muscles of the breathing tubes behave, or may influence susceptibility to allergic inflammation of the airways. Perhaps these hormones also influence the actions of the inflammatory cells and chemicals that participate in asthmatic reactions. Understanding these possible hormone effects might help explain the changes women experience in their asthma at times of hormonal fluctuation—such as during puberty, pregnancy, and before menstrual periods.

In this chapter we will focus on three aspects of asthma management that are particularly germane and in some cases unique to women: asthma during pregnancy, asthma in relation to menstrual periods and hormonal therapy, and asthma and osteoporosis risk.

ASTHMA DURING PREGNANCY

Women with asthma who are pregnant, or hoping to become pregnant, are naturally concerned about how pregnancy will affect their asthma. Unfortunately, we cannot predict whether the severity of your asthma will change when you become pregnant. In fact, when you become pregnant, you stand about an equal chance of experiencing improvement, worsening, or no change in your asthma. However, for some women the change is dramatic. For the first time ever, they struggle with troublesome asthma throughout their pregnancy, or they experience a miraculous improvement in previously difficult-to-control asthma. Generally speaking, your experience with asthma during a previous pregnancy tends to predict a similar course the next time around, but this rule does not always hold true. Mild asthma during one pregnancy does not guarantee mild asthma in a subsequent pregnancy. By the same token, if your asthma gave you a lot of trouble during your first pregnancy, it might bother you less the next time.

Of equal concern to many women is how their asthma will affect the outcome of their pregnancy. Fortunately, studies suggest that with good asthma control during pregnancy, the likelihood that a woman with asthma will have a healthy pregnancy and a healthy baby is the same as it is for a woman who does not have asthma. The greatest risk to the developing baby is a severe asthma flare-up that causes the mother to have low blood oxygen. The fetus is dependent on the mother's oxygen for its development and suffers if deprived of oxygen. The key to a successful outcome is to work with your primary care doctor and appropriate specialists to maintain good asthma control throughout your pregnancy.

In general, the risk of asthma flare-ups is greatest in the third trimester, between weeks 24 and 36; flare-ups after week 37 are uncommon. Women who have had a difficult time with asthma during pregnancy occasionally worry that they won't be able to breathe and push effectively during labor and delivery. We are able to reassure them that asthma flare-ups are uncommon during labor and delivery. Still, it is wise to plan to deliver your baby in a hospital, where both of you will be sure to get the care you need in the event that your asthma does act up. Discuss your labor and delivery plans with your doctors in advance of delivery. Your asthma should not preclude any type of delivery that you may choose, including natural childbirth. Regardless of how your asthma behaves during your pregnancy, it is likely to return to "normal" (the way it was before your pregnancy) about three months after your baby is born.

NORMAL CHANGES TO EXPECT DURING PREGNANCY

Many changes in the normal functioning of your body take place during pregnancy. For example, your heart rate increases, your blood pressure decreases, and you develop a mild anemia. Increases in the hormone progesterone will cause you to breathe more deeply. The amount of air that you move in and out of your lungs each minute increases, although you probably won't notice this difference. Most women—about 70 percent—experience shortness of breath at some point during their pregnancy. This often occurs as early as the first trimester, before the fetus and uterus enlarge. This shortness of breath is probably due to normal hormonal changes. Still, if you are feeling short of breath during your pregnancy, you should talk with your health care provider. It is important to make sure that there is no reason for your breathlessness other than your pregnant state.

Keep in mind that these pregnancy-related breathing changes do not affect your peak flow or other tests of how fast you can force air from your lungs. If your peak flow drops, it is not because you are eight months pregnant and your baby is pushing up on your diaphragm. It is probably because your asthma is flaring up.

ASTHMA TREATMENT GOALS DURING PREGNANCY

When you are pregnant, you are "breathing for two," so it is doubly important to keep your asthma under good control. When you are breathing well, your baby is getting enough oxygen. But if your peak flows are down and you need to use your quick-acting bronchodilator inhaler more often than usual, it is not good for you or for your baby.

> "*Until you are pregnant and have a child, until another life is in jeopardy, that's when you really take stock and say, 'Wait a minute—wow, I'm not breathing perfectly. I have to take these medicines, etc.' It was also the best thing that could have happened to my asthma—having a baby—because now I really pay attention to my own health. What I learned with the pregnancy is that it really snaps you into shape as far as your own care. You have to take care of your body and be able to breathe in order to make the baby breathe.*"
> —SHELLEY, 36

The treatment goals for asthma are the same when you are pregnant as when you are not. Of course, there is the additional goal of enabling you to have a normal birth experience and a healthy baby, the most likely outcome when your asthma is well controlled during pregnancy.

If you are not already under the care of a specialist for your asthma, you and your obstetrician should consider referral to a pulmonary or allergy specialist to help you manage your care during your pregnancy. We often find that care providers who do not specialize in asthma tend to undertreat pregnant women with asthma. Some health care providers (physicians, nurses, and pharmacists) who are not knowledgeable about the treatment of asthma during pregnancy may be fearful about harmful medication side effects during pregnancy. We feel strongly that poorly controlled asthma is a greater risk to you and your unborn baby than the medications used to control it. A specialist will be familiar with the medications that are safe and effective both for you and your baby. Your active participation in keeping your asthma under control is important. You, your asthma specialist, and your obstetrician are equal partners in a team effort. Close communication is very important, so that your obstetrician is well informed about how your asthma is doing, and your asthma specialist is well informed about your pregnancy.

> *Tiffany, 20, was diagnosed with asthma when she was 7 or 8, after awakening from a deep sleep in severe respiratory distress and having to be rushed to the hospital. Once stabilized with medications, her asthma "wasn't too bad," she says, until she became pregnant.*
>
> *"Around the sixth month, I started having a hard time breathing and had to go to the hospital for nebulizer treatments pretty often—maybe four or five times until I delivered my son." The baby was delivered by cesarean section because his heart rate had dropped, but Tiffany's asthma didn't give her trouble during the delivery.*
>
> *"I got a break for a few months after my first baby was born," she says, noting that her asthma worsened again during the sixth month of her second pregnancy, just as it had during the first one.*
>
> *"If possible, wait till you have your asthma under good control before you get pregnant," advises Tiffany. "Take all your meds, and talk to your asthma doctor about being pregnant, so your asthma can be monitored. Before I first saw an asthma doctor when I was pregnant for the second time, I knew I had asthma but I didn't know anything about it. I'd been raising myself since I was 13 and didn't have any guidance. Now I know to take my meds and avoid the things that set my asthma off, like smoke, and markers, and nail polish remover, and a bunch of other things. It's important to educate yourself about asthma, and an asthma doctor can help you do that."*
>
> —TIFFANY, 20

We recommend a three-pronged approach to achieving the goals of good asthma control during your pregnancy: avoiding your asthma triggers, treating your asthma with safe medications, and monitoring for any signs of a flare-up of your asthma.

AVOIDING YOUR ASTHMA TRIGGERS DURING PREGNANCY

It is not always easy to avoid your asthma triggers, but pregnancy is the time to be especially careful. Wash your hands more often than usual, to reduce the chances of catching infections that can cause your asthma to flare up. Viral respiratory infections can lead to bronchitis and sinusitis, common causes of severe episodes of asthma.

As for tobacco smoke, not only is it an asthma trigger, it is loaded with poisons that are dangerous to you and to your unborn baby. Women who smoke cigarettes or who are repeatedly exposed to secondhand tobacco smoke during pregnancy are more likely to have a miscarriage. Infants of mothers who smoked cigarettes during pregnancy are more likely to be stillborn or born prematurely, or to have lower birth weights. These infants are also at increased risk of sudden infant death syndrome (SIDS). If you smoke, now is the time to quit. If you need help quitting smoking, ask your doctor for assistance, including help finding a good smoking cessation program near you.

ASTHMA MEDICATIONS DURING PREGNANCY

Women often tell us that when they learned they were pregnant, they stopped their asthma medications out of concern for their baby. Our response, invariably, is to emphasize that medications are frequently an important part of good asthma control. Well-controlled asthma greatly improves the likelihood of a healthy pregnancy and a healthy baby.

> *Diagnosed when she was 5, Martha's asthma got worse when she was in her twenties, requiring her to take a short course of prednisone tablets as often as five or six times a year, often when she had a sinus infection. Martha, 38, who is an allergist, also has "horrible allergies"—to cats, seasonal pollens, dust, and other substances—which have contributed to her difficult asthma. Her asthma and allergies are under better control since she moved into a house with no carpeting about five years ago.*
>
> *Asked about her asthma during her pregnancy several years ago, Martha says, "I did fairly well until a period during my second trimester when I was short of breath a lot." As is often the case, "everything started to get better at around 32 weeks," she says. She swam regularly, right up to when the baby was born, did fine during delivery, and gave birth to a healthy baby girl.*
>
> *"Even though I'm a doctor, I wouldn't make any important treat-*

*ment decision about my asthma without consulting my pulmonologist,"
she says. "For example, if I thought I needed prednisone, I wouldn't start
taking it without first talking with her."*

*Adds Martha, "When you have asthma and you're pregnant, you
wonder, 'Am I short of breath because of my asthma or because I'm pregnant?' It's useful to talk with someone who knows about asthma and
pregnancy and can help differentiate between the normal shortness of
breath from pregnancy and shortness of breath related to asthma."*

— MARTHA, 38

During your pregnancy it is very important for you to work closely with a
physician who knows what medications can be most safely used. He or she will
work with you to decrease your medication to the lowest dose needed to control your symptoms, and when choosing between two medications that are
similarly effective will select the one thought to be safest during pregnancy.

Determining the safety of any medication in pregnancy is a difficult task.
Out of respect for the safety of developing fetuses, research experiments are almost never performed in which one group of pregnant women is given a new
medication while another, similar group receives a placebo. Safety information must be collected indirectly, usually in one or more of the following ways.
First, the medication can be given to pregnant animals, often in amounts
much greater than would be used in humans, and harmful effects monitored
in the offspring of these animals. Medicines that can be given in very high
doses to pregnant animals without evidence of harmful effects are thought
likely to be safe in humans at far smaller doses.

Second, records can be kept of the medicines women are taking during
their pregnancy, and the pregnancy outcomes can be tracked. When data are
collected on large numbers of women, the outcomes of their pregnancies can
be compared with those of healthy women taking no medicines. Careful statis-
tical comparisons can then be made to determine whether more complications were found in the women taking a particular medication and whether
their newborn babies were equally healthy. In one particularly important
study, the Boston Collaborative Drug Surveillance Program, information was
collected in just this way on the medication use of thousands of pregnant
women. Similarly, more and more often now, pharmaceutical companies are
supporting registries that track pregnancy outcomes in women taking newly
released medications.

Finally, there is the physician's judgment about safety, which comes from
long-term experience with a medication. We feel more confident about the

safety of medicines that have been available for use by pregnant women for decades than we do about the safety of medicines released only a year or two ago. Asthma is a very common illness among women of childbearing age. Every year many thousands of pregnant women take antiasthma medications. If some of these medications were dangerous to the developing child, there would be ample opportunity to observe harmful effects. We would expect that at least a suspicion of harm would be raised among doctors and patients after years of direct experience.

The Food and Drug Administration uses a rating system for suggesting to doctors and patients the relative safety of medicines during pregnancy. The system uses the letters A through D. Category A indicates that a medicine has proved safe in human studies of pregnant women. Virtually no medications receive this label, because of the lack of controlled studies of medications in pregnant women. Category D indicates that a medicine is known to cause harmful effects in the developing fetus. No asthma or allergy medicines are included in this category. Most asthma and allergy medicines receive either a B or a C rating. Category B indicates that a medicine is probably safe, based on animal studies and the absence of negative human studies. Category C indicates less certainty as to safety, not because of any known harmful effects in humans, but because of bad outcomes in some animal species at ultrahigh medication doses. If two medications—one with a B rating, the other with a C rating—generally work equally well, your doctor will most likely select the medication with the B rating.

Some of our preferred asthma and allergy medicines and their FDA safety ratings are listed in the following table.

Drugs and Dosages for Asthma and Associated Conditions Preferred for Use During Pregnancy

DRUG CLASS	SPECIFIC DRUG (FDA CLASSIFICATION)	DOSAGE
Anti-inflammatory	Cromolyn (Intal, Nasalcrom) (B)	2 puffs four times daily (inhalation) 2 sprays in each nostril two to four times daily for nasal symptoms
	Budesonide (Pulmicort, Rhinocort) (B)	1–4 inhalations twice daily for asthma 1–2 sprays once daily for nasal symptoms

	Beclomethasone (QVAR, Vancenase, Beconase) (C)	2–5 puffs twice daily (inhalation) 2 sprays in each nostril twice daily for allergic rhinitis
	Prednisone, prednisolone, methylprednisolone (not classified)	Steroid course: for example, 40 mg a day for 4 days, then the dose is reduced to zero over 1–2 weeks If prolonged course is required, single morning dose on alternate days may minimize adverse effects.
Bronchodilator	Inhaled beta-2 agonists Terbutaline (Brethine) (B) All others (including albuterol and long-acting inhaled beta-agonists) are category C	2 puffs every 4 hours only as needed
	Theophylline (Uniphyl, Theo-24, Theolair) (C)	Oral: Dose to reach serum concentration level of 6–8 µg/ml
Antihistamine	Chlorpheniramine (Chlor-Trimeton and others) (not classified)	4 mg by mouth up to four times daily 8–12 mg sustained-release twice daily
	Tripelennamine (B)	25–50 mg by mouth up to four times daily 100 mg sustained-release twice daily
Cough medicine	Guaifenesin (not classified)	2 tsp by mouth four times daily
	Dextromethorphan (not classified)	Note: Avoid all cough medicines containing alcohol
Antibiotics	Amoxicillin Erythromycin (for patients allergic to penicillin) (B)	2–3 weeks therapy for sinusitis using 250–500 mg four times daily

This table presents our preferred drugs and suggested dosages for the home management of asthma and associated conditions during pregnancy.

TREATING YOUR ASTHMA DURING PREGNANCY

Most often, asthma begins before the childbearing age, so that most pregnant women with asthma will already be taking, or at least will already have been prescribed, medications for their asthma. The first question that usually comes to mind is, "Should I stop my asthma and allergy medications, for the safety of my baby?" The same question is pertinent to couples who are seeking to conceive a child. "Could my asthma and allergy medicines do harm to the early stage embryo, even before I know that I am pregnant? Should I stop these medicines while we are trying to conceive?"

Potentially Harmful Medications

Fortunately, none of the asthma and allergy medicines are in Category D, the category of medicines considered "teratogenic," meaning that they can cause serious birth defects and developmental abnormalities in a high percentage of unborn babies. Other medicines, such as isotretinoin (Accutane), used to treat severe acne, are highly teratogenic and should be avoided by any woman engaging in unprotected sexual intercourse. Two types of antibiotics are also in this category and should be avoided during pregnancy: the tetracyclines (which can affect the teeth of the developing baby), and antibiotics of the family that includes ciprofloxacin (Cipro) and levofloxacin (Levaquin) because they can affect cartilage development in the joints of the fetus.

Although no asthma medications pose this type of threat to the fetus, there are some asthma and allergy medications that are best avoided during early pregnancy. Early pregnancy (the first trimester) is a time when many of the major organs in the body are forming, and as such it is a time for particular caution. One group of medicines to avoid in early pregnancy are those that tend to constrict blood vessels and might deprive the developing baby of adequate blood supply. This group includes nasal decongestant tablets such as pseudoephedrine (Sudafed and others) and phenylephrine (in Entex LA and others). By analogy, we would also recommend avoiding adrenaline, also called epinephrine. This medicine, given as an injection, used to be the mainstay of the emergency treatment of asthma flare-ups. Now equally effective alternatives are available, as discussed in Chapters 5 and 16.

One type of medicine poses a particular dilemma. It has been suggested that steroids in tablet form (such as prednisone [Deltasone and others] and methylprednisolone [Medrol]) can increase the risk of your child's being born with cleft lip and/or cleft palate. The evidence for this effect comes mainly from experiments performed in pregnant rabbits. Observations in humans have provided variable results, but at least some studies have reached similar conclusions. This potential risk relates only to the first trimester of pregnancy. No increased risk for cleft lip/palate has been reported with the *inhaled* corticosteroids.

The dilemma comes when a pregnant woman suffers a severe flare-up of her asthma. Sometimes only steroids in tablet form can restore her breathing, first to safe levels and then to normal. In that event, the small risk of an infant's being born with cleft lip/palate is clearly outweighed by the beneficial effects of the medicine—namely, restoring comfortable breathing, ensuring adequate oxygen to mother and baby, reducing the risk of miscarriage, and, during very severe attacks, keeping mother and baby alive. In severe asthma episodes, the dangers of withholding oral steroids during the first trimester are far greater than the dangers of taking the medicine. Remember, in virtually all studies of pregnancy outcomes among women with asthma, the greatest risk for poor outcomes, including birth defects, has been poorly controlled asthma and severe asthma episodes during pregnancy.

Safe Medications

Central to managing asthma are the inhaled beta-agonist bronchodilators and the inhaled steroids. Fortunately, it is safe for you to continue both types of medicines throughout your pregnancy. Albuterol (Ventolin, Proventil) is the most commonly prescribed inhaled beta-agonist bronchodilator; others include metaproterenol (Alupent, Metaprel) and pirbuterol (Maxair). These medicines have been used in the treatment of asthma for many years, and only minuscule amounts of medicine enter the bloodstream, so only minuscule amounts can be carried to the unborn baby. Most physicians consider them fully safe in pregnancy. One beta-agonist bronchodilator, terbutaline, has received a category B rating for use in pregnancy because of its known safety in treating premature labor. Once available as a metered-dose inhaler called Brethaire, terbutaline is now available only in tablet or injectable formulations (Brethine), a major drawback to its routine use.

You can use your quick-acting bronchodilator as needed during your pregnancy, but remember: if you are using it frequently (several times each week), your asthma is poorly controlled, and you (and your doctor) should be considering additional therapies to achieve better control.

Among the inhaled corticosteroids, two preparations (of the five that are available) have the longest and best studied safety records: beclomethasone (previously Beclovent or Vanceril, now available as QVAR) and budesonide (Pulmicort). Budesonide has recently been given a category B rating from the

FDA because of the lack of any harmful effects observed in three large registries of pregnant women maintained in Sweden. This is not to say that the other inhaled steroids, namely triamçinolone (Azmacort), flunisolide (Aerobid), and fluticasone (Flovent), are harmful for pregnant women. It simply says that their safety has not been as clearly established. As you will recall, when taken in the usual doses only a very tiny amount of any of these inhaled steroid medications actually enters the bloodstream, and even less escapes being broken down in the liver to be carried unchanged to the uterus and the developing fetus.

The leukotriene-blocking drugs montelukast (Singulair) and zafirlukast (Accolate) are among the newest antiasthmatic medications. Nonetheless, they too are considered safe in pregnancy and have been given a category B rating by the FDA. Animal studies using very high doses of medicine have shown no harmful effects in a variety of species tested, and no increased risk of miscarriages or birth defects has been observed in humans. We remain somewhat cautious about their use in pregnancy, mainly because of their newness (first introduced worldwide in 1996).

ALLERGY MEDICINES DURING PREGNANCY

Severe narrowing of the bronchi, the air passageways in the lungs, can be dangerous and even life-threatening. Narrowing of the nasal passageways, even to the point of complete obstruction, is not dangerous and is never life-threatening, but it can be mightily annoying. The nasal tissues normally tend to swell during pregnancy, and if you are prone to nasal allergies (allergic rhinitis), you are in double jeopardy during your pregnancy. A constantly stuffy nose may make your mouth dry, make it difficult to sleep, and make your breathing feel uncomfortable.

Because the newer antihistamines, such as loratadine (Claritin; Alavert), fexofenadine (Allegra), cetirizine (Zyrtec), and desloratadine (Clarinex), are of unproven safety during pregnancy, we recommend returning to the older generation of antihistamines when you are pregnant. We would favor chlorpheniramine (Chlor-Trimeton) or diphenhydramine (Benadryl). For many allergy sufferers, this choice leaves you between "a rock and a hard place": on the one hand, you have a miserably stuffy or drippy nose, but on the other hand, you may become intolerably sleepy from these first-generation antihistamines.

Don't despair; you have some other options. First, you can safely use nasal steroid sprays during pregnancy. In particular, budesonide, the same steroid preparation recommended for treating asthma during pregnancy, is available as a nasal steroid spray, either from a pressurized canister (Rhinocort) or as a liquid aerosol (Rhinocort AQ). Irrigation with a nasal saline spray (available over the counter) is always safe. It can help rinse out mucus, pollens, and chemical irritants and can be used numerous times each day with absolute confidence in its safety.

We do not have the same sense of certainty about two other types of therapy for nasal symptoms—the leukotriene blockers montelukast (Singulair) and zafirlukast (Accolate), and the anticholinergic nasal spray ipratropium (Atrovent). The leukotriene blockers are of some benefit in allergic rhinitis and have a category B rating for use during pregnancy. However, they are only mildly effective, and they are too new for us to feel confident that their benefits for nasal symptoms outweigh their potential for harmful effects. As for ipratropium nasal spray (Atrovent Nasal Spray), there is insufficient information about its use in pregnant women. However, because it is applied topically in minute doses rather than taken internally, it is probably safe.

Monitoring Your Asthma During Pregnancy

Your peak flow meter is an especially valuable tool during pregnancy (see Chapters 2, 3, 10, 11, 12, 16, and 17 for more on the use of peak flow meters). Peak flow measurements are simple and safe. You can do them at home at no cost (other than the cost of obtaining a peak flow meter). Monitoring your lung function—whether or not you are having symptoms—becomes particularly important during pregnancy, when you are breathing for two. Even though you feel fine, you could have narrowing in your airways and an asthma episode in the making. When your peak flow drops, a puff or two of your quick-reliever medication may help stop an asthma episode before it worsens. If using your quick-reliever does not cause your peak flow to improve, you need to consult with your doctor and perhaps have your medications adjusted.

If you suspect that you are having a flare-up of your asthma, because you are coughing more, feel short of breath, or hear yourself wheezing, you can quickly judge the severity of the flare-up with your peak flow meter. You can judge how serious this episode is and how urgently you will have to get help. We discuss the management of asthma attacks in Chapter 16. Suffice it to say here that the peak flow meter provides you the means to confirm that your symptoms are due to an asthma flare-up, to judge the severity of that flare-up, and to communicate effectively when you speak with your health care provider. Because preventing asthma attacks is the key to the successful outcome of your pregnancy, you have an excellent ally in your peak flow meter.

OTHER MEDICAL CONDITIONS THAT MAY AFFECT PREGNANCY AND YOUR ASTHMA

Even when you are doing your best to avoid your asthma triggers, carefully adhering to you medication plan, and monitoring your asthma closely, other conditions may complicate your pregnancy and affect your asthma. Among the most common are high blood pressure, diabetes mellitus, rhinitis, and gastroesophageal (acid) reflux. You and your doctor can work together to manage these conditions so they do not cause serious problems.

If you have asthma and high blood pressure, also called hypertension, or develop high blood pressure during your pregnancy, in general it is best to avoid the so-called beta-blockers sometimes used to treat this condition. Beta-blockers are a class of medications that in people with asthma are known to cause constriction of the muscles around the airways and therefore aggravate asthma. Another common group of antihypertensive medications, the angiotensin-converting enzyme inhibitors, such as enalapril (Vasotec) and lisinopril (Zestril, Prinivil), should be avoided because of harmful effects to the developing baby. Many other choices are available, from a variety of drug categories, such as diuretics, vasodilators, and calcium channel blockers. If you need medication to reduce your blood pressure, your physician will be able to suggest an alternative treatment.

Hormonal changes cause a small percentage of women who did not previously have diabetes mellitus to develop it during pregnancy. This so-called gestational diabetes is usually temporary and frequently goes away when hormones return to their prepregnancy levels. Steroids in tablet form, such as prednisone, can make diabetes worse by causing your blood sugar to rise. If you have gestational diabetes or diabetes that began before your pregnancy, close communication with your asthma specialist, obstetrician, and the primary physician managing your diabetes is important in optimizing your treatment.

As noted, changes in your blood vessels during pregnancy can cause the nasal passageways to become sensitive and swollen, especially during the second half of pregnancy. They become dilated (larger) due to increased blood volume and the effects of hormones. If you have nasal congestion in the absence of a cold or an allergic reaction, you may have pregnancy-related rhinitis, or swelling of your nasal passageways. As you probably know from having had head colds and perhaps allergies, rhinitis can make your breathing feel worse. If you are experiencing nasal congestion and postnasal drip, talk with your doctor about how best to treat these symptoms. Some suggestions are mentioned above ("Allergy Medicines During Pregnancy").

Gastroesophageal reflux (see Chapter 15) is the regurgitation of stomach contents up into the esophagus (swallowing tube). Acid reflux often causes the burning pain behind the breastbone known as heartburn. If you have gastro-esophageal reflux, it may get worse during your pregnancy. If you don't normally have reflux, you may develop it while you are pregnant. Hormonal changes in pregnancy can cause the sphincter, the muscular connection between your stomach and esophagus, to relax inappropriately. Add the pressure of the baby in your abdomen to this and you can see how stomach juices and acid can be pushed up into your esophagus. Reflux usually improves and often goes away entirely after you have delivered your baby.

Besides being unpleasant, reflux can make your breathing worse. When stomach acid travels up the esophagus and into the back of your throat, it is possible to inhale the acid into your windpipe and airways. There the acid will further irritate airways already inflamed by asthma.

Without having to take more medicine, there are many things you can do to lessen acid reflux. Adjusting your diet is one of them. Avoid caffeine (tea, coffee, caffeinated sodas, chocolate), carbonated beverages, and fatty or spicy foods. Raise the head of your bed six to eight inches by placing bricks or blocks under your bed frame or box spring. When you are lying at a slightly upward incline rather than completely flat, it is not as easy for stomach contents to roll back up from the stomach into the esophagus. On the other hand, simply sleeping on stacked pillows may make reflux worse by putting your body into a folded-up position that increases pressure in your abdomen.

Over-the-counter antacids can be helpful and are often sufficient to control reflux. The over-the-counter histamine type-2 blockers like ranitidine (Zantac), cimetidine (Tagamet), and famotidine (Pepcid) are safe in pregnancy. If you are receiving treatment for reflux disease with a proton pump inhibitor such as esomeprazole (Nexium), pantoprazole (Protonix), lansoprazole (Prevacid), or rabeprazole (Aciphex), you will be reassured to know that these drugs (but not omeprazole [Prilosec]) are rated by the FDA as category B for use in pregnancy. Some of our obstetrical colleagues feel comfortable about their safety in pregnancy; others do not, so we would encourage you to discuss treatment with these medicines with your obstetrician and asthma specialist.

Frequently Asked Questions About Asthma and Pregnancy

1. *Can I exercise as usual?*

   Yes, if you are otherwise healthy and feeling well, you should be able to participate in all the activities you were involved in before you became pregnant. Although pregnancy is not the best time to start a vigorous new exercise program, exercising during pregnancy is good for your health.

   If exercise makes your asthma flare up, do the things you would normally do before exercising. These might include using your albuterol inhaler before you begin exercising, and making sure to warm up before exercising and to cool down afterward. Jogging in cold weather is less likely to bother your asthma if you keep your nose and mouth covered with a scarf to warm and humidify the air you breathe. If necessary, your doctor can help you adjust your medications to allow you to exercise. You should also let your obstetrician know about the exercise program you are planning during your pregnancy.

2. *If I get a flu shot, will it harm my baby?*

   There is no need to skip your flu shot if you are pregnant. In fact, there is all the more reason to get it. The vaccine contains a killed virus that cannot make you sick and will not harm you or your baby. Influenza, or the flu, can be quite serious during pregnancy. It is especially important to get a flu shot if you are pregnant and you have asthma, because the flu can make your asthma worse. Also, people with asthma and other diseases affecting the airways are especially susceptible to complications from the flu, including pneumonia.

   It is best to wait until after the first trimester of your pregnancy before receiving your flu shot. Although not linked to flu shots, first-trimester miscarriages are common, and when possible, you don't want to give your body anything new to react to during this period.

3. *Is it safe to get allergy shots while I am pregnant?*

   If you were on a stable dose of immunotherapy (allergy shots) before you became pregnant and did not experience any related problems, it is fine to continue with the therapy. However, it is best not to *start* immunotherapy while you are pregnant because, at the start of therapy, you are at increased risk for adverse side effects. These can include anaphylaxis, a severe allergic reaction that could cause potentially life-threatening low blood pressure and put you and your baby at serious risk.

4. *Can I safely breast-feed my baby, even though I am taking asthma medications?*

   Yes. The amount of asthma medication that gets into your breast milk is not enough to adversely affect your baby. Breast milk provides wonderful, cost-free nutrition, protects your baby against infection, and may even decrease the risk of diabetes later in life. Be sure to talk with your doctor about breast-feeding your baby as you determine your postpartum asthma care plan.

As for the relationship between breast-feeding and asthma, the information we have so far is conflicting: some studies have found that breast-feeding babies protects them against developing asthma and against early wheezing, whereas other studies have described the opposite effect. You will want to discuss the pros and cons of breast-feeding with your doctor to help you decide if it is for you.

HOW YOUR MENSTRUAL CYCLE, BIRTH CONTROL PILLS, AND HORMONE REPLACEMENT THERAPY MAY AFFECT YOUR ASTHMA

As we noted earlier, pregnancy is not the only circumstance in which women's hormones can affect their asthma. The effects of hormonal fluctuations before each menstrual period, oral contraceptives, and hormone replacement therapy can all influence the course of asthma.

PREMENSTRUAL ASTHMA

In as many as 30 percent of women, asthma predictably worsens several days before or at the start of every menstrual period. This is called premenstrual (or perimenstrual) asthma. Some women who have premenstrual asthma may not be aware of it. When we ask women to watch closely to see if their asthma changes each month in association with their menstrual cycle, many come back surprised to say, "Yes, my peak flows go down just before I get my period; I use my albuterol more, and I feel more tightness in my chest." Although premenstrual asthma is a well-described phenomenon, the exact physiological mechanisms that cause it are not well known. It is probably linked somehow to changes in hormone levels, but further study is needed to work out the precise details.

If you observe that your asthma gets worse around the time of your menstrual period, you can anticipate and perhaps head off the problem. You can work with your doctor to adjust your medication regimen every month to minimize perimenstrual symptoms. If you are prepared for this change in the pattern of your asthma, you will probably be able to prevent asthma exacerbations related to your menstrual period. Some women find relief only when they suppress their menstrual cycles, as, for example, with oral contraceptives.

BIRTH CONTROL PILLS

Not all women report that their asthma improves when they begin oral contraceptives. Some women find that their asthma worsens on the pill; others note no difference. If you are starting oral contraceptives for the first time, find out how they affect you: use your peak flow meter to monitor any possible change in the severity of your asthma.

HORMONE REPLACEMENT THERAPY

Another important hormonal life change for women occurs at menopause, often referred to as the change of life. It usually occurs in middle age, or at any age if the ovaries are removed surgically, when estrogen production falls and menstrual periods stop. Until recently, a large number of postmenopausal women have chosen to take hormone replacement therapy—that is, estrogen via a skin patch or tablets, sometimes in combination with progesterone. As with oral contraceptives, we generally can't predict how hormone replacement therapy will affect asthma in postmenopausal women. You may have heard of or read about the Nurses' Health Study, based at Brigham and Women's Hospital and Harvard Medical School, a large study that has been looking at women's health issues since 1976. Data on postmenopausal estrogen replacement therapy showed that menopausal women in the study who were currently using or who had used estrogen replacement therapy had a 50 percent greater risk of developing asthma than those who did not take hormonal replacement therapy. Still, the likelihood of any woman developing asthma after menopause remains low, and only a *very small* percentage of women taking hormone replacement therapy ever develop asthma.

As with oral contraceptives, if you begin hormone replacement therapy, it is important to monitor your asthma closely for change in its severity, particularly if you have difficult-to-control asthma.

Clearly, we need additional large studies to understand better the effects of reproductive hormones (estrogen, progesterone, and testosterone) on the airways. But the fact that pregnancy, menstrual periods, birth control pills, and hormone replacement therapy can all affect asthma, at least in some women, is strong evidence for the conclusion that female hormones are a key factor in some of the differences in asthma between women and men.

ASTHMA AND SEXUALITY

A few words here about asthma and sexuality: asthma need not interfere with an active sex life any more than it need interfere with participation in sports—

which is to say, not at all. Asthma medications do not affect sexual function, unlike some medications that are used to treat depression or high blood pressure. It is true that for some people, sexual activity, like athletic activity, can be an asthma trigger. If you are one of these people, work closely with your doctor to optimize your asthma treatment plan so that you can be as fully sexually active as you want to be without being limited by asthma symptoms.

ASTHMA THERAPIES AND OSTEOPOROSIS

Osteoporosis is a serious disorder characterized by thinning of the bones: the word means, literally, "porous bone." An estimated 28 million Americans have osteoporosis, which causes the bones to become fragile and to break more easily than normal. What is the connection with asthma? The steroid medications used to treat asthma (see Chapter 6), when taken in tablet form and distributed throughout the body, promote calcium loss from bones and the development of osteoporosis. To a lesser extent, the inhaled steroids, when taken in high doses and over a period of many years, can also contribute to the development of osteoporosis. Women are at particular risk. In general, osteoporosis occurs more commonly in women: approximately 80 percent of people with the disease are women.

Osteoporosis can affect bones all over the body, but fractures most often occur in the hips, spine, wrists, and ribs. Men and women can get osteoporosis at any age, but in women it usually begins around the time they reach menopause, when estrogen, which protects the bones from thinning, decreases significantly. Osteoporosis is a *silent* disease. Bone loss occurs gradually, without pain or any other symptoms—until a fracture occurs. In many cases, a fracture is the first sign of the disease; another indication is curvature of the spine in the upper back. Early detection and intervention can help you fight back against bone loss.

Because there are no symptoms to tell you whether you are at risk of fracture from osteoporosis, screening for this disease becomes critically important. If you have taken moderate to high doses of inhaled steroids for your asthma for a period of several years, or if you have taken oral steroids, such as prednisone, for flare-ups of your asthma more than once a year, we recommend that you have a full assessment of your osteoporosis risk, including a bone density scan (bone densitometry). This test is a quick, painless, noninvasive, low-dose X ray that shows whether or not your bones are thinning, and if so, to what degree. Talk with your doctor about getting a bone density scan. Once you have the study, initiation of treatment and further monitoring of your bone density over time may be indicated.

In addition to steroids, there are many known risk factors for the development of osteoporosis. These include, importantly, tobacco smoking and immobility. If you are currently smoking, the risk of osteoporosis is one more reason to quit.

Minimizing the possibility of osteoporosis is an important reason to step down, or gradually reduce (see Chapter 10), your inhaled steroid medication to the lowest dose necessary to control your asthma. We would emphasize, however, that it is not a reason for stopping inhaled steroids altogether. To reiterate: inhaled steroids improve your breathing capacity, reduce your asthma symptoms, reduce your need for "rescue" asthma medicines, lessen your chances of asthma flare-ups, and protect you from dangerous, potentially life-endangering attacks of asthma. They also reduce the chance that you will need oral steroids to control your asthma—and without doubt, steroids in tablet form are worse for your bones than inhaled steroids, where the effect is slight. So work with your doctor to find the lowest dose of inhaled steroids that you need, and work to minimize all your other risk factors for osteoporosis.

Maintaining your bone health involves adequate intake of calcium and vitamin D and regular weight-bearing exercise. Numerous medications are available to prevent significant bone loss while taking systemic steroids, and to restore bone mass once osteoporosis has been diagnosed.

CHAPTER 14

Asthma in the Elderly

While out walking on a fall day a few years ago, Marjorie, 68, found her-
self suddenly very short of breath. "I had no clue what it was," she says.
"I stopped and rested for a minute and got my breath back. I said to my-
self, 'I wonder what that was?'"

A month or so later, she got a cold that settled in her chest. "I began
having a hard time breathing and was coughing up a lot of phlegm," she
says, noting that these symptoms persisted for the duration of the cold.
When Marjorie visited a friend who has asthma, the friend recognized
her symptoms and suggested that Marjorie had asthma too.

"When my friend told me she thought I had asthma, I didn't take it
seriously," says Marjorie. "I wasn't familiar with what asthma really
was, and no one in my family ever had it. I am the youngest of five sisters
and always watched to see what they got. None of them ever got asthma,
so it never entered my mind that I would get such a thing. It was the
most remote thing that could happen to me."

Marjorie got better and forgot about asthma until she caught an-
other cold a few months later and wound up in the hospital. "I was
coughing terribly, and I couldn't believe how my breathing had become
so labored," she says. There, in the hospital emergency department, the
diagnosis of asthma was made.

Now under the care of a specialist, Marjorie needs her quick-acting
bronchodilator whenever she gets a cold, which predictably leads to
wheezing and coughing and shortness of breath. "I always take my al-
buterol with me when I leave the house," she says, "but when I have a
cold, it is never out of my sight. If you've ever had a scare, you keep it
close by." She also takes a controller medication and medicines for aller-
gies.

— MARJORIE, 68

IF YOU ARE IN YOUR SEVENTIES OR EIGHTIES and have been diagnosed with asthma in recent years, or if your elderly parent or grandparent was recently diagnosed, the news may have come as a surprise. Most people tend to think of asthma as a childhood disease, for good reason: most asthma is diagnosed by the age of 5, and many children "outgrow" their asthma around puberty. Nonetheless, adults of any age may develop asthma, although the new onset of asthma becomes increasingly rare the older we get. If you *are* an adult with asthma, you will likely take your asthma with you into old age.

Often there is no identifiable cause of adult-onset asthma. That being said, there are a few exceptions: some adults with no previous asthmatic symptoms develop asthma from exposure to substances in the workplace. Cigarette smoking is a risk factor for developing asthma in adulthood. Some older patients describe the onset of their asthmatic symptoms after a particularly nasty respiratory tract infection. Their chest cold went away but their asthmatic tendency persisted. Among postmenopausal women, hormone replacement therapy has been identified as a risk factor for new-onset asthma (see Chapter 13).

Since asthma develops late in life only rarely, most elderly people known to have asthma have had it for a long time. Studies indicate that as many as 10 percent of people over 65 have asthma, higher than the prevalence of asthma in childhood. It is easy for doctors to overlook a diagnosis of asthma in the elderly. Even doctors associate asthma with childhood more than with old age. In addition, asthma shares symptoms with other diseases that are common in old age—for example, emphysema, chronic bronchitis, and congestive heart failure. These diseases are more likely than asthma to develop late in life and may quite easily be mistaken for asthma. In considering an older person's complaint of shortness of breath with exertion, asthma may not be a diagnosis that quickly comes to mind. Also, older people with shortness of breath may think the cause is simply old age and assume that everyone at their age must experience breathing difficulties with exertion. Alternatively, they may be inclined to attribute their symptoms to bronchitis or another respiratory infection, assume it will go away, and decide not to consult their doctor.

DIAGNOSTIC CHALLENGES IN THE ELDERLY

If you ask a child what brings on his or her symptoms of asthma, exercising and allergen exposures (such as to the pet cat at home or the rabbit at school) often head the list. Many older people have given up demanding physical exercise, at least exercise that will cause them to breathe heavily, especially in cold air. And although allergies may be present at any age, in general the tendency to make allergic reactions declines with age. Fewer people at age 60 exhibit atopy (the tendency to make allergic reactions in the skin, nose, eyes, and bronchial tubes) than do children at age 6.

Still, we have diagnostic tools at our disposal to identify asthma in the elderly, if the diagnosis comes under consideration. Using a stethoscope, we will listen to the chest for the typical widespread musical wheezes of asthma—and to exclude findings such as a localized wheeze or crackling sounds in the lungs when a patient takes a deep breath that might suggest alternative diagnoses, such as a tumor of the lung or heart failure. Most helpful are breathing tests (see Chapter 2), which can usually be performed by people of virtually any age who remain mentally clear. Because breathing tests require the understanding and cooperation of the patient, people who suffer from a mental disorder such as dementia or psychosis may not be able to perform them. Much less often, people cannot perform the tests because of a physical disability, such as an injury to their chest that makes forceful breathing painful. Asthma is likely 1) if the air comes out more slowly than normal when you are asked to blow air rapidly and forcefully out of your lungs, and 2) if the air comes out significantly faster 10 to 15 minutes after you use a quick-acting bronchodilator. On occasion, these breathing test results can be seen in someone with chronic bronchitis, but they almost always signify asthma.

IS IT ASTHMA, EMPHYSEMA, OR BOTH?

A particular diagnostic challenge has to do with the possibility of confusion among asthma, emphysema, and chronic bronchitis. We have often been asked to evaluate older people with lung disease who come to us having been told, at various times, that they have asthma, emphysema, chronic bronchitis, and asthmatic bronchitis! Their confusion reflects ambiguity on the part of the medical profession, some of which is based in diagnostic uncertainty and overlap, and some in well-meaning biases about diagnostic labels.

Emphysema is the most feared among the *obstructive* lung disease, diseases that cause the emptying of air from the chest to slow. It conjures up images of desperate breathlessness, dependence on a wheelchair, and the need for a continuous supply of extra oxygen breathed through plastic tubes in the nostrils. With rare exceptions, emphysema is the result of long-term cigarette smoking. (A disease called alpha-1 antitrypsin deficiency can also cause emphysema in the absence of cigarette smoking.) Emphysema typically develops in one's fifties and sixties. It does not in fact cause narrowing of the bronchial tubes; rather, it is a destructive process that breaks down the elastic substances in the walls of the air sacs. When the lungs lose their elasticity, they are easily expanded (during inhalation) but have difficulty recoiling back to their resting size (during exhalation). Like a rubber band that has lost its stretchiness, the lungs can be pulled open without difficulty but have no spring to push the air back out.

Chronic bronchitis is a persistent inflammation of the bronchial tubes. It is different from acute bronchitis (a chest cold or a deep respiratory tract infection) in that it is present month after month and year after year, not for a week or two when one is sick with a "bug." Chronic bronchitis manifests as daily coughing with white or clear sputum production. Almost always, the cause of chronic bronchitis is cigarette smoking. Not surprisingly, after years of inhaling the smoke from burning tobacco leaves, the bronchial tubes become irritated and secrete extra mucus. The "smoker's cough" of chronic cigarette smokers is a manifestation of chronic bronchitis.

Because they share cigarette smoking as their common cause, both emphysema and chronic bronchitis often develop in the same person. It is difficult to separate out exactly to what extent emphysema or chronic bronchitis is causing a smoker's shortness of breath. As a result, physicians often use the term chronic obstructive pulmonary disease (or COPD) to describe the presence of one or the other or a combination of the two in the lungs of a long-term cigarette smoker.

COPD is the fourth leading cause of death among Americans, and it is likely to remain a common problem as long as cigarette smoking does. In 2002, for the first time, as many women as men died of COPD, a deadly consequence of the societal acceptance of women's cigarette smoking some 40 to 50 years ago.

Sometimes when people with COPD suffer a respiratory tract infection, they develop chest congestion and their airways become further narrowed by mucus. They may have wheezing that sounds indistinguishable from asthma, and their bronchial narrowing improves with some of the same medications that are used to treat asthma. They suffer recurrent asthma-like flare-ups and for this reason are sometimes said to have "chronic asthmatic bronchitis."

The easiest distinction between asthma and COPD in the elderly is that people with asthma should have normal or near-normal lung function (on their breathing tests) when they are well. People with COPD, even at their best, have permanent and irreversible lung damage that never goes away. In Chapter 1 we described asthma as "reversible airway narrowing"; COPD is considered *irreversible* obstructive lung disease (or diseases). However, the entire story is not that simple. As you may recall from the discussion of "airway remodeling" in Chapter 3, some people with asthma develop scarring around their bronchial tubes and permanent airway narrowing. It is our impression that this scarring develops most often when asthma has been undiagnosed or under-treated for many years. You can imagine that it might be difficult to distinguish asthma with permanent airway narrowing from COPD, especially if the person with asthma ever smoked cigarettes (or if the person with COPD ever had childhood allergies and wheezing before taking up cigarette smoking).

To further complicate the picture, for many years physicians tended to show a bias when applying diagnostic labels to people with obstructive lung disease. If you were a cigarette-smoking man who complained of coughing, sputum production, and shortness of breath, your doctor was likely to call your disease COPD, whereas if you were a cigarette-smoking woman with ex-actly the same symptoms, your doctor was more likely to diagnose asthma! This bias was probably a leftover from the days when smoking and smoking-related lung diseases were male problems. In our modern world, smoking and its medical consequences have become more clearly gender neutral.

MORE CAUSES OF WHEEZING IN THE ELDERLY

While COPD is at the top of the list of diseases not easily distinguished from asthma in the elderly, it is not alone. Another contender is congestive heart failure. When the heart muscle fails to pump efficiently (such as when it has sustained multiple heart attacks), fluid can build up in the lungs. As the fluid collects in the lungs, including around the bronchial tubes, it can cause cough-ing and shortness of breath and sometimes even wheezing. These symptoms can come and go, and they are often worse at night when the person is lying down. You can see how these symptoms might be mistaken for asthma. One cardiac center reported that as many as 20 percent of their patients with congestive heart failure had been started on bronchodilator treatments for asthma—which they turned out not to have—over the years prior to their re-ceiving a cardiac diagnosis.

In an older population, chest tumors are much more likely than they are in young people and are another possible cause of wheezing. The same is true of blood clots in the lungs. Elderly people are also more susceptible to problems with swallowing than younger people and are thus more likely to aspirate food into their bronchial tubes; this can cause wheezing, just as aspiration of a coin or peanut may cause wheezing in an infant or toddler. We recommend a chest X ray for every older person with the new onset of asthmalike symptoms, to help evaluate whether the coughing, wheezing, or shortness of breath is asthma or something else mimicking asthma.

MEDICINES THAT CAN MAKE ASTHMA WORSE

Older people are more likely to be on medicines for various chronic conditions. Some of these medicines can make asthma worse, in people of any age. In particular, people with asthma are uniquely sensitive to beta-blockers, medications used to treat a variety of illnesses, including heart disease, high blood pressure, migraine headaches, hyperthyroidism, cirrhosis, and tremors. Some beta-blockers have particularly strong effects on the bronchial tubes, causing constriction. These include propranolol (Inderal), nadolol (Corgard), timolol (Blocadren, Timoptic eyedrops), and sotalol (Betapace).

Other beta-blockers, called cardioselective or beta-1-selective beta-blockers, act mainly on the heart and have less of an effect on the lungs. Examples of cardioselective beta-blockers are metoprolol (Lopressor, Toprol), atenolol (Tenormin), bisoprolol (Zebeta), and betaxolol (Betoptic eyedrops). People with mild to moderate asthma can often safely take a cardioselective beta-blocker without triggering an asthma attack. However, some individuals with asthma appear to be uniquely sensitive to any kind of beta-blocker. For example, severe and even fatal asthma attacks have been described following the use of nonselective beta-blocker eyedrops, despite the minuscule amount of medication that is absorbed from the surface of the eye and carried in the bloodstream to the bronchial tubes. If you have asthma and need a beta-blocker for another serious medical condition, we encourage you to receive a test dose of the beta-blocker in your doctor's office, where your breathing can be closely monitored (for example, with a peak flow meter or spirometer) and any flare-up of your asthma promptly treated.

Asthma flare-ups can also be triggered by intravenous agents used in some cardiac stress tests to stimulate the heart. Sometimes used as part of a pharmacological stress test, adenosine (Adenoscan) and dipyridamole (Persantine) can trigger bronchospasm. If you require a cardiac evaluation of this sort, alternative methods are available. You need only take the precaution of reminding your doctor, or telling your cardiologist, that you have asthma.

THE EFFECT OF ASTHMA MEDICATIONS ON THE REST OF THE BODY

Just as some medications used for other conditions can make asthma worse, medications used to treat asthma can sometimes make various chronic medical conditions worse. Such chronic conditions are more likely to occur in older people. The quick-acting bronchodilators tend to have stimulatory side effects similar to those of adrenaline (see Chapter 5). Even though modern inhaled bronchodilators are designed for maximal effect on the bronchial tubes and minimal effect on the heart, occasionally people with certain heart diseases may be sensitive to even these minor effects of selective beta-agonist bronchodilators.

If you have very active angina (chest pains due to inadequate blood supply to the heart) or cardiac arrhythmias with rapid heartbeat, then even the minor cardiac stimulation from inhaled bronchodilators might aggravate your heart condition. No perfect alternative is available. You might try another type of bronchodilator, ipratropium (Atrovent). It is neither as strong nor as quick-acting as the beta-agonist bronchodilators (such as albuterol [Ventolin, Proventil]), but it has fewer stimulatory side effects on the heart. Or you might try the single-isomer form of albuterol, called levalbuterol (Xopenex), as discussed in Chapter 5. It too may cause slightly less cardiac stimulation than albuterol; however, at present it is only available as a solution for nebulization.

Because so little drug enters the bloodstream when medications are inhaled, drug interactions from inhaled bronchodilators or steroids are almost nonexistent. The bronchodilator theophylline (see Chapters 5 and 7) is different. It is taken in tablet or capsule form and has numerous interactions with other medications, including common antibiotics such as erythromycin and ciprofloxacin. If you take theophylline as part of your asthma treatment, it is good to be cautious about adding new medications. Check with your doctor or pharmacist about possible interactions that might cause the amount of theophylline in your bloodstream to increase or decrease.

One particular drug-drug interaction is relevant to some of the leukotriene-modifying drugs. Both zafirlukast (Accolate) and zileuton (Zyflo) affect the function of warfarin (Coumadin) such that the dose of warfarin should be reduced to maintain the same anticoagulant, or blood-thinning, effect.

INHALERS AND ARTHRITIS

Many older people (and some younger ones) have arthritis that affects their hands. Clever inhalational aids have been developed for this situation. Arthritis involving the thumbs and fingers can result in loss of motor strength in the hand, which precludes the usual method of depressing the metal canister located within the metered-dose inhalers. That makes it hard to actuate these devices. Alternative, plastic handgrip devices are available, designed on the principle of a simple lever. After the metered-dose inhaler is placed in one of these holders, a light handgrip motion is all that is needed to fire off the inhaler.

One of these devices, called Vent-Ease, fits all inhalers that are the shape and size of the albuterol metered-dose inhaler. Another device, called MDI Ease, accommodates the slightly shorter ipratropium (Atrovent) and combination albuterol-plus-ipratropium (Combivent) inhalers.

SIDE EFFECTS OF STEROIDS ON THE ELDERLY

Another treatment issue in the elderly has to do with the long-term harmful effects of steroids. Diabetes, high blood pressure, cataracts, glaucoma, osteoporosis, and easy bruising of the skin are all relatively common in older people who do not take steroids; their development is hastened by long-term (many months to years) use of oral steroids. In an older person requiring steroid tablets to control his or her asthma, we are especially eager to reduce the dose of steroids and whenever possible to stop them altogether. Because of concern about the absorption into the bloodstream of high doses of inhaled steroids (more than 1,000 micrograms a day), we work hard to minimize the dose of inhaled steroids as well.

Finally, we are particularly vigilant about steroid-induced side effects in the elderly, screening patients with eye exams, blood pressure monitoring, blood glucose testing, and bone density measurements (bone densitometry X rays). Where appropriate, we treat with protective medications, such as calcium, vitamin D, and bisphosphonates (for example, alendronate [Fosamax] or risedronate [Actonel]) to protect against osteoporosis.

CHAPTER 15

When Asthma Doesn't Get Better

As we have described in earlier chapters (see especially Chapters 3 and 10), the spectrum of asthma severity is wide. You may know of many people with asthma who have mild disease that requires only occasional use of a quick-acting bronchodilator for relief of infrequent symptoms. You may also know of other people with asthma who require one or more daily medicines to stay well and to stay free of asthma symptom. On occasion they are troubled by coughing or shortness of breath, such as during the allergy season, or when suffering from a respiratory tract infection (a "bad cold"). You, or your child, or someone in your family may have asthma that fits either of these descriptions. However, there may be a type of asthma that you haven't encountered: unusually severe, difficult-to-control asthma.

At one end of the range of asthma severity is a group of people disabled by their asthma. Nothing seems to help. They have tried multiple different medications. They have suffered multiple complications from their asthma medications, some simply unpleasant (like shakiness), others devastating (like a 40-pound weight gain, fractured bones, or diabetes). They continue to suffer coughing, wheezing, and shortness of breath. Climbing a flight of stairs is a huge effort, and sleeping through the night without disturbance due to coughing or chest heaviness seems a distant memory.

They are all too familiar with their local hospital and its emergency department. Unpredictable flare-ups of their asthma have landed them there many times. Perhaps on one of those occasions they turned blue (from low blood oxygen), passed out, or stopped breathing. They are alive today because their doctors and other health care providers restored their breathing with the help of a tube placed into their windpipe and the use of an attached breathing machine (mechanical ventilator). As you might imagine, many such people with difficult-to-control asthma become frightened, frustrated, confused, and sometimes overwhelmed by hopelessness.

Another group of patients have difficult asthma because of persistent narrowing of their breathing tubes, narrowing that is present even when they arc feeling generally well. Most people with asthma have normal or near-normal lung function when well. Unlike the cigarette-smoking-related lung diseases, emphysema and chronic bronchitis, asthma *usually* does not cause any permanent loss of breathing capacity. However, exceptions to this rule exist. Occasionally we see patients with asthma who, even when they are not in the midst of an asthma flare-up and when their lungs are free of wheezes or congestion, have reduced lung capacity, sometimes quite severely reduced. We spoke of this condition in Chapters 3, 8, and 14 as a kind of scarring of the bronchial tubes from long-standing, often inadequately treated asthma and called the phenomenon airway remodeling. People with this kind of permanent damage to their airways often have difficulties similar to someone with emphysema, despite never having smoked cigarettes.

At the Partners Asthma Center, we see many people with difficult-to-control asthma. They are referred to us because they have daily or nearly daily asthmatic symptoms. They often miss work, school, and social activities, and they have to limit their physical activities. Many need to take steroid tablets to control their asthma. After taking these tablets on a regular basis for months or even years, they now have two severe diseases: difficult-to-control asthma and the syndrome of steroid toxicity (called Cushing's syndrome, after the renowned surgeon Dr. Harvey Cushing at the Peter Bent Brigham Hospital in Boston). Long-term use of steroid tablets may have caused them one or more of the manifestations of steroid excess: weight gain, diabetes, high blood pressure, cataracts, glaucoma, skin bruising and stretch marks, thinning of the bones (osteoporosis), and muscle weakness—and this is an incomplete list of the potential complications. (For more on complications from steroid tablets, see Chapter 6.)

Our mission is to help restore people with difficult-to-control asthma to health and full functioning. We seek to accomplish this while reducing their dose of oral steroids and, if possible, stopping them altogether. The process requires a persistent, sustained effort on the part of the patient and the physician. It is often a team effort that requires the resources of other specialists, especially those concerned with the ears, nose, and throat (ENT physicians, also called otolaryngologists); the stomach and intestines (gastroenterologists); the heart (cardiologists); and the mind (psychiatrists and psychologists). We may call on the expertise of nutritionists, physical therapists, speech therapists, and social workers.

In this chapter we discuss our general approach to helping people with difficult-to-control asthma. We recognize that each patient with difficult-to-control asthma is somewhat different and that individualized detective work is often needed to determine why asthma in a particular person is so much more severe and resistant to treatment than it is in the vast majority of other people with asthma. Nonetheless, we believe strongly that this discussion is pertinent to virtually everyone with asthma. Our approach is the same as with everyone whom we see with asthma, just more intensive and comprehensive.

We employ a systematic approach that begins with ensuring that the diagnosis of asthma is correct. We explore with our patients the stimuli and aggravating conditions that may be fueling such severe asthmatic inflammation and twitchy airways, and then seek ways to reduce the stimuli. We work to optimize the medication program, minimize oral steroid use, and overcome barriers to good adherence to the treatment plan. We develop a plan of action in case asthmatic symptoms worsen—an asthma "action plan" (see Chapter 16). To a greater or lesser extent, all patients with asthma could benefit from such a systematic review of their care.

Diagnosed with asthma at age 5, Andrew, 40, can recall several hospitalizations for asthma when he was a young child. "I had severe attacks from age 5 to age 11," he says. "It's like a blur, but I can remember not being able to breathe and going to the hospital and being put in an oxygen tent. Then when I turned 11, boom, it just stopped. No more asthma attacks until I was 28."

Then he started having severe attacks every six weeks that kept him away from his job as a supervisor in the annuities department of a bank. Among Andrew's asthma triggers are pets, cigarette smoke, and perfume. "One time I had an attack from laughing too hard," he says. "I don't even know all the triggers. Sometimes I can go from one room to another and have an attack that quickly." Adds Andrew, "The main thing that makes me know it's coming is a hard, dry, persistent cough."

From about 1990 to 1993, Andrew was hospitalized nearly every month for asthma exacerbations. "If my family didn't hear from me, they would check the hospital," he says. In 1994 he went on permanent disability.

Since he has been under a specialist's care, Andrew has had just "minor flare-ups," he says. "No hospital admissions for four to five years, no emergency room. The key is taking your medications.

"I try not to let asthma limit me any more than I can help," says Andrew. One thing that he still cannot do, he notes, is walk upstairs without getting short of breath. "I don't know what it is about stairs, but they sap

the energy right out of you." On level ground he does much better, he says. "I don't run as much as I used to, but I try to play basketball and baseball with my sons. I ride my stationary bike three or four times a week, and I think it's helpful."

—ANDREW, 40

TAKING CONTROL OF DIFFICULT ASTHMA

If your asthma has felt out of control, there are many steps you can take to make it better. Through careful detective work, you may be able to identify asthma triggers at home or at work that have previously escaped your notice. You can review your medication plan with your doctor to be sure that you are taking the most effective medications for you at dosages that meet your needs. Your doctor can also help you discover whether another medical condition, or a medication you may be taking for another condition, could be making your asthma worse. It may also be worth exploring the possibility that you don't have asthma after all but another medical problem that causes wheezing, coughing, or shortness of breath, mimicking asthma. Finally, if your asthma remains stubborn despite your best attempts, you and your doctor may decide that you would benefit from consulting an asthma specialist.

ARE YOU AVOIDING EXPOSURE TO YOUR ASTHMA TRIGGERS?

You may find that a renewed effort to identify and then avoid environmental exposures will improve your severe asthma. Although you can't change your allergic tendencies, you can protect yourself from breathing in large amounts

Questions to Ask When Asthma Doesn't Get Better

- Is it something in the environment?
- Is it the way I am taking my medications?
- Is a medication I am taking for another condition making my asthma worse?
- Is another medical condition making my asthma worse?
- Is it possible that I don't have asthma after all but another medical condition with symptoms that mimic those of asthma?

of substances to which you are allergic. Similarly, you can limit your exposure to inhaled irritants such as cleaning chemicals, tobacco smoke, and air pollution, to cite only a few examples of substances that make people's asthma worse. Cigarette smoking and secondhand smoke exposure are particularly important—and avoidable—contributors to difficult asthma. Like the home, school and workplace are also good locations to search for the stimuli that may be aggravating your troublesome asthma. (We cover environmental stimuli of asthma—and tips for avoiding them—in more detail in Chapter 4.)

In some cities around the country, community asthma coalitions are helping people reduce their exposure to environmental triggers. For example, the Boston Urban Asthma Coalition is focusing its efforts on enhancing the quality of life for people with asthma by improving their living conditions within the inner city. This organization works with public officials to reduce common asthma triggers, such as cockroach debris, in public housing developments.

Community asthma coalitions like the one in Boston have sprung up in many cities in recent years in response to the increasing problem of asthma, especially in urban areas. These coalitions have different focuses but share the common goal of working with schools, health care clinics, housing officials, and other groups and individuals to increase awareness of asthma as a serious public health problem and to improve the quality of life of people with the disease. To find out if there is an asthma coalition near you, contact the National Heart, Lung, and Blood Institute's Web site (www.nhlbi.org). Such a coalition could be a valuable resource for helping you reduce your exposure to asthma triggers or assisting you with other asthma issues.

IS IT HOW YOU TAKE YOUR MEDICATIONS?

While avoiding the stimuli for asthmatic inflammation of the airways is an essential part of keeping your asthma under control, it is usually not sufficient by itself. A carefully developed—and carefully followed—medication plan is also needed. We often find that people who are referred to our asthma center with poorly controlled asthma are not taking the proper medications they need to control their asthma, or are not taking them in the prescribed fashion.

It is easy to see the origin of the problem. Because your asthma remains troublesome, your doctor adds another medication, and another, and another. After a time you are bewildered by the array of tablets, inhalers, and nebulizers. Some are meant to be taken once a day, some twice, some four times a day, some only if needed. Some of the medicines don't make you feel any better immediately after taking them; do you still need to take them? Others make you shaky, give you a hoarse voice, or disturb your sleep; how important is it that you continue them? One inhaler makes you cough each time you use it, so you doubt that any medicine gets into your lungs. Another inhaler has no taste or visible plume, so you can't tell whether any medicine is actually being released. No wonder you feel uncertain about your asthma treatments, or perhaps ready to toss out the whole lot.

With patients in these circumstances who are taking prednisone or methylprednisolone (Medrol) every day, we focus our efforts at reducing this medicine first, because of its attendant harmful effects. We then look at the medicines that we consider least effective (for example, cromolyn inhaled four times a day) or of insufficient benefit to justify their common side effects (for example, slow-release albuterol tablets). It may be possible to simplify the treatment program without reducing its effectiveness.

You need to identify the key elements of your program of preventive medicines: the controllers. For difficult asthma these usually include a potent inhaled steroid and a long-acting inhaled beta-agonist bronchodilator. You may also need to take a third controller medicine, a leukotriene blocker. The controllers may not give immediate relief when you use them: some do (the long-acting inhaled beta-agonists begin to work quickly); some don't (the inhaled steroids and leukotriene blockers are not expected to cause immediate improvement). Regardless, you need to take them every day, whether you feel well or ill. They are the core of your treatment program. Even when your asthma is not bothering you, take your controller medicines faithfully. Generally, these medicines will cause at most only minimally uncomfortable side effects. (For more on the inhaled steroids, see Chapter 6; for the other controllers, see Chapter 7.)

If you find that when using your inhaler you cough out the medicine each time you try to inhale it, tell your doctor. To overcome the problem, he or she may recommend the use of a spacer device (see page 81), a different type of inhaler (for example, a dry-powder inhaler or a metered-dose inhaler with a different propellant), or a nebulizer. If you doubt that you are actually getting medicine out of your dry-powder inhaler, cover the mouthpiece with a thin, colored cloth. Inhale medicine through the cloth, then examine it to see whether a thin layer of white powder is actually deposited there.

Probably most important of all, have your doctor or someone knowledgeable in the office review the proper use of your inhaler with you. Even if you have been taking medicine by inhaler for years, it can't hurt, and may help a great deal to check that you are using it properly. The most effective asthma medicine in the world won't help you if it gets no farther into your system than the back of your throat. Again and again we find that difficult asthma becomes well-controlled asthma when faulty inhaler technique is corrected. No one expects you to know intuitively how to juggle three balls in the air, and you shouldn't be expected to know how properly to use an inhaler device without (repeated) instruction. (For more on delivery devices and using them effectively, see Chapters 6 and 7.)

Some people tell us that they don't use the inhaled steroids or other controller medications prescribed for them because they are leery of taking daily medications, or because the only thing that stops their wheezing and coughing is their quick-relief inhaler. We remind them that their albuterol (or other quick-acting bronchodilator) puffer is for quick relief of symptoms only. It will not reduce the underlying airway inflammation that is always present in asthma. Relying on quick relief dooms you to continued difficulty with your asthma, to more symptoms, and to greater dependence on the quick reliever. Taking your preventive medicine every day is not only safe, it is smart. It helps bring your asthma under control so that you don't find yourself needing the quick reliever as often. It helps make your bronchial tubes less asthmatic.

DOES YOUR TREATMENT FIT YOUR LIFESTYLE?

If you are taking your controller medication or medications on a daily basis, a medication schedule that involves dosing four times a day will be hard to sustain. Many people who are on such a frequent dosing schedule forget to take many of their doses and may simply decide not to bother with them. (It can be especially hard to remember to take your medications when you are feeling well.) Fortunately, recent advances in asthma medications and in our understanding of how best to use them have greatly simplified most asthma treatment regimens. Most often your doctor will be able to prescribe a schedule of once- or twice-daily medication use. Here are some of the developments and guidelines that have led to more convenient dosing schedules:

- **Inhaled steroids twice a day.** All of the inhaled steroids are now FDA-approved for twice-daily dosing, instead of the former four times a day. Also, with the newer inhaled steroids, larger amounts of medication are available in a single puff, so fewer puffs are necessary.

- **Once-daily dosing.** In mild asthma some people who have gained good control with their inhaled steroid can, with their physician's guidance, switch from the usual twice-daily dosing to once a day (same total daily dose) without loss of benefit. This approach has gained FDA approval specifically for the inhaled steroid budesonide (Pulmicort), but the same will probably soon be the case with all of the inhaled steroids.

- **Combination medications.** As noted previously (see Chapters 7 and 10), it is now possible to take an inhaled steroid and a long-acting bronchodilator at the same time using a single dry-powder inhaler device. The medication Advair is a combination of the long-acting bronchodilator salmeterol (Serevent) and the inhaled steroid fluticasone (Flovent). Advair comes in three different strengths (reflecting three different concentrations of fluticasone in each inhalation) and is taken as one inhalation, two times daily. Advair is approved for adults and for children age 12 and up. Studies of its use in children age 4 to 11 are underway. Outside the United States, Advair is already used in younger children.

- **Once-a-day tablets.** Montelukast (Singulair), one of the leukotriene-blocking drugs (see Chapter 7), is an effective controller medication for some people; it is taken as a once-a-day tablet. For children as young as 2, a chewable tablet is available, offering a more appealing option than cromolyn, the former mainstay of long-term control medications for children, which requires inhaler or nebulizer treatments four times a day. A new form of montelukast (oral granules) has been approved for children 1 year and older.

- **Quick reliever as needed.** You may at one time have been advised to use your quick-reliever medication four times a day. While this was once our recommendation, we have learned from scientific research that using your quick reliever only when you need it to relieve your asthmatic symptoms, even if this is just once a week, is equally effective.

- **Injections for severe allergic asthma.** A new option for the treatment of severe allergic asthma is once- or twice-monthly injections of anti-IgE antibody, called omalizumab (Xolair). By removing the allergy protein, IgE, from the blood, omalizumab helps to reduce asthma symptoms, protect from asthma flare-ups, and in many cases permit the reduction of other asthma medications.

If you find your present medication schedule burdensome, you may want to consult with your physician about the possibility of reducing the number of times a day you take your asthma medications. At the same time, it is important to make sure that you are taking your controller medication at a sufficiently strong dose to keep your asthma under control.

COULD IT BE A MEDICATION YOU ARE TAKING FOR ANOTHER CONDITION?

It is not only your asthma medications and how you take them that can influence your asthma. Some medications that you take for other conditions can make your asthma worse.

Everyone with asthma should avoid the group of medicines called beta-blockers. These are used to treat heart disease, high blood pressure, glaucoma, and other common medical conditions. While beta-agonists—the class of medications your quick-reliever medication belongs to—open your bronchial tubes wider, beta-blockers will cause them to narrow and are known to exacerbate asthma. This caution pertains even to beta-blocker eyedrops used to treat glaucoma. Most often your doctor will have an alternative drug that he or she can choose. (See Chapter 14 for more on this subject.)

Sometimes it is particularly important that you take a beta-blocker, and no equally good substitute is available. One example would be a person with asthma who suffers a heart attack, in which case beta-blocker therapy is one of the best protections against future heart attacks. In this case, we would encourage you to take your first dose of beta-blocker, one that is selective for its effects on the heart and not the bronchial tubes, under direct medical supervision. Extreme caution is particularly important in people with difficult-to-control asthma.

Medications called ACE (for angiotensin converting enzyme) inhibitors, which lower blood pressure and take stress off the heart, don't appear to worsen asthma. However, in some people ACE inhibitors cause a persistent cough that can be mistaken for asthma.

You may be one of the 3 to 5 percent of people with so-called aspirin-sensitive asthma. If so, you should avoid aspirin and NSAIDs (nonsteroidal anti-inflammatory drugs), such as Advil, Motrin, Aleve, and many others that are commonly used for headaches and other pain. People with aspirin-sensitive asthma are likely to have severe asthma attacks within one to two hours of taking these medications. (For reasons we don't understand, aspirin sensitivity is rarely encountered in children.) The only way to know for sure if you are sensitive to aspirin and related medications is if you have a bad reaction after taking one of them. If you have avoided aspirin and NSAIDS as an adult (as many people have), you have two choices: continue to avoid these medications, or take a small dose in a safe place—your doctor's office—and have your breathing observed for three hours afterward. (See Chapter 11 for more on aspirin sensitivity and asthma.)

As a group, people with aspirin-sensitive asthma have more difficult-to-control asthma than people with asthma who are aspirin tolerant. A unique feature of people with aspirin-sensitive asthma is their tendency, as part of their asthmatic inflammation, to make excessive amounts of the inflammatory chemicals called leukotrienes. If you have aspirin-sensitive asthma, the leukotriene-blocking medications (see Chapters 7 and 11) may be particularly effective for you. These include montelukast (Singulair), zafirlukast (Accolate), and zileuton (Zyflo). This last, zileuton, has a unique mechanism of action and is sometimes effective even when the former two have not been. However, its manufacture will soon be stopped.

A WORD ON ADDICTIVE SUBSTANCES, LEGAL AND ILLEGAL

While it goes without saying that everyone, with and without asthma, should avoid illegal drugs for the sake of his or her health and well-being, certain street drugs are particularly bad for people with asthma. Those that are breathed in, such as crack cocaine and inhaled heroin, are especially dangerous. People with asthma who take these drugs often wind up in hospital emergency departments with severe asthma exacerbations. If you have a drug problem and asthma, making the decision to seek treatment for your addiction can keep you out of the emergency department with a dangerous asthma attack and can potentially save your life.

Perhaps no less addictive than street drugs and, in the long run, definitely just as bad for asthma, are cigarettes. We have emphasized elsewhere (see Chapters 4 and 13) the serious effects of both firsthand and secondhand smoke on asthma. If you are a smoker and your asthma is not under good control, stopping smoking may be the answer. If you want to quit, consider a smoking cessation program. Nicotine replacement in the form of skin patches, gum, nasal spray, or a cigarettelike inhalational device helps prevent nicotine withdrawal symptoms. The medication bupropion (Wellbutrin, Zyban) helps control the craving for cigarettes.

Compelling evidence about the beneficial effects of reducing exposure to secondhand smoke comes from a study on inner-city asthma: when parents of children with asthma stopped smoking at home, their children's asthma got better. The children's use of quick-reliever medications dropped 40 percent, and their lung function improved significantly. The children coughed and wheezed less and had more nights free of nighttime awakenings due to asthma and more days when they could participate in all their normal activities.

COULD ANOTHER MEDICAL CONDITION BE PREVENTING YOUR IMPROVEMENT?

If your asthma is not getting better despite appropriate medications and careful avoidance of your asthma triggers—including any medications or addictive substances that could make your asthma worse—the difficulty may be due to some other medical condition that can complicate asthma. For many people with asthma, sinus disease is just such a condition. Nasal congestion and sinus pressure can sometimes be almost as disabling as asthma itself, and active sinus disease is sometimes an important contributor to difficult-to-control asthma.

As you know if you are prone to sinus infections, blowing yellow or green mucus from the nose is a sign of sinus infection, as the mucus from the infected sinus drains through the nose. Sinusitis usually clears up with a course of antibiotics that kill the germs, and a nasal decongestant (spray or tablets) that reduces nasal swelling so the infected mucus can drain from the sinuses.

Sometimes a four-to-six-week course of antibiotics is needed to treat recurrent or lingering sinus infection. Occasionally, even prolonged medical treatment doesn't work, sometimes because of nasal polyps that block the nose and prevent mucus drainage from the sinuses. A CT scan of the sinuses can identify a persistent accumulation of mucus in the sinuses. Surgery may sometimes be necessary to remove the nasal polyps and to open larger drainage pathways from the sinuses. Inadequately treated allergic rhinitis is another common cause of recurrent sinusitis. If ongoing sinus problems are keeping your asthma from getting better, you may want to consult with an otolaryngologist, a physician who specializes in sinus disease.

Another common complicating factor in asthma is gastroesophageal reflux disease, commonly referred to as GERD (pronounced as one word) or simply as "reflux" for short. We sometimes see people with difficult asthma who turn out also to have gastroesophageal reflux, and once their reflux is under control, their asthma gets better too. In reflux, the muscle that forms a ring around the lower end of the esophagus, called the lower esophageal sphincter, fails to do its job of relaxing when food is passing down into the stomach and tightening to prevent food from regurgitating back up from the stomach into the esophagus. The sphincter muscle does not always contract with sufficient force to keep stomach contents in the stomach. Stomach juices can roll back up into the esophagus and sometimes into the throat.

Stomach juices contain hydrochloric acid and digestive enzymes. You can imagine that if stomach contents are inhaled (aspirated) into the airways, they can cause a lot of irritation and worsened asthma. Some physicians believe that just the presence of stomach acid in the esophagus can trigger a reflex via nerves in the chest that in turn leads to narrowing of the bronchial tubes and coughing.

If you have frequent heartburn and sometimes have a sour taste in your mouth, reflux may be the reason. Effective medications are available to treat reflux (see Chapter 13). Sometimes you can control it with lifestyle changes: modification of your diet (cutting down on caffeine, carbonated beverages, and spicy and fatty foods), avoiding late meals close to bedtime, and raising the head of your bed six inches or so (with a foam wedge under the mattress or with bricks or cinderblocks under the headboard).

Gastroesophageal reflux is very common in children. Almost every infant throws up or has wet burps from time to time. Most children outgrow their reflux, generally by the time they can stand or walk upright. Some children have both asthma and reflux. We recommend treating reflux in children when they have their sleep regularly disturbed by reflux, develop pneumonia from reflux, or do not gain weight well. The first treatment to try is simple: don't feed the child just before napping or sleeping. If that doesn't work, we prescribe medicines that reduce the acid production in the stomach.

Two other medical conditions that may complicate asthma—and that are as rare as sinusitis and gastroesophageal reflux are common—are Churg-Strauss syndrome and allergic bronchopulmonary aspergillosis. You will probably never have to concern yourself with either one of them, but they are worth knowing about, just in case.

Common and Rare Conditions That May Complicate Asthma

COMMON

- Allergic rhinitis (allergies of the nose)
- Sinusitis (inflammation or infection of the sinuses)
- Gastroesophageal reflux disease (GERD)

RARE

- Churg-Strauss syndrome
- Allergic bronchopulmonary aspergillosis

Churg-Strauss syndrome (see also Chapter 7) involves allergic inflammation in the blood vessels. As an inflammatory disease of blood vessels, a vasculitis, it can involve many different organs throughout the body, most commonly the lungs (as an allergic-type pneumonia as well as severe asthma), heart (causing heart failure), skin (rashes), and nerves (nerve weakness or tingling, called neuropathy). Recently, there has been a renewed interest in this extremely rare condition, because of its emergence in people with very severe asthma dependent on daily steroid tablets for control who have recently started montelukast (Singulair) or zafirlukast (Accolate) while their oral steroids were being reduced or discontinued. It is impossible to say whether these patients would have developed this allergic inflammation even in the absence of the leukotriene-blocking medication.

The extremely small risk of this unusual complication is estimated to be less than the chance of anaphylactic shock from penicillin. Nonetheless, in our own practice, when using montelukast (Singulair) or zafirlukast (Accolate) in people with severe asthma who are attempting to withdraw from daily prednisone, we monitor their symptoms and certain blood tests especially closely. Churg-Strauss syndrome is treated with oral corticosteroids, usually prednisone, and sometimes with an immunosuppressant drug, such as cyclophosphamide (Cytoxan).

Allergic bronchopulmonary aspergillosis is caused by a common fungus found in water and soil. We all breathe in spores from the aspergillus fungus, and for most of us these spores are harmless. However, in a very small percentage of people with asthma (less than 1 percent), aspergillus can grow along the surface of the bronchial tubes and cause a major allergic reaction. (On rare occasions, other types of fungus can cause a similar condition.) Coughing up thick plugs of heavy, discolored mucus is a sign of this condition. A chest X ray will reveal an inflammatory reaction to the presence of the fungus in the lungs, and a blood test will reveal very high levels of the allergy immunoglobulin, IgE (IgE is discussed in Chapters 1 and 8). The treatment for allergic bronchopulmonary aspergillosis is steroid tablets for the allergic response caused by the fungus, and now the newer, oral antifungal medications such as itraconazole (Sporanox) and voriconazole (Vfend) to kill the fungus.

Both Churg-Strauss syndrome and allergic bronchopulmonary aspergillosis warrant treatment by an asthma specialist. They are sufficiently rare that even your local allergist or pulmonologist may seek referral to a specialized asthma center for consultative advice.

COULD YOUR DIAGNOSIS OF ASTHMA BE WRONG?

You have done everything right. You have worked hard to identify your asthma triggers and to reduce or eliminate your exposure to them. You consistently take your asthma medications. You don't work in a setting where inhaled irritants are likely to cause your asthma to flare up. You don't have any of the complicating conditions described above. Yet you still have trouble with shortness of breath, coughing, and wheezing. Why? It may be time for you and your doctor to consider the possibility that you do not have asthma after all.

A number of other diseases and conditions that cause some combination of wheezing, coughing, and shortness of breath are sometimes mistaken for asthma.

EMPHYSEMA AND CHRONIC BRONCHITIS

Like asthma, emphysema and chronic bronchitis (referred to collectively as chronic obstructive pulmonary disease, or COPD) cause narrowing of the bronchial tubes that leads to wheezing, coughing, and shortness of breath (see also Chapters 2 and 14). In asthma the airway narrowing is usually reversible, while in emphysema and chronic bronchitis it is permanent. Asthma is often associated with allergy and typically begins early in childhood. Emphysema and chronic bronchitis are almost always the result of long-term cigarette smoking and become apparent in middle age or later. Despite these general rules, the distinction can sometimes be difficult. A person with asthma may also have smoked cigarettes for many years. Is he or she now developing COPD as well? A cigarette smoker may report having had hay fever and eczema as a child and now starts wheezing and coughing in middle age. Is this adult-onset asthma or emphysema?

If It's Not Asthma, What Might It Be?

- Emphysema and chronic bronchitis (chronic obstructive pulmonary disease)
- Heart failure
- Gastroesophageal reflux disease (GERD)
- Foreign body aspiration (when something goes down "the wrong pipe" and gets stuck in the airways)
- Cystic fibrosis
- Vocal cord dysfunction
- Congenital abnormalities of the windpipe or esophagus

FOREIGN BODY ASPIRATION

Foreign body aspiration is an alternative diagnosis that can mimic asthma in both adults and children. (See also Chapter 2.)

In one child seen at the Partners Asthma Center, the onset of asthmalike symptoms was coincident with the disappearance of a shoe belonging to her sister's Barbie doll. An X ray revealed an abnormality in the right lung. The shoe was found and then removed from the child's airway. An adult patient with persistent wheezing who came to us with suspected asthma turned out to have vegetable debris lodged in one of her major bronchial tubes. Once the vegetable matter was removed, the wheezing stopped (and our chest surgeon boasted that he had cured a case of "asthma"!).

VOCAL CORD DYSFUNCTION

Another unusual cause of asthmalike symptoms is vocal cord dysfunction, which is a "functional" abnormality of the upper respiratory tract, specifically of the vocal cords (with which you produce speech and song). It is called functional because it does not involve any structural abnormality or disease process of the vocal cords themselves. When people with this disorder breathe, their vocal cords come together, leaving only a narrow opening through which air can flow. This drawing together of the vocal cords (at a time when they should be held wide apart to allow easy passage of air) is the cause of their wheezing.

Vocal cord dysfunction is most often seen in the context of psychological stress or psychiatric illness. For example, in our pediatric population, we encounter adolescents with vocal cord dysfunction who are caught up in high-pressure athletic programs. Perhaps as a way out of an overly demanding situation, these young people unconsciously bring their vocal cords together, causing wheezes and perhaps an associated high-pitched cough that can be mistaken for asthma. People with both asthma and this functional upper airway wheezing pose especially difficult diagnostic dilemmas.

Your doctor may suspect the possibility of vocal cord dysfunction if he or she hears loud wheezes when listening with a stethoscope near the neck, but no wheezes or only very distant ones when listening over the chest. The diagnosis is most often confirmed when during a period of active upper airway wheezing an ear, nose, and throat specialist examines the vocal cords with an angled mirror or flexible tube inserted through the nose and into the back of the throat (a laryngoscope). Psychological counseling can be very helpful for people with vocal cord dysfunction, as can speech therapy exercises that promote proper coordination of muscle function in the upper airway.

CYSTIC FIBROSIS

Also possible to confuse with asthma is the genetic disease called cystic fibrosis, which affects about 30,000 children and adults in the United States. Children whose asthmalike respiratory symptoms are not improving even with good asthma treatment sometimes turn out not to have asthma but cystic fibrosis. We are particularly likely to consider this diagnosis if there is a family history of cystic fibrosis or if the child has some of the other common manifestations of the disease, such as nasal polyps or chronic diarrhea. In cystic fibrosis, the airways are filled with sticky mucus and become home to bacteria, usually in the first few years of life. Children develop a chronic cough and, because of associated involvement of the digestive system, frequently have difficulty gaining weight. The majority of people with cystic fibrosis are diagnosed by the time they are 2. In the Partners Asthma Center we occasionally diagnose someone over 40—most often someone with an unusually mild form of the disease that had previously been overlooked.

People with cystic fibrosis have abnormal concentrations of salt in their sweat. The "sweat test," which measures the salt content of sweat, is the traditional method of diagnosing cystic fibrosis. Nowadays a blood sample can be sent to specialty laboratories for direct genetic testing, which looks for the abnormal genes involved in causing the disease. No cure currently exists for cystic fibrosis, but antibiotics are used to treat respiratory infections, and physical therapy for the chest, as well as mucus-thinning drugs, can reduce the frequency of respiratory infections and improve lung function.

DEVELOPMENTAL ABNORMALITIES OF THE TRACHEA AND ESOPHAGUS

Finally, in very young children, developmental disorders of the trachea (windpipe) and esophagus are sometimes mistaken for asthma. In tracheomalacia, the trachea is soft and has a tendency to collapse. In bronchomalacia, the lower airways are similarly floppy and prone to collapse. If the trachea or bronchi narrow to a critical diameter, wheezing develops (particularly during exhalation) and it becomes hard to breathe, just as in asthma. In a related condition, tracheal stenosis, there is a localized pinched or narrowed area of the trachea, often just below the vocal cords. Infants with these conditions will have coughing and noisy breathing. These are congenital conditions (present at birth) that usually go away over time as the trachea and bronchial tubes naturally stiffen and widen with age. An adult can develop tracheal stenosis or tracheomalacia after a prolonged period of mechanical ventilation in an intensive care unit, generally after a breathing tube has been passed through a surgically created hole in the neck (a tracheostomy). The pressure caused by the tracheostomy tube where it seals along the inner wall of the trachea can weaken the wall of the trachea (tracheomalacia) or cause a tight band of scar tissue to form (tracheal stenosis).

Also in the category of rare developmental abnormalities are so-called vascular rings and slings, both of which involve blood vessels that may squeeze the trachea from the outside, causing narrowing. These blood vessels are normal in a fetus and usually go away before birth; the problem occurs when they do not go away and remain present after birth. Treatment usually involves surgical correction of the abnormal pattern of blood flow.

Last on our list of rare birth defects that are sometimes mistaken for asthma in very young children are tracheoesophageal fistulas. A fistula is a hole, and a tracheoesophageal fistula is a hole between the trachea and the esophagus. The trachea and the esophagus normally start out as a single structure and then separate during the course of normal fetal development. When development is not normal, a fistula—or even more rarely, a canal—may develop between them. Children born with these fistulas often cough, have difficulty swallowing, and may choke while eating or drinking. When they swallow food or liquids, some of the material can make its way from the swallowing tube (esophagus) into the windpipe (trachea) through this abnormal connection. They literally inhale the food. The consequence is coughing, inflamed and irritated airways, and recurrent respiratory infections. The association made between eating and coughing may raise suspicion of the diagnosis. Confirmatory tests include specialized X-ray studies (in which material visible on X ray is swallowed and followed down into the stomach or lungs) and direct visualization of the trachea and esophagus by endoscopy (which employs a tiny camera mounted on a flexible tube). The problem is resolved by surgical repair of the fistula.

WHEN TO SEE A SPECIALIST

If you are doing everything you know to be possible in terms of environmental control and medical treatment to manage your asthma and you are still not getting better, a specialist may be able to help you discover the reason and improve your asthma management.

If you decide to consult with a specialist on your own or your child's behalf, you may wonder whether an allergist or pulmonologist is best. Both allergists (allergy specialists) and pulmonologists (lung specialists) are trained as asthma specialists, so either is a good choice.

As we noted earlier (see Chapter 4), allergists are perhaps more expert in immunology and allergic diseases in addition to asthma, while pulmonologists have more specialized training in diseases of the chest and in the function of the lungs. If you are considering allergy shots, or immunotherapy, to try to reduce your allergic sensitivities, an allergist would be the appropriate specialist. (See Chapter 4 for more on this long-standing but still controversial treatment approach.) A pulmonologist is a particularly good choice if specialized pulmonary testing is needed or if other lung diseases are being considered. The criteria recommended by the National Asthma Education and Prevention Program for when to seek specialist consultation are listed below.

You may have the good fortune to live in an area where a group of physicians including allergists, pulmonologists, and other specialists work collaboratively in the care of patients who have, or may have, asthma. An asthma center will have consultants from various specialties whom they can call on, such as an otolaryngologist who is expert in sinus disease, a psychiatrist who is familiar with the emotional issues often involved in vocal cord dysfunction,

When to See an Asthma Specialist

It is recommended that you see a specialist if any of the following apply to your situation:

- Two or more emergency department visits for asthma exacerbations within the past six months.
- Daily oral steroid tablets or more than two courses of oral steroids for asthma exacerbations in the past six months.
- Severe persistent asthma (daily symptoms, frequent nighttime awakenings, limited physical activities, peak flow values less than 60 percent of your personal best, or highly variable peak flows).
- Life-threatening asthma flare-up within the past two years.
- Child under age 3, with moderate or severe persistent asthma.
- Special circumstances:
  1. Uncertain diagnosis; atypical signs or symptoms; complicating illnesses (for example, severe rhinitis and/or nasal polyps, gastroesophageal reflux, allergic bronchopulmonary aspergillosis, or vocal cord dysfunction).
  2. Need for specialized testing (for example, allergy skin testing, full lung function tests, provocation challenge, or bronchoscopy).
  3. Intensive education and counseling needed.
  4. Assessment for occupational or environmental asthma or food allergy.

and a gastroenterologist skilled in the management of severe gastroesophageal reflux disease. An asthma center will also offer the opportunity for specialized diagnostic testing, such as exercise and methacholine challenge tests when the diagnosis of asthma is uncertain (see Chapter 2).

These centers have nurse educators who can take the time to help you explore and identify possible asthma triggers and ways to reduce or eliminate them; they can also help you perfect your inhaler technique. Asthma centers also often offer asthma support groups, an opportunity you would not expect in a general medical practice.

If you have difficult-to-control asthma and are within easy traveling distance of such a center, you may want to consider receiving at least some of your asthma care there. Asthma centers such as these have reported their experience in managing difficult-to-control asthma, and the results are encouraging. A majority of patients who were initially dependent on daily steroid tablets to control their asthma were able to discontinue their use. Patients who had suffered near-fatal asthma attacks no longer had such life-endangering attacks. In most instances, difficult-to-control asthma became manageable asthma, through the intensive use of conventional medications and conventional treatment methods.

You may have heard of experimental medications used to treat particularly difficult asthma, especially "steroid-dependent" asthma. As in patients with rheumatoid arthritis, methotrexate, which suppresses the immune system, has been used in severe asthma as a potential alternative to daily steroid tablets. So has inhaled lidocaine (the topical anesthetic agent akin to Novocaine), the antibiotic troleandomycin, gold injections, and cyclosporin, the medicine used to prevent rejection of transplanted organs. Desperately severe illness sometimes prompts extreme therapeutic measures. We would only emphasize that these are still very much experimental treatments. Their value is unknown, and they are not without potential harm, sometimes quite serious. We suggest that treatment with these experimental agents be undertaken only by experienced physicians, and preferably in the context of a carefully designed research study. It is our belief that the great majority of people with difficult asthma can be successfully treated without resorting to these unproven therapies.

CHAPTER 16

Developing Your Asthma Action Plan

"You can live with asthma. You can do a lot of things. But you have to deal with your asthma straight up. You can't fool yourself. You can't play with it. You can't forget to take your medicines with you. It's your life. This is what is keeping you breathing. Even if you think you are not going to have an attack, you don't know that. Why take the chance? Keep the medicine with you, please."
—HAZEL, 56

ONE OF THE MAJOR REASONS for learning more about asthma—and thus one of the purposes of this book—is to help you manage your asthma effectively on a day-to-day basis. Another purpose, the focus of this chapter, is to help you make good decisions if and when you are having a flare-up of your asthma.

Preventing and managing asthma attacks are part of living with asthma. Even if you have only very mild asthma, you are not immune. Flare-ups of asthma, sometimes quite severe and frightening ones, can complicate the course of even mild asthma. People with more severe asthma are more vulnerable. Being scrupulous about taking your medications and avoiding your asthma triggers is good protection against asthma flare-ups, but it is not foolproof. It is best to be prepared with the information and skills you need to help yourself or your child if a breathing crisis occurs. It is best to have a plan.

"A team effort between you and your doctor is the way to keep your asthma under control. You have to formulate a game plan and stick to it. When you feel better, it's tempting to let the game plan go by the wayside, but that would be a mistake. You need to be faithful to your plan. My regular medications are Advair and Singulair. I add Pulmicort when I get a cold or feel uncomfortable in my chest. It's like insurance and usually gets me out of trouble. I also use my peak flow meter, and I know it

> *shouldn't get below 190 [liters per minute]. If I start using Pulmicort and don't get better, it's time to call and check with the doctor to see if it's time for prednisone."*
> — MARGARET, 60

If you find yourself having trouble breathing, and even gasping to catch your breath, the best thing you can do is not to panic, but to take calm action to restore your breathing to normal. You will be much more likely to remain calm if you have considered in advance what you would do in the event of an asthma attack. Based on what you have learned about asthma from the previous sections of this book, together with your own experiences, you are ready to plan a strategy, or Asthma Action Plan, for handling a mild, moderate, or severe asthma attack. It is important to discuss your plan of action with your doctor and then to write your Asthma Action Plan down and keep it someplace handy. (In the next chapter you will find some made-up examples of asthma attacks that provide opportunities to practice your decision making.)

Remember, though, that your Asthma Action Plan is meant to help you be prepared for an asthma attack; it is not meant to make you into your own doctor or to make you feel that you need to manage your care alone. You may have friends and family nearby. (It is a good idea to share your Asthma Action Plan with your family and friends so they will know how to help you.) Medical advice from your doctor or, after hours, from a covering doctor, is only a phone call away. We recommend that you discuss with your doctor what phone numbers to call and which health care provider you should expect to be able to reach after hours and on weekends. Don't hesitate to call if you have any doubt about what to do. Remember also that if nothing you do seems to be working, you can always get emergency help by dialing 911.

PREVENTING ASTHMA ATTACKS

A wise physician once said, "The best treatment of a severe asthma attack begins three days before it occurs." Here's an example of what he meant:

A patient recently came to see one of us for an urgent visit because of wheezing and shortness of breath. Her asthma had become quite severe in the previous few days. She was coughing incessantly. She had difficulty lying down at night because of coughing and chest congestion, and found it necessary to sit in a chair for most of the night. Her breathing had become so labored that walking to and from her car was difficult. She got some relief from her quick-acting bronchodilator (albuterol by metered-dose inhaler), but her symptoms recurred after only an hour or two. She found herself using her albuterol five to six times a day, and again once or twice overnight.

She had been doing well at a routine checkup six months earlier. She thought that maybe a recent trip to Chicago and exposure to cold winter air there had worsened her asthma. In addition, she felt as though she might be coming down with a cold. Of note, she had run out of her inhaled steroid medication two months earlier and had not renewed it. She had also stopped taking her preventive, long-acting inhaled bronchodilator because of muscle cramps that she felt it was causing.

In the office, her breathing appeared labored. Throughout both lungs she had loud wheezes audible with a stethoscope. Her peak flow, which had been 410 liters per minute at her last visit, was now only 180 liters per minute. She was in the midst of a severe asthma attack.

In this example, the best treatment of the asthma attack would have been, and could have been, prevention. Had the patient renewed her preventive inhaled steroid medication when she ran out two months earlier, the attack might never have happened—and if it did occur, it would probably have been milder. Stopping her preventive inhaled steroid medicine allowed her bronchial tubes to become inflamed and hypersensitive once again. Triggers of bronchial muscle constriction, like the cold winter air in Chicago, would not have bothered her asthma nearly as much had she continued to keep this airway inflammation in check with her steroid inhaler. It is likely that her bronchial tubes had become progressively more "twitchy" over the two months since she ran out of her medicine and didn't renew it. Her breathing may have become slowly and subtly worse. Cold air exposure, and possibly a viral respiratory tract infection, then tipped her over the edge.

In addition, it is likely that she could have seen this attack coming. Perhaps she might have noted some early warning signs:

- Starting to waken from her sleep on occasion with coughing and chest tightness (whereas she had previously slept the night through)

- Starting to need her albuterol inhaler once or twice during the day (whereas before she had not needed it for weeks at a time)

- Starting to feel her breathing more labored at the top of a flight of stairs (whereas during the summer she could climb up and down stairs repeatedly without thinking about it)

Even better, she could have checked her peak flow with a portable peak flow meter (see Chapters 2 and 3 for details about peak flow monitoring). After stopping her steroid inhaler, she would have noticed a gradual decline in her peak flow numbers. Instead of her usual 400 to 410 liters per minute, she would have found a gradual downward trend. Starting approximately two weeks after stopping the preventive steroid medication, she might have noted that her peak flow values were more often 300 to 350 liters per minute. Perhaps she would have found that the numbers started to fluctuate more than usual: 280 liters per minute after first awakening, 380 liters per minute late in the afternoon, 250 liters per minute if she woke in the middle of the night, and 370 liters per minute after using her albuterol inhaler at night. This sort of variability in peak flow numbers is a warning sign of poor asthma control.

The point here is that had she been able to recognize signs of worsening asthma control, she would have been able to act to get things back under control *before* her asthma deteriorated into a full-fledged attack. The seeds of this flare-up had been planted weeks earlier; it did not burst forth as suddenly and unexpectedly as it seemed. The best treatment of this asthma attack would indeed have been prevention: in this case, restarting the preventive steroid inhaler and addressing the muscle cramps caused by the long-acting inhaled bronchodilator. If the solution to getting your worsening asthma back under control does not strike you as being as obvious as in this case, ask for help in problem solving. Contact your doctor . . . *before* an asthma attack necessitates urgent attention.

RECOGNIZING AN ASTHMA ATTACK AND JUDGING ITS SEVERITY

Still, not all asthma attacks are preventable. Viral respiratory tract infections that settle into the chest ("bad chest colds") can trigger severe asthma attacks. Intense allergic exposures can occur unexpectedly, such as to the in-laws' cat or to outdoor mold spores on a windy autumn day. In this chapter we address how you should manage an asthma flare-up once it has occurred. How best to deal with an asthma attack depends in large part on how severe the attack is. Your first task in managing an asthma attack is assessing how severe it is—just how sick are you? Of utmost importance is that you do not *underestimate* a severe attack. The greatest mistake that you can make is to minimize your symptoms and dismiss their importance even though your breathing is quite limited and you are truly in danger.

Sometimes you can easily recognize a severe attack based on how you feel. You know you are having a severe attack if you become short of breath even when walking slowly on level ground, if when speaking you have to interrupt yourself to catch your breath, and if you are perspiring and cannot lie down because of difficulty breathing.

When the symptoms of an asthma attack are not so overwhelming, it can be tempting to minimize them—to attribute them to a cold or an allergy and convince yourself that you will be better in the morning and that there is no need to "bother" the doctor. This sort of denial can lead to trouble, causing some people to delay taking the necessary steps to bring their breathing under control, and to wind up in the hospital emergency department with dangerous breathing problems. However, even if you are very attentive to your symptoms, you can easily misjudge the severity of an asthma attack. It is possible to have severe narrowing of your breathing tubes but be unable to detect it based on how you feel. If you are only somewhat short of breath, you might naturally conclude that your asthma attack is mild, when in fact the underlying airway narrowing may be considerable, and if it gets even a little bit worse, you may soon be gasping for air. (Studies have shown that it is not uncommon for physicians as well as patients to misjudge the severity of an asthma attack based on symptoms alone, either overestimating or underestimating the severity.)

Fortunately, symptoms are not the only measure of the severity of an asthma attack. Your home peak flow meter can tell you how well or poorly your lungs are functioning and can provide you with important information and guidance in the event of an asthma attack. Think of your peak flow meter like a thermometer. You may not check your temperature every day, but at the onset of a bad infection it is good to make a measurement. You know that you feel warm, but is your temperature 99 or 104 degrees Fahrenheit? It is hard to tell with the back of your hand applied to your forehead; it is easy to measure with a thermometer.

So too with your peak flow meter: it takes just a few seconds to measure exactly how narrowed your breathing passages have become. It is useful both to you and to any health care provider with whom you communicate about your asthma if you can indicate exactly what your peak flow value is and how that number compares with your usual or best value. In general, your asthma attack is mild if the value that you measure with your peak flow meter is greater than 80 percent of your normal value. It is moderate if the value is 50 to 80 percent of normal, and it is severe if your peak flow is half or less of its normal value.

Infants and young children will not be able to make peak flow measurements or to tell you just how short of breath they feel. You will need to use other signs to assess the severity of their asthma flare-ups. As we discussed in

Your Peak Flow Zones

Your peak flow zones are based on your personal best peak flow* number. The zones will help you assess your asthma and take the right actions to keep it controlled. The colors used with each zone come from traffic lights.

Green zone (80 to 100 percent of your personal best) signals a mild asthma attack. Use your quick-acting bronchodilator for relief of your asthma symptoms. Take your usual daily long-term control medicines, if you take any.

Yellow zone (50 to 80 percent of your personal best) signals caution—you are having a moderate asthma attack. Besides taking your quick-relief bronchodilator, you will probably need to increase your other asthma medicines as directed by your doctor or as written in your Asthma Action Plan.

Red zone (below 50 percent of your personal best) signals medical alert! Besides taking your quick-relief bronchodilator and increasing your preventive medicines, you should contact your doctor now. You may need to begin oral steroid tablets. Keep monitoring your peak flow until there is improvement or until you are in a safe place (doctor's office or urgent care setting).

*Your *personal best peak flow* is the peak flow that you have been able to achieve when you are feeling well and your asthma is at its best. You can prepare to manage an asthma attack by finding out what your personal best peak flow is. Check your breathing with a peak flow meter on several days when you are feeling perfectly well and write the number down somewhere where you can easily find it again.

FROM: NATIONAL INSTITUTES OF HEALTH ASTHMA ACTION PLAN

Chapters 3, 10, and 12, you should look for the following signs of a *severe* asthma attack:

- very rapid breathing rate (especially if more than 60 breaths per minute)

- bluish discoloration of the lips or fingers (cyanosis)

- retraction of the skin at the top of the breastbone with every breath in

- able to talk only in single words

- need to sit upright to breathe

- agitated behavior

- infants stop feeding

USING YOUR MEDICINES TO RELIEVE YOUR ASTHMA ATTACK

The first steps to relieve an asthma attack of any severity are to get away from the triggers, such as furry animals, cigarette smoke, or strong fumes, that may be causing the attack and to use your quick-acting bronchodilator. The usual bronchodilator dose is two puffs, breathed slowly and deeply one at a time. In a sudden, severe crisis of breathing, you can safely use as many as four puffs spaced just a few seconds apart.

Although under normal circumstances we usually recommend that you use your quick-relief bronchodilator no more than four times a day, a flare-up of asthma changes the rules. To treat an asthma flare-up, you can safely use your bronchodilator as often as every 20 minutes for up to two hours, if needed. If you have a nebulizer at home for administering your inhaled bronchodilator as a wet aerosol or mist, you can use it with the same frequency. Increasing your bronchodilator dose may increase the jitteriness and racing heart that many people experience when taking these medications, but these side effects are not considered dangerous and are worth putting up with under the circumstances. Two cautions: do not use more theophylline than usual—doing so could cause severe toxic reactions—and do not use your long-acting bronchodilator (salmeterol or formoterol) more than once in the morning and once at night.

As you know, the quick-relief bronchodilators treat only part of an asthma attack, the part due to constriction of the muscles surrounding the bronchial tubes. The other part, the swelling of the walls of the bronchial tubes and the overproduction of mucus, requires the anti-inflammatory steroids.

If your asthma attack is relatively mild and is getting better with your quick-relief bronchodilator, you can take steroid medication by inhalation. If you use an inhaled steroid every day as your controller medicine, double your daily dose (take twice as many puffs as usual) for as many days as needed until you are back to normal. If you don't use a steroid inhaler year-round but have one at home for use when your asthma acts up during the pollen season or in emergencies, now is the time to break it out and use it. As long as your asthma attack remains under control—that is, as long as you are getting relief from your symptoms and your peak flow is improving—this is a sound strategy. Often the improvement will be gradual, and until the steroid medication takes effect, usually after a day or two, you should continue to use your bronchodilator regularly (approximately every four to six hours).

For more severe attacks, or for attacks when your breathing and your peak flow get progressively worse instead of better, you'll need to take a short course of oral steroids (tablets or liquid). The definition of *short* in "a short course of oral steroids" will vary from practitioner to practitioner and from one asthma attack to another, depending on its severity and response to treatment. We will have more to say on the subject in a moment, but in general we are talking about somewhere between 4 and 21 days of treatment with oral steroids. If you already take oral steroids on a regular basis, the dose will need to be increased. If you have had a short course of oral steroids in the past, your physician may have provided you with a prescription for prednisone (Deltasone), prednisolone (Prelone, Pediapred), or methylprednisolone (Medrol) to have at home for use in an asthma crisis. If not, you'll need to call your doctor and ask for a prescription. In either case, be sure to keep your doctor informed if you are having serious breathing difficulty.

Some people are reluctant to take oral steroids for fear of side effects. The side effects we worry about—such as osteoporosis, glaucoma, and thinning of the skin—are of concern only when oral steroids are taken at high doses over several weeks to months. The side effects that may occur with a short course—increased energy and appetite, stomach upset, fluid retention, insomnia, nervousness, and mood swings—are in general not dangerous and go away when you stop taking the medication. Two exceptions are worth mentioning. If you have diabetes, oral steroids can drive up your blood sugar dramatically. It is important that you monitor your blood sugar closely while on oral steroids and adjust your diabetic medicines appropriately to prevent dangerously high blood sugar levels.

The second complication of even a short course of oral steroids is very rare: aseptic necrosis, or injury to the long bones, such as the thighbone (femur) or upper arm bone (humerus). Aseptic necrosis means death of bone tissue caused not by infection but by lack of blood flow (it's also called avascular necrosis). It can cause hip or shoulder pain and permanent injury. Fortunately, it is exceedingly rare.

In general, the side effects of a short course of oral steroids, *if* you experience them, are unpleasant but tolerable. Oral steroids are used to treat severe asthma attacks, and in that context maintaining your breathing should become your absolute priority. As we tell our patients, half jokingly, "Breathing is important!" When only steroids taken systemically will restore your breathing capacity, you need to take the medicine and deal with side effects if they occur. You can minimize stomach upset by taking steroid tablets with food or with over-the-counter acid blockers such as famotidine (Pepcid), ranitidine (Zantac), or cimetidine (Tagamet). You can reduce swelling and bloating by keep-

Guidelines for Managing an Asthma Attack at Home

- Use your peak flow meter to assess the severity of the asthma attack.
- Take two puffs of your **quick-relief bronchodilator.** You can safely use your bronchodilator as often as every 20 minutes for up to two hours, if needed.
- In the event of a mild-to-moderate asthma attack that is improving with your quick-relief bronchodilator, double your daily dose of **steroid inhaler** (take twice as many puffs as usual) for as many days as needed until you are back to normal. If you do not usually take inhaled steroids but have them on hand in case of an asthma attack, take them as directed by your doctor.
- A more severe asthma attack requires **oral steroids** (prednisone [Deltasone], prednisolone [Prelone], or methylprednisolone [Medrol]). If you have steroid tablets at home in case of a severe asthma attack, take them according to your doctor's instructions. Otherwise, call your doctor's office and arrange to have a prescription called to your pharmacy.
- In the event of a severe asthma attack that does not improve with home measures, seek help. Go to a nearby hospital emergency department or acute care facility.

ing your salt intake down. And you can try various approaches to combat insomnia—a sedating antihistamine (such as in over-the-counter Benadryl) or a sleeping pill prescribed by your doctor. (For more on oral steroids and their side effects, see Chapter 6.)

When you are having a severe asthma attack, promptly starting oral steroids may be your best approach to staying out of your local urgent care center, emergency department, or hospital intensive care unit. There you will surely be given systemic steroids in very high doses. If you need oral steroids, better to take them and get well rather than delay, put your self (or child) at risk, and then receive them in larger doses on an emergency basis. Beginning oral steroids immediately is often the most effective means of avoiding getting worse and needing to be hospitalized for your asthma. Don't put it off.

WHAT IS A "SHORT COURSE OF ORAL STEROIDS"?

Physicians who do not specialize in asthma often ask us what is the best dosing schedule for a course of oral steroids. The answer is that there are a variety of ways to prescribe oral steroids, and no single one is best for every individual, or even for every asthma attack in the same individual. A common approach in adults, and the one we often use for severe exacerbations, is to prescribe prednisone for approximately two weeks, gradually reducing the dosage every four days: 40 milligrams a day for the first four days, then 30 milligrams a day for four days, then 20 milligrams a day for four days, and finally 10 milligrams a day for the last four days. In children weighing less than approximately 90 pounds, the dose of oral steroids is adjusted for weight. A typical dose is 1 milligram for every kilogram of weight (which works out to approximately one-half milligram for every pound of weight). Very severe attacks are treated with 2 milligrams per kilogram (approximately 1 milligram per pound), up to a maximum of 60 milligrams a day.

There is no "right" schedule for taking oral steroids. No particular schedule has been proved preferable to another. In the absence of clear-cut advantages of one regimen over another, many different approaches are used by different physicians. For example, we recommend that the full daily dose of oral steroids be taken all at once, usually in the morning. Other physicians recommend divided doses, taking half of the total amount in the morning and the other half at night.

You may have heard of a "steroid taper"—a gradual reduction of the steroid dose over one to two weeks. One pharmaceutical company sells a prepackaged six-day tapering course of the steroid drug methylprednisolone (Medrol). It is clearly laid out in the package: the first day you take six of the 4-milligram Medrol tablets, the second day you take five of these tablets, the third day you take four, and so on. Although commonly practiced, a steroid taper is not necessary. Some physicians prefer a steady regimen of 40 or 60 milligrams a day for four or more days, then stopping without a taper.

One rationale for a taper is to ensure that asthma does not flare up again as the dose of oral steroids is reduced. As long as the triggering stimulus is no longer present and a suitable program of controller medications is begun, a recurrent flare-up is unlikely. Another rationale is that side effects may be fewer when the dose of oral steroids is gradually reduced rather than abruptly stopped, but this is an unproved assumption.

Probably the most logical schedule is one in which you follow your improvement with daily peak flow measurements. Once your peak flow is back to your usual (back to your personal best or close to it), you can stop (or cut back over a day or two) the steroid tablets or liquid, *as long as you continue on regular inhaled steroids to prevent a recurrence of the attack*. You can then continue to monitor your peak flow to ensure that the improvement in your breathing achieved with the oral steroids is maintained in the days and weeks after stopping them.

Developing Your Asthma Action Plan

In the previous section we outlined in broad, general terms how you might intensify your asthma treatments to recover from an asthma attack. The general message is this: *recognize* that your (or your child's) breathing symptoms (coughing, shortness of breath, wheezing, chest tightness) may be due to an asthma attack, *assess* how severe the attack is, and *act* to restore your breathing to normal. The actions you take will depend on the medicines you usually take for your asthma, the additional medicines and equipment you have available at home, and your self-confidence in making good judgments about adjusting your treatments before speaking with your physician.

Find the time when you are not acutely ill to sit with your physician and discuss how you should respond to an asthma attack. What should you do first in the event of a mild or moderate asthma attack? What should you do if you do not get better after taking these actions? What should you do in the event of a severe asthma attack, and what if there is no improvement after you do these things?

We hope that you are like a good airplane pilot. We hope that you are never faced with a crash landing but that you are fully prepared to deal with one if it were to occur. We encourage you and your doctor to think about what actions you can take before calling to get help, and when you should rush to the emergency department without waiting for telephone advice. Best of all, write your plan down. In time of crisis, it's better to have a written Asthma Action Plan to which you can refer than to try to recall the details of a conversation you had with your doctor months earlier.

Many different forms are available for written asthma action plans. One is the Partners Asthma Center action plan card. It is printed on two sides of one thick sheet of paper and has creases so it folds to the size of a credit card, for easy placement in your wallet. Another was prepared specifically for children by a collaborative organization called the Massachusetts Health Quality Partners (www.mhqp.org). It uses the model of green, yellow, and red zones for categorizing asthmatic symptoms, as discussed above. It is 8½ by 11 inches in size, for posting on a bulletin board or refrigerator door. Other examples of action plan records are available through the National Asthma Education and Prevention Program (www.nhlbi.nih.gov/guidelines/asthma/asthgdln.htm).

We cannot say exactly how your particular Asthma Action Plan might look. We offer a couple of models here not to recommend them to you—they may or may not be applicable to your particular circumstances—but to try to give examples of what might otherwise seem like a vague concept. The specific actions chosen for these plans are far less important than the fact of your having

PARTNERS
ASTHMA CENTER

My Asthma Action Plan

Name: _____

My Physicians' Names:

Primary: Dr. _____

Asthma: Dr. _____

My Asthma Medications: _____

_____

_____

_____

_____

My Other Medications: _____

_____

_____

_____

_____

_____

Medication Allergies: _____

_____

_____

_____

_____

Peak Flow Values

My BEST PEAK FLOW is _____ liters/minute.

When my peak flow is less than _____ liters/minute (less than half of my best value), I am having a severe attack.

A: In the event of a **MILD OR MODERATE** asthmatic attack I would first:_____

_____

_____

_____

If there is no improvement, my next step would be to: _____

_____

_____

B: In the event of a **SEVERE** asthmatic attack, I would first: _____

_____

_____

_____

_____

_____

If there is no improvement, my next step would be to: _____

_____

_____

_____

If there is still no improvement,

SEEK EMERGENCY HELP IMMEDIATELY

EMERGENCY PHONE NUMBERS

My Asthma Doctor:_____

(ask to page your asthma doctor or the covering fellow)

Ambulance: _____ or 911

Example #1: The plan on the following page might be appropriate for an adult who has mild persistent asthma for which she uses as her controller medicine an inhaled steroid (for example, fluticasone [Flovent] 44 micrograms per puff, two puffs twice daily). She has an albuterol metered-dose inhaler for quick relief, used as needed. The plan is organized according to the layout of the Partners Asthma Center action plan card.

271

PARTNERS
ASTHMA CENTER

My Asthma Action Plan

Name: *John Smith*

My Physicians' Names:
Primary: Dr. *Jane Doe*
Asthma: Dr. *Henry Hill*

My Asthma Medications: *Flovent, 2 puffs morning and night. albuterol, 2 puffs up to 4 times a day, as needed*

My Other Medications: *None*

Medication Allergies: *None*

Peak Flow Values

My BEST PEAK FLOW is **440** liters/minute.
When my peak flow is less than **220** liters/minute (less than half of my best value), I am having a severe attack.

A: In the event of a MILD OR MODERATE asthmatic attack I would first: *Use my albuterol inhaler, 2-4 puffs as one treatment, up to a treatment every hour.*

If there is no improvement, *within 2 hours* my next step would be to: *Increase my steroid inhaler (fluticasone [Flovent]) to 4 puffs morning and night.*

B: In the event of a SEVERE asthmatic attack, I would first: *Use my albuterol inhaler, 2-4 puffs as one treatment, up to a treatment every 20 minutes for 2 hours; and increase my steroid (fluticasone [Flovent]) inhaler to 4 puffs morning and night.*

If there is no improvement, *within 2 hours* my next step would be to: *Take prednisone 40 mg (regardless of the time of day) and notify my doctor that I have begun a course of oral steroids.*

If there is still no improvement,
SEEK EMERGENCY HELP IMMEDIATELY
EMERGENCY PHONE NUMBERS
My Asthma Doctor: **555-9876**
(ask to page your asthma doctor or the covering fellow)
Ambulance: **555-1234** _____ or 911

a plan that you and your doctor have agreed on. You can always modify the details of the plan at some future date, as your asthma changes or as new medicines become available. Most important is that you have a clear-cut, organized plan for how to deal with an asthma attack.

Massachusetts Asthma Action Plan

Name:	Date:

Birth Date:	Doctor/Nurse Name	Doctor/Nurse Phone #

Patient Goal:	Parent/Guardian Name & Phone

Important! Avoid things that make your asthma worse:

The colors of a traffic light will help you use your asthma medicine.

Green means **Go Zone!** Use controller medicine.

Yellow means **Caution Zone!** Add quick-relief medicine.

Red means **Danger Zone!** Get help from a doctor.

Personal Best Peak Flow: _____

GO — You're Doing Well! ➡ Use these daily controller medicines:

You have _all_ of these:

- Breathing is good
- No cough or wheeze
- Sleep through the night
- Can go to school and play

Peak flow from _____ to _____

MEDICINE/ROUTE	HOW MUCH	HOW OFTEN/WHEN

CAUTION — Slow Down! ➡ Continue with green zone medicine and add:

You have _any_ of these:

- First signs of a cold
- Cough
- Mild wheeze
- Tight chest
- Coughing, wheezing, or trouble breathing at night

Peak flow from _____ to _____

MEDICINE/ROUTE	HOW MUCH	HOW OFTEN/WHEN

CALL YOUR DOCTOR/NURSE: _____

DANGER — Get help! ➡ Take these medicines and call your doctor now:

Your asthma is getting worse fast:

- Medicine is not helping
- Breathing is hard and fast
- Nose opens wide
- Ribs show
- Can't talk well

Peak flow from _____ to _____

MEDICINE/ROUTE	HOW MUCH	HOW OFTEN/WHEN

GET HELP FROM A DOCTOR NOW! Do not be afraid of causing a fuss. Your doctor will want to see you right away. It's important! If you cannot contact your doctor go directly to the emergency room and bring this form with you. **DO NOT WAIT.**

Make an appointment with your doctor/nurse within two days of an ER visit or hospitalization.

Doctor/NP/PA Signature: _____ Date: _____

I give permission to the school nurse, my child's doctor/NP/PA, or _____ to share information about my child's asthma.

Parent/Guardian Signature: _____ Date: _____

ADAPTED FROM NIH PUBLICATION (7/20/00)

Special Considerations

You may wonder whether you should buy a nebulizer system to use in the event of an asthma attack. Nebulizers (see also Chapters 5 and 12) are commonly used in many emergency departments to administer quick-acting bronchodilators for treatment of asthma flare-ups. A liquid form of the medicine, such as albuterol or levalbuterol (Xopenex), is put into the nebulizer cup and a continuous mist is generated. You (or your child) are asked simply to breathe in and out, continuously inhaling the medication-containing mist. A full treatment takes approximately ten minutes. Various names for these nebulizer treatments include "updraft" treatment, handheld nebulizer, and continuous-flow nebulizer.

You can obtain the same equipment for use at home. In the home system, the nebulizer is driven by compressed air. The compressor runs on electricity and is about the size of a small toaster. Compressor and nebulizer systems can be rented from respiratory home-care companies or purchased at many pharmacies (or Web sites) for $100–$120. Battery-operated systems (to bring, say, on a camping trip) and systems that can be run from your automobile's battery are also available but are considerably more expensive.

People with difficult-to-control asthma and frequent severe asthma attacks may choose to have a nebulizer system at home rather than rely on urgent trips to the doctor's office or emergency department. Anyone who has ever had a very severe, potentially life-threatening asthma attack should probably have a nebulizer system at home to use while awaiting additional emergency care. This is the same system many parents rely on to administer asthma medicines to their young children. No method for delivering inhaled bronchodilators is more powerful or reliable.

However, as we noted in Chapter 5, it turns out that other methods are just

Example #2: The example on the following page might pertain to a 10-year-old boy, four feet two inches tall, with mild persistent asthma. He takes the leukotriene blocker montelukast (Singulair) once daily and carries as his quick-acting bronchodilator pirbuterol (Maxair). His doctor and his parents have worked out a plan for managing his asthma attacks. Available at home for use when his asthma worsens are a dry-powder steroid inhaler (Pulmicort Turbuhaler) and a liquid form of the systemic steroid prednisolone (Prelone), containing in this particular formulation 15 mg of prednisolone in each teaspoonful of syrup. This plan is organized to match the layout of the Massachusetts Asthma Action Plan (green-yellow-red zones).

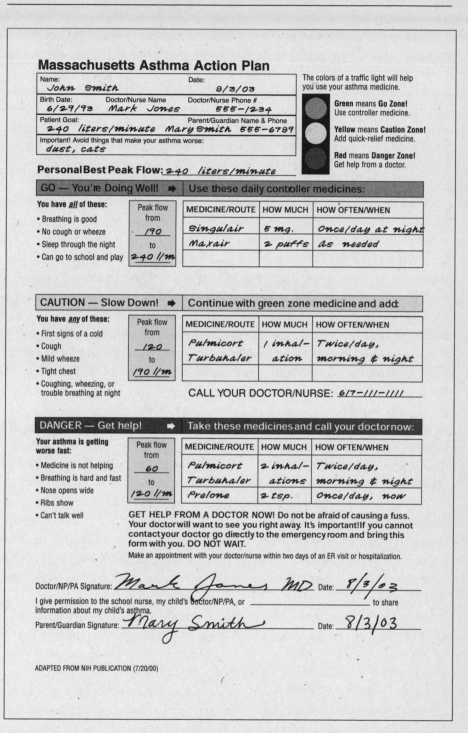

Massachusetts Asthma Action Plan

Name: John Smith
Date: 8/3/03
Birth Date: 6/29/93
Doctor/Nurse Name: Mark Jones
Doctor/Nurse Phone #: 555-1234
Patient Goal: 240 liters/minute
Parent/Guardian Name & Phone: Mary Smith 555-6789
Important! Avoid things that make your asthma worse: dust, cats

The colors of a traffic light will help you use your asthma medicine.

Green means **Go Zone!** Use controller medicine.
Yellow means **Caution Zone!** Add quick-relief medicine.
Red means **Danger Zone!** Get help from a doctor.

Personal Best Peak Flow: 240 liters/minute

GO — You're Doing Well! ➡ Use these daily controller medicines:

You have all of these:
- Breathing is good
- No cough or wheeze
- Sleep through the night
- Can go to school and play

Peak flow from 190 **to** 240 l/m

MEDICINE/ROUTE	HOW MUCH	HOW OFTEN/WHEN
Singulair	5 mg.	Once/day at night
Maxair	2 puffs	As needed

CAUTION — Slow Down! ➡ Continue with green zone medicine and add:

You have any of these:
- First signs of a cold
- Cough
- Mild wheeze
- Tight chest
- Coughing, wheezing, or trouble breathing at night

Peak flow from 120 **to** 190 l/m

MEDICINE/ROUTE	HOW MUCH	HOW OFTEN/WHEN
Pulmicort Turbuhaler	1 inhalation	Twice/day, morning & night

CALL YOUR DOCTOR/NURSE: 617-111-1111

DANGER — Get help! ➡ Take these medicines and call your doctor now:

Your asthma is getting worse fast:
- Medicine is not helping
- Breathing is hard and fast
- Nose opens wide
- Ribs show
- Can't talk well

Peak flow from 60 **to** 120 l/m

MEDICINE/ROUTE	HOW MUCH	HOW OFTEN/WHEN
Pulmicort Turbuhaler	2 inhalations	Twice/day, morning & night
Prelone	2 tsp.	Once/day, now

GET HELP FROM A DOCTOR NOW! Do not be afraid of causing a fuss. Your doctor will want to see you right away. It's important! If you cannot contact your doctor go directly to the emergency room and bring this form with you. DO NOT WAIT.

Make an appointment with your doctor/nurse within two days of an ER visit or hospitalization.

Doctor/NP/PA Signature: Mark Jones MD **Date:** 8/3/03

I give permission to the school nurse, my child's doctor/NP/PA, or _____ to share information about my child's asthma.

Parent/Guardian Signature: Mary Smith **Date:** 8/3/03

ADAPTED FROM NIH PUBLICATION (7/20/00)

as good—so that even in the absence of a nebulizer you can deliver bronchodilator medicine that is just as strong and quick acting. If you use your albuterol (or other quick-relief bronchodilator) carefully, attached to a spacer chamber, and inhale four to six puffs, with a slow breath in and a brief holding of breath at the end of each inhalation, you get just as much benefit as from a ten-minute nebulizer treatment. This is good news, because it means that if you carry a beta-agonist bronchodilator inhaler with you and have good inhalational technique, you are prepared for most acute emergencies of your asthma.

Finally, one other option for those who have experienced life-threatening attacks of their asthma is a needle and prefilled syringe containing epinephrine. An injection of epinephrine works as well as a nebulizer treatment of beta-agonist bronchodilator and at one time was standard treatment for asthma in most emergency departments. It remains the treatment of choice for allergic reactions characterized by throat swelling or low blood pressure, such as severe bee sting or food reactions. It is made available as a self-injectable system (Epi-Pen), about the size of fountain pen. Its virtue is that it is easily transported anywhere in a purse or fanny pack. Bronchodilator relief from epinephrine lasts from 20 minutes to three to four hours (depending on the severity of the asthma attack), buying you some time while you seek emergency help.

Another special consideration for some people is what to do in an acute attack of asthma if your controller medicine is Advair (see Chapter 7), a fixed-dose combination of the inhaled steroid fluticasone and the long-acting inhaled bronchodilator salmeterol.

A good strategy for dealing with a mild to moderate attack of asthma is to double your dose of inhaled steroids for several days. But if your inhaled steroid is combined with a long-acting bronchodilator, doubling the dose of steroids means also doubling the dose of the long-acting bronchodilator. If your Advair dose is one inhalation twice daily, is it safe to increase to two inhalations twice daily?

We believe the answer is yes, it is safe to double the dose and for a few days to use twice the usual recommended dose of the long-acting inhaled bronchodilator salmeterol (Serevent). Even at twice the usual dose, salmeterol has few adverse side effects. However, if you are very sensitive to the adrenaline-like stimulatory effects of the beta-agonist bronchodilators, you might decide on another option. Continue the same dose (one inhalation twice daily) of Advair, and add another inhaled steroid that you may have available—for instance, you could add two puffs of fluticasone (Flovent) twice daily. It is also okay to add a different steroid preparation (for example, to add two inhalations of budes-onide [Pulmicort Turbuhaler] twice daily). Finally, since Advair comes in three different strengths, reflecting three different doses of fluticasone (Flovent) combined with the same amount of salmeterol (Serevent), you may be able to switch to a more potent Advair inhaler (Advair 250/50 or Advair 500/50 in place of Advair 100/50), still taken as one inhalation morning and night.

WHEN YOU NEED EMERGENCY CARE

"By the time you start wheezing, your asthma attack has already started. If I take three [bronchodilator] treatments, and it doesn't go away—hospital, here I come. You don't take chances."
—HAZEL, 56

If home measures are not working, you should go to your nearest emergency room or acute care facility for help. Make sure that you indicate on your written Asthma Action Plan where you will go in an asthma crisis and how you will get there. If your asthma attack is serious enough to require emergency care, clearly it is not a good idea to drive yourself. If someone else is not available to drive you, call 911.

If you are not seriously ill, the first thing you can expect in the emergency department is a wait, sometimes up to several hours. Everyone arriving in the emergency department is assessed by the "triage" nurse, and the sickest patients are treated first, regardless of order of arrival. No one likes to wait in the emergency department, but you can rest assured that if you are in any danger because of your asthma, you will be taken care of promptly. (If good medical care is not being practiced and you are kept waiting despite severely distressed breathing, speak up on your own behalf. Sometimes severely impaired breathing is not as apparent as, for instance, bleeding or a very high fever.)

When you are taken into the treatment area, you will be asked about the history of your asthma, about any allergies you may have, and about medications you take for your asthma and for any other medical conditions. A physician will examine you, and ideally your lung function will be measured, with, for example, a peak flow meter. A nurse or a respiratory therapist will administer a quick-relief bronchodilator treatment by nebulizer or metered-dose inhaler, and you may simultaneously receive extra oxygen. Sometimes extra oxygen is given routinely as a precaution; in some facilities extra oxygen is given only if a measurement of the oxygen in your blood indicates a low level. Children usually receive oxygen through the same face mask used to administer bronchodilator treatments; in adults, oxygen is usually delivered by way of plastic tubing that fits in your nostrils, called nasal cannulas or nasal prongs.)

To monitor your progress, your care providers may choose to check your peak flow following the initial bronchodilator treatment (you're likely to receive more than one treatment), and at intervals thereafter, the frequency depending on how well you respond to the treatment. If your asthma flare-up is moderate to severe, or if the initial bronchodilator treatment doesn't make you better, you will probably be given oral or intravenous steroids.

Your medical team will probably place on your finger a painless probe, part of a device called a pulse oximeter that monitors the level of oxygen in your blood. If your asthma flare-up is very serious, you may also have blood drawn for a test called an arterial blood gas, which will indicate the level of carbon dioxide in your blood. In a very severe asthma attack, carbon dioxide can build up in your blood. It is important for your doctor to know if your breathing has become so severely impaired that you cannot rid your body of carbon dioxide normally. This is a dangerous stage of an asthma attack that may indicate need for treatment in a special setting, such as the hospital's intensive care unit.

Once you are better, you should still expect to stay in the emergency department for several hours of observation. Before discharging you home, the physician in charge of your care will want to make sure that your improvement is not just temporary. Most people go home with prescriptions for more medication than they were taking previously. It's often the case that an asthma attack that is bad enough to send you to the emergency department reflects a need for a medication adjustment.

If you do not require overnight hospitalization and are discharged from the emergency department, you will probably be sent home with a short course of oral steroids. Medical experiments have shown that patients who are prescribed a course of oral steroids following emergency department treatment are less likely to have recurrent asthma attacks in the two weeks following discharge than those sent home on bronchodilating medications only. Sometimes an intramuscular injection of an oil-based preparation of steroids that seeps out of the muscle into the bloodstream over a week or two can substitute for a course of oral tablets or a liquid preparation.

In addition to the oral steroids, it is a good idea to use a steroid inhaler after you have had a severe asthma attack requiring emergency department care. Studies clearly demonstrate that use of a steroid inhaler in the months following emergency department treatment for an asthma attack reduces the likelihood of repeat emergency department visits for asthma.

AFTER AN ASTHMA ATTACK: FOLLOW-UP CARE

An asthma attack serious enough to require care in the emergency department also requires follow-up care with your regular doctor. Your follow-up visit is a good opportunity for you and your doctor to explore what may have caused your asthma attack in the first place (if the cause is not clear) and how to reduce the likelihood that you will have another attack under similar circumstances. You can also explore what, if anything, you might have done differently to keep your breathing from getting bad enough to require emergency care. You may go home with a revised Asthma Action Plan, one that directs you, for example, to take a higher dose of inhaled steroids when or if you have another asthma attack, or one that includes having a supply of oral steroid tablets available at home. Don't hesitate to take advantage of your follow-up visit, or any office visit, to work with your physician on the most effective plan to keep you safe and healthy.

CHAPTER 17

Testing Your Skills for Dealing
with an Asthma Flare-up

OUR GOAL, LIKE YOURS, is that you never have an asthma attack—or, at most, very rarely. At the same time, as we have emphasized in Chapter 16, we want you to be prepared and to know what to do to help yourself if an asthma attack occurs. In collaboration with your doctor, you need to develop your own Asthma Action Plan, and perhaps share some of this information with family members or close friends.

Having read this book, you should have—and it is important that you do have—a clear idea of what steps to take in the event of an attack of asthma. For example:

- What would you do first for a mild or moderate attack?

- What would you do if you didn't quickly get better?

- What would you do if you were suffering a severe asthma attack?

- What if the initial treatment didn't work?

Here we invite you to practice your responses to a flare-up of asthma by giving you some made-up case examples and asking what you would do. Some of these examples may mirror your own situation closely. Others may not be relevant to your asthma, or may involve treatments that you do not have available to use at home, at least today. Going through these situations will give you confidence that you can deal effectively with an asthma flare-up under various circumstances, should one occur.

Part of that decision making is knowing when to seek help. Remember that, as we emphasized in Chapter 16, managing asthma attacks does not mean having to stay at home and care for your asthma by yourself. Rather, it means two important things: first, knowing what initial steps you can take to get better, and second, knowing when, where, and how to get help quickly when you need it.

SITUATION #1: THE HEAD COLD

Imagine that your asthma has been generally well controlled. You take a steroid inhaler (two puffs twice daily) to keep it under control. Most days you do not need your quick-relief bronchodilator (albuterol) inhaler at all. Other days you use it perhaps once or at most twice in a day, although you always carry it with you.

Last week you had a head cold, as did other members of your family. You had a low-grade fever for two days, with a sore throat and nasal congestion. Earlier this week your cold seemed better, but you started coughing a lot. Last night you were awakened repeatedly with coughing and slept poorly. You used the albuterol inhaler twice during the night, with some relief.

Today you are still coughing and raising clear phlegm (resembling egg white). In addition, you find yourself short of breath with even light exertion, such as walking 50 feet. You use your albuterol inhaler again, but it doesn't seem to help for more than about five minutes. You check your peak flow with your peak flow meter. You are dismayed to find that your peak flow is only 180 liters per minute, less that half your usual (400 liters per minute).

Sizing Up the Situation

This episode is more than just a bad cold. It is a severe asthma attack. It is not normal for a routine chest infection to cause shortness of breath when you walk only a short distance. In this example, a head and chest cold has caused a flare-up of underlying asthma. The low peak flow value, less than half the usual value, confirms that this is a severe attack, in the "red zone" (see Chapter 16).

Important Things to Know and Do

- If you have a compressor and nebulizer system at home (see Chapter 5), this would be a good time to use it to deliver a quick-relief bronchodilator (such as albuterol) by continuous mist.

- If you don't have a compressor and nebulizer, use your quick-relief bronchodilator inhaler with a spacer (to maximize delivery of the medication to the airways) and take four puffs, spaced one minute apart.

- If you don't have a spacer with you, use the inhaler as carefully as you can without one. You can continue to take your quick-relief bronchodilator (by nebulizer or by inhaler) every 20 minutes for one to two hours if needed. We ask parents of children with asthma flare-ups to call us if they have had to give their child two consecutive treatments.

- If you continue to have intense symptoms of asthma after using your bronchodilator two to three times, you can be certain that a major part of the problem is swelling of the bronchial tubes and filling up of the bronchial tubes with mucus. The air passageways are severely inflamed, and no amount of bronchodilator alone will treat this part of the problem. You need corticosteroids (steroids for short) to treat the swelling and inflammation of your bronchial tubes (see Chapter 6).

- When you are having a severe attack like this one, it is generally necessary to take steroids by mouth as tablets. Your doctor will probably want to prescribe prednisone, prednisolone (Prelone, Pediapred), or methylprednisolone (Medrol). You should call your doctor (or covering physician) immediately to discuss your condition and possibly get a prescription for steroid tablets or liquid. Be sure to measure your peak flow before calling. Reporting your peak flow value to your health care provider will help him or her gauge how severe the attack is and how best to respond to it.

- If you have previously had a severe attack of asthma, your doctor may have given you some steroid tablets to have at home; this would be a good time to take some, perhaps 30 to 60 milligrams. You should also plan to notify your doctor that you are ill and that you have begun a course of steroid tablets.

- Steroid tablets usually take several hours (two to six hours) to begin to exert an effect. You can continue to use your bronchodilator (for example, albuterol inhaler) as often as every hour while waiting for the tablets to take effect. You should rest and relax as much as possible. As long as your breathing (and peak flow) are steady or improving during this time, you will do fine.

- On the other hand, if your breathing is getting worse, you will need to seek emergency help. Quickly get to a nearby urgent care center or emergency room. **A severe asthma attack can be dangerous, especially if you are getting worse despite frequent use of your bronchodilator.**

- Here are the things that would make you or a family member want to call 911 for an emergency rescue team:

Being unable to speak more than a word or two because of shortness of breath

Passing out or nearly passing out

Developing a bluish discoloration of the lips and skin due to lack of oxygen

Having a peak flow of less than 100 liters per minute

SITUATION #2: THE NEIGHBORS' CAT (PART ONE)

Imagine that as part of your asthma you have multiple allergic sensitivities, including to cats. Nonetheless, you have been feeling well this fall, taking two inhalations twice a day of your steroid medication (except when you fall asleep without remembering your evening dose!). You are active and enjoy working out at the gym. You routinely use your bronchodilator inhaler before exercising but otherwise rarely seem to need it. Sometimes you wonder whether you still have asthma at all.

Today you are invited to your neighbors' home for dinner. They took in a stray cat last month, but because of your allergies they promise to keep the cat outside or in the basement during your visit.

The evening seems to be going fine, until you sit on a certain sofa. Soon thereafter you begin to sneeze and to develop watery, itchy eyes. You feel a tightening in your chest and itching below your chin. You use your bronchodilator inhaler once but get only minor relief. You start coughing and raise some clear mucus. Your neighbors offer you some water.

Sizing Up the Situation

Most likely, you're allergic to something in your neighbors' house, probably cat dander on the sofa and elsewhere (see Chapter 4). The best first step in treating an asthma attack caused by an allergic or irritant trigger is to remove yourself from exposure to the trigger, if possible. So step one in this situation would be to leave the neighbors' house.

Important Things to Know and Do

- In this situation, it is safe to use your bronchodilator inhaler more often than the usual limit of four to five times a day (see Chapter 5). If necessary, you can take it every 20 to 30 minutes for one to two hours or until you feel more comfortable.

- If it's available, use your peak flow meter to check your peak flow (see Chapters 2, 3, and 16). It will help you judge how severe this attack is. You may be able to estimate its severity by how you feel, especially by how breathless you are as you walk around. However, sometimes you can be fooled. The greatest concern is that you might underestimate just how sick you really are. Many people tend to minimize their symptoms, not wanting to admit that something might be seriously wrong.

- If you check your peak flow and find it to be more than half of your personal best value, you can be reassured that this is a mild-to-moderate attack (green or yellow zone). If your peak flow is less than half of your personal best value, you are having a severe attack (red zone), in which case you will need to exercise greater caution and seek more intensive treatment.

SITUATION #2: THE NEIGHBORS' CAT (PART TWO)

When you arrive back home from your neighbors' house, you find that you can walk up to your second-story apartment without much shortness of breath. You continue to experience some coughing and wheezing. You use your quick-relief bronchodilator again, and soon thereafter you check your peak flow. It is 400 liters per minute, whereas normally your peak flow is quite steady at 500 liters per minute.

SIZING UP THE SITUATION

A good strategy for treating a mild-to-moderate asthma attack, such as this one, is to double your usual daily dose of inhaled steroids. In this example, you would begin taking four puffs twice daily (or two puffs four times a day) of the steroid inhaler. The results are usually not as rapid and dramatic as with steroids in tablet form, but side effects are far fewer.

IMPORTANT THINGS TO KNOW AND DO

- Sometimes the asthma response to an allergic stimulus (such as breathing in cat dander) can be delayed, reaching its maximum 6 to 12 hours after the initial exposure. Even after initial improvement, there may be subsequent worsening, referred to as a "late asthma response." Be on your guard during this time frame.

- By removing yourself from the cat dander and increasing your dose of inhaled steroids, your asthma will most likely come back under control over the next day or two. During this time, keep extraclose watch on your asthma symptoms and, if possible, your peak flow.

- If you are not getting better, contact your medical provider. If you *are* improving, continue the extra puffs of the inhaled steroid for three to four more days, and if you are then all better, resume your usual dose.

- This example illustrates a good general strategy for using your inhaled steroids: increase the dose when your asthma is poorly controlled, and decrease the dose to the lowest amount sufficient to control symptoms and prevent attacks when your asthma is well controlled. Choosing the appropriate doses should be done with your doctor.

SITUATION #3: HOME IMPROVEMENTS

You have exercise-induced asthma, meaning that you have asthma and that exercise is the main trigger that brings on narrowing of your airways.

Your doctor has given you a pirbuterol (Maxair) inhaler to take before you exercise in order to prevent your symptoms of coughing, wheezing, and chest tightness. If you develop any of these symptoms at any other time, you use the inhaler (usually one puff is sufficient) and obtain rapid relief.

This week the workmen have come to begin long-awaited renovations on your bedroom. There is a lot of plaster dust in the air, and you find yourself coughing at night. You don't think much about it (your spouse, who doesn't have asthma, has also had some coughing) until you develop a low-grade fever and a miserable "head cold." Your coughing now keeps you (and your spouse) up most of the night. You can't lie down in bed without becoming short of breath. Each breath is accompanied by an uncomfortable rattling in your chest. It is difficult to talk or do any light physical exertion without provoking long bouts of coughing.

You suspect that this severe coughing and chest congestion may be a sign of your asthma. You borrow your daughter's peak flow meter to measure your breathing capacity. The peak flow result, 300 liters per minute, is only two thirds of the value measured when you were in your doctor's office. You use your quick-relief pirbuterol inhaler and it helps. The coughing lessens and your peak flow increases to 330 liters per minute. However, 30 minutes later you are again coughing severely, and your peak flow is now 280 liters per minute.

SIZING UP THE SITUATION

Get help! You are having a serious asthma attack, and the medication you have available to treat asthma, the pirbuterol inhaler, is not providing more than very temporary relief. You will need stronger therapies both to get better and to prevent getting worse, possibly dangerously ill.

Important Things to Know and Do

- Many people in these circumstances report that their quick-relief bronchodilator "stopped working." In fact, what has probably happened is that the bronchial tubes have become swollen and filled with mucus. The problem is no longer just spasm of the muscles surrounding the bronchial tubes, and the solution can no longer be just a medicine that causes those muscles to relax. You now need an anti-inflammatory medicine—a steroid medicine—to reduce the swelling and excess mucus production (see Chapter 6).

- The action that you take will depend on the health care resources available to you at that moment. You might call your doctor and get advice immediately, make an urgent visit to your doctor's office, or go to a nearby emergency department or other urgent care facility. Do not delay. The danger in waiting is that your asthma may worsen quickly, perhaps to the point that every breath becomes an effort and that even walking slowly seems like an impossible task.

- While you await a callback from your doctor or during your trip to a medical facility, you can continue to use your quick-relief bronchodilator inhaler. It will probably continue to help a little bit for short periods. You can take up to four puffs at a time, every 20 to 30 minutes for the next hour or two, until other medical treatments are begun (see Chapter 5).

- However, don't rely solely on the temporary improvement that your pirbuterol (or albuterol) inhaler provides. This is the most common mistake made in severe asthma attacks, the very bad attacks that end in hospitalization or even death. The brief, minor help in breathing that the quick-acting bronchodilator gives can fool you into thinking that you are getting better. Or it may convince you that you will start getting better soon. All the while your bronchial tubes continue to swell and become plugged up.

- Steroid treatment for swelling of the bronchial tubes works better and faster when started early. In this example, with the help of the peak flow meter, you can tell that you are getting worse, not better. There is no need to wait longer. Avoid the excuses, such as "I hate to bother the doctor," or "I'm sure that I will get better if I just rest for a little bit." Start now to get the medical treatments you need.

SITUATION #4: BLOWING IN THE WIND

This spring has been particularly difficult for your asthma. The grass and tree pollens to which you are allergic seem to coat every surface, indoors and out. Your asthma, more troublesome over the last year or two, has become particularly severe in the last week. You have been coughing up pale yellow sputum, wheezing off and on, and feeling breathless when climbing stairs.

When you go to bed everything seems okay, but you wake up at three in the morning with the feeling that an elephant is sitting on your chest. It is difficult to pull in air. Every breath seems an effort. You sit up in bed, reach for your quick-relief bronchodilator on your bedside table, and then wait for some relief. You begin to think about what options you have if the inhaler does not help.

You take a lot of medicines on a regular basis for your asthma. You take an inhaled steroid twice daily, theophylline twice daily, a leukotriene blocker in the evening, and prednisone, currently 10 milligrams every other day. You also have an over-the-counter antihistamine-and-decongestant combination that you use twice daily.

After 20 minutes you feel only a little bit better. You get out of bed, walk slowly to the kitchen, and make yourself some tea. Even though the doctor specifically mentioned that if you needed help you could call at any time, you are reluctant to call at this hour of the morning. You consider what else you might take for your asthma.

SIZING UP THE SITUATION

With so many asthma medicines at your disposal, you may be tempted to take extra doses of some or all of them. Consider carefully. Some (for example, the leukotriene blocker, such as montelukast [Singulair]) won't help in a crisis; others (such as theophylline) are potentially dangerous if you take too much. In this situation you will need more of the anti-inflammatory steroids, most likely more of your prednisone.

IMPORTANT THINGS TO KNOW AND DO

- You should never feel hesitant to call your doctor late at night in an emergency, especially if he or she has told you to do so. A severe asthma attack is a medical emergency, and your doctor, or another doctor covering for your doctor, is there to help in a crisis.

- In an asthma attack, your best options are a quick-acting bronchodilator (see Chapter 5) to open the constricted muscles surrounding the breathing tubes, and steroids to reduce the swelling (inflammation) in the walls of the tubes.

- Extra theophylline, a long-acting bronchodilator (see Chapter 7), may help somewhat, but it is risky to take without knowing how much theophylline is already in your bloodstream. Too much theophylline can cause unpleasant side effects (headache, nausea, vomiting, nervousness, and heart pounding). A very high level of theophylline in the blood can even lead to seizures and serious irregular heart rhythms. It's best not to take extra doses of theophylline without first discussing it with your doctor.

- Extra doses of a leukotriene-blocker medicine (see Chapter 7) such as zafirlukast (Accolate) or montelukast (Singulair) won't effectively treat an asthma attack. These medications are "controllers" of asthma; they are not in the category of "relievers."

- Taking more than the usual dose of your antihistamine-decongestant combination won't help your asthma. It is prescribed for allergy symptoms in your nose and eyes, not as treatment for your asthma.

- If you have one of the long-acting inhaled bronchodilators—salmeterol (Serevent) or formoterol (Foradil)—in your medicine cabinet, do *not* use it now for quick relief. The effects of these medicines last such a long time that it is not appropriate to use them repeatedly in a crisis.

- For this attack you can take more steroids either by increasing the number of puffs of the inhaled steroid that you take each day (take twice as many as before) or by increasing the dose of prednisone. Which approach you choose will depend on how severe this attack is (time to check your peak flow with your peak flow meter!), your past experiences treating similar attacks, and your discussions with your doctor.

- Often patients who have taken steroids in tablet form for many years try to avoid increasing the dose so as to avoid more of the serious side effects they cause. However, remember that breathing is the priority! It may be necessary to increase the dose of prednisone to 10 or 20 milligrams *every* day for a time, then decrease it again when you're feeling better (and when your peak flow has returned to your normal value). Be sure to notify your health care provider if you need to adjust your prednisone dose.

- It will take time (at least several hours) for the increased dose of steroids to start to reduce the inflammation of the breathing tubes. In the meantime, you can use your quick-relief bronchodilator more frequently than is usually recommended (that is, more often than the usual limit of four times a day). If necessary, you can take two to four puffs every 20 minutes for up to two hours, and then two to four puffs every hour. If you find that you do indeed need the inhaled bronchodilator that often, you are having a very severe attack. You should notify your health care provider so that you can get help and advice.

- While you wait for your breathing to return to normal, stay relaxed and breathe slowly and deeply.

- Think about how you can reduce your exposure to springtime pollen in the future (see Chapter 4). A good first step might be to keep the windows closed and to filter the indoor air with an air conditioner or window fan with attached filter. Have someone else do the dusting and vacuuming. If you must do it, clean with a damp cloth, use special filter bags on your vacuum cleaner, and, if necessary, wear a face mask while cleaning.

SITUATION #5: TROUBLE IN THE NURSERY

Your 2-year-old son, Robert, has had a difficult night, and so have you. Yesterday he had a runny nose and a low-grade fever. His older brother, now 4 years old, has had a cold, as have many of his preschool playmates, so you weren't surprised when Robert showed signs of the same thing. His nose dripped a thick, greenish discharge, he complained that his throat was hurting him, and he had a rattling-sounding cough. As usual, he was superactive throughout the day; not even the beginnings of a head and chest cold slowed down this ball of energy.

However, around midnight he crawled into your bedroom and into your bed. The poor guy couldn't stop coughing. Sometimes he would cough so hard that he gagged and had dry heaves. He would fall off to sleep for five or ten minutes, then wake again, coughing and fussing. He couldn't get comfortable. You could hear his breathing even while he slept. He breathed through his mouth, and at times he seemed to breathe very fast. While he slept, you counted his breaths, using the bedside clock with its second hand to time exactly one full minute. His breathing rate was 30 breaths in a minute. You recall that a breathing rate of 40 or more breaths a minute while sleeping was meant to trigger an alarm for you. He—and you—sleep fitfully.

Dealing with Robert's asthma is a new experience for you. None of his older siblings has had asthma, and his father's asthma went away before you met him, so it has not been part of your married life. It was just six months ago that the pediatrician diagnosed Robert's asthma. She said that his lingering cough with each cold was an indication of asthma, and on several occasions she heard wheezing when listening to Robert's lungs with her stethoscope. She gave you some medicines and instructions, but until now you have not needed them. She even talked to you about possible flare-ups of asthma. You search your memory to recall what she advised for just such an event as this.

SIZING UP THE SITUATION

Having a *written* Asthma Action Plan can help you remember exactly your doctor's advice for how best to handle an asthma attack, even when you are feeling agitated or sleep-deprived. Despite having a written Asthma Action Plan and following its recommendations, if at any time you are uncomfortable about whether what you are doing to treat your child's asthma is the best thing, consult with your doctor or other health care provider.

IMPORTANT THINGS TO KNOW AND DO

- Robert's severe coughing, chest rattling, and rapid breathing suggest that with this chest cold, which is probably a viral infection like his brother's, he is suffering a flare-up of his asthma. Viral respiratory infections are the most common cause of asthma attacks in young children. Unlike his older siblings, he needs antiasthmatic medications to be included in the treatment of his colds. He should receive his quick-acting bronchodilator and possibly other asthma medicines for his chest symptoms.

- The pediatrician probably gave you albuterol (Ventolin, Proventil) or levalbuterol (Xopenex) as his quick reliever. She may have given you an albuterol metered-dose inhaler with a spacer and face mask, or an albuterol or levalbuterol solution to be administered by a compressor-driven nebulizer. Now is the time to give your child a dose of this quick-relief medication. Even if it may make him a little bit jittery, don't hesitate to give it to him, even in the middle of the night. If his coughing and distress get better, it is likely that he, and you, will sleep better, despite the stimulating side effects of these adrenaline-derived bronchodilators.

- As their descriptive name implies, these quick-acting bronchodilators (see Chapter 5) bring relief quickly. If they are going to help, they will probably do so within five to ten minutes. However, their effect also wears off relatively quickly, usually within three to four hours. If your child continues to have troublesome coughing and seems listless or just not himself, it may be necessary to repeat the dose in three to four hours, and again three to four hours thereafter, continuing throughout the day.

- Your Asthma Action Plan may indicate that when more than one or two doses of the quick-acting bronchodilator are needed, you should begin a controller medicine. You may have a leukotriene-blocker tablet that you can give him (for example, montelukast [Singulair Chewtab]), a steroid spray with spacer and face mask (for example, fluticasone [Flovent] with an Optichamber spacer and face mask), or a steroid solution for your nebulizer (budesonide [Pulmicort Respules]). Continue to give your child the inhaled bronchodilator *in addition* to this controller medicine.

- It is possible that your child will not get better, even when you and he follow your Asthma Action Plan to the letter. No asthma plan, no matter how well thought out, is 100 percent successful every time. If your child's condition seems to be deteriorating despite your taking all the appropriate measures, seek help. There are more powerful treatments available for his asthma, such as a steroid liquid to be swallowed (for example, prednisolone [Prelone]). It may be that he needs to be more closely monitored in a hospital setting, where the oxygen in his blood can be measured and where experienced nurses and doctors can attend to his breathing difficulties, day and night if necessary. Part of your Asthma Action Plan should be getting your child quickly and safely to a medical facility when treatments at home are not working.

CHAPTER 18

Wrapping It Up

YOU CAN CONTROL YOUR ASTHMA, AND YOUR LIFE

If you could only take one thing from this book, we hope it would be the understanding that no matter how severe your asthma, you can control it and live your life to the fullest. You may need to take some precautions and medications, but asthma needn't stop you from doing most everything you want to do. That said, it's important to remember that asthma can be a serious condition with dangerous flare-ups. It's also a chronic condition, which means it doesn't go away when you're feeling well—and neither should your attention to prevention.

The symptoms of asthma—coughing, wheezing, shortness of breath, and chest tightness—come on when the bronchial tubes become narrowed in response to an asthma trigger, such as exercise, viral respiratory infections, and allergens. But even when symptoms are not present and the bronchial tubes are wide open, their sensitivity, or "twitchiness," is still there.

To determine the severity of your asthma, you and your doctor will look at the frequency of these symptoms, how often you need medicine to control them, and how often you experience the serious symptoms of an asthma flare-up. Your peak flow (as measured by your peak flow meter) can also help you make this judgment. The type of asthma you have (mild intermittent, mild persistent, moderate persistent, or severe persistent) also affects the kind of treatment you need. Remember, with asthma care, one size does not fit all.

MEDICATE TO ALLEVIATE—AND PREVENT

Everyone with asthma—no matter the severity—is going to need medication at some point to continue breathing freely. You can take "quick relievers" like inhaled beta-agonist bronchodilators to ease symptoms fast. So if you run for the bus on a cold morning and find yourself in the midst of a mild asthma flare-up once you get on board, a quick reliever can help. These medications relax the muscles around the bronchial tubes, allowing the air passageways to open wider. True to their name, quick relievers begin to work within one to two minutes.

If your symptoms come on more than just once in a while, or if they're particularly severe, you'll probably also need a controller medication. Some of these act on the underlying problem of inflamed bronchial tubes, others target the related bronchial muscle constriction, and still others work on both problems. They're taken every day, whether or not you have symptoms, to reduce the likelihood of a flare-up. The controller medications include:

- **Inhaled steroids.** These medicines are the mainstay of treatment in most people with asthma. They reduce the bronchial inflammation that is central to asthma. Taking steroids by inhalation avoids most of the side effects associated with steroids in tablet form, and inhaled steroids do not lose effectiveness over time. (By the way, these steroids should not be confused with the illicit drugs used by some bodybuilders and competitive athletes to build up their muscles.)

- **Long-acting beta-agonist bronchodilators.** These are best used in combination with anti-inflammatory therapy, such as inhaled steroids. They work to keep the muscles surrounding the bronchial tubes relaxed day and night, and they have proven to be a highly effective way to keep asthma under control without having to resort to very high doses of inhaled steroids.

- **Mast cell stabilizing medications.** These are virtually without side effects, but are less effective as controller medications in most people than inhaled steroids or long-acting beta-agonist bronchodilators.

- **Leukotriene blockers.** Medications in this new class act as both bronchodilators and anti-inflammatory medicines. They can be used alone to control mild asthma or in combination with inhaled steroids to maximize improvement while keeping the dose of inhaled steroids relatively low. The response to the leukotriene blockers has been variable among people with asthma, with some benefiting much more than others. At present no test allows one to predict who will benefit from this group of medicines and who will not.

- **Anti-IgE antibody.** This novel form of therapy for moderate and severe allergic asthma involves injections administered once every two to four weeks. Initial results are highly promising, with improved control of symptoms, fewer asthma flare-ups, and less need for other controller medica-

Goals of Asthma Treatment

No matter how severe your asthma or what kind of medication you need, the goals of your treatment are to:

- Prevent troublesome symptoms
- Maintain normal or near-normal lung function
- Maintain normal activity levels
- Prevent asthma flare-ups (exacerbations)
- Minimize medication side effects

tions. Given the enormous cost of this therapy, it is probably best initiated only under the guidance of an asthma specialist.

Once your asthma is under good control, it is a good idea for you and your doctor to find the lowest dose of controller medication that's effective for you (called "stepping down" your treatment).

AN OUNCE OF PREVENTION . . .

Besides trying to optimize your day-to-day functioning, an important part of your asthma treatment plan is avoiding serious flare-ups ("attacks") of your asthma. These are the steps you can take to reduce the chance of asthma flare-ups:

- **Avoid allergens.** If you're allergic to something, being near it can cause your bronchial tubes to become inflamed and more sensitive. If you know you're sensitive to common allergens such as dust mites, cockroaches, furry animals, birds, molds, or pollens, you can successfully reduce your asthma symptoms by trying to stay away from these things. Your doctor can give you allergy tests to help pinpoint exactly what you're allergic to.

- **Keep away from other asthma triggers.** For example, if you have aspirin-sensitive asthma, avoid all aspirin-containing medications and nonsteroidal anti-inflammatory drugs (NSAIDs).

- **Stay smoke free.** Smoking or even being around cigarette smoke makes asthma worse. Children of cigarette-smoking parents are particularly vul-

How to Become "Asthma Smart"

1. Learn all you can about asthma.

2. Get the most out of your doctor's visit by asking any questions you have.

3. Prevent asthma problems before they occur.

4. Know when you are getting into trouble with your asthma.

5. Be ready to respond to worsening of your asthma.

nerable. Though quitting smoking may not be easy, it is possible: there are more former smokers in the United States today than there are smokers.

- **Exercise caution.** Heavy exercise causes asthma symptoms in many people with the disease. But that doesn't mean you should stop being active. Instead, take some precautions, such as exercising inside when it's cold, warming up and cooling down, and using your quick-acting bronchodilator shortly before working out.

- **Get to know your asthma.** Know as much about your asthma as you can. You are as important as your doctor in controlling your asthma. This book can help you learn about your asthma—how to assess its severity, identify triggers, and work with your doctor to get the best treatment you can. Use your peak flow meter to measure what normal breathing is for you, and what it is during a flare-up. Create your personalized Asthma Action Plan so you can figure out—and remember—what to do when a flare-up strikes.

WHAT ABOUT ALTERNATIVE MEDICINE THERAPIES?

Think carefully before you turn to unorthodox treatments or untested supplements. If you do try them, evaluate their effects, both good and bad. Most important, if you use a nontraditional therapy, use it to supplement, not to replace, standard treatment. Some other precautions:

- Tell your doctor if you're taking supplements or visiting an alternative medicine practitioner.

- Do your homework and read up on the potential side effects of any nontraditional therapy.

- Be skeptical. If promises and claims sound too good to be true, they probably are.

- Make sure that any alternative-medicine healer you might want to see has appropriate credentials.

- Remember that products labeled "all natural" or "organic" are not necessarily safe, and the purity and safety of such products have not been validated by the Food and Drug Administration, unlike with regular medicines.

SEEING INTO THE FUTURE

Though most people with asthma can control their asthma symptoms and successfully prevent asthma flare-ups or manage them quickly when they occur, there's still room for improvement in available treatments. Here are some things to look for on the medical horizon.

- Better bronchodilators, new inhaled steroids, and new types of inhalation devices are all under development.

- New techniques in molecular biology will probably lead to additional tailor-made medications (biotherapeutics) aimed at specific chemical steps in the allergic response.

- And, of course, we all continue to hope for a cure for asthma. As the genetics of asthma is unraveled in the next 10 to 20 years, this possibility will most likely be brought nearer and nearer.

In the meantime, a major challenge for the American health care system is to ensure that the highly effective, convenient, and safe medications currently available to treat asthma are both available to and used by all those who would benefit from them. A well-informed medical consumer is a good first step toward that goal.

ASTHMA GUIDELINES FROM THE
NATIONAL INSTITUTES OF HEALTH: 2002 UPDATE

The National Asthma Education and Prevention Program is a health initiative of the National Institutes of Health. Since 1990, a panel of experts has created guidelines for the diagnosis and treatment of asthma and updated these guidelines as new scientific studies were published. The recommendations for diagnosing and treating asthma in this book are all consistent with these guidelines.

The most recent revision to the guidelines occurred in 2002. These updates are grouped into three categories: medications, monitoring, and prevention. We summarize the new recommendations as follows:

MEDICATIONS

- **Use of inhaled steroids in children:** Prior to 2002, the guidelines indicated that inhaled steroids are the most effective controller medication for adults. In 2002 this recommendation was extended to include children. The evidence now shows that inhaled steroids in children improve lung function, reduce symptoms, reduce the need for courses of oral steroids (prednisone or prednisolone), and lessen the risk of asthma attacks requiring urgent care.

  Inhaled steroids are appropriate for infants and young children with repeated episodes of wheezing and disturbed sleep; with symptoms requiring quick-relief bronchodilators more than twice a week; or with severe asthma attacks less than six weeks apart.

  The experts found that low-to-medium doses of inhaled steroids are safe, even in children. In particular, it is unlikely that inhaled steroids in these doses have long-term effects on bone growth and a child's final height. Likewise, the risk of harmful effects of inhaled steroids on other organs, particularly the eyes, was deemed insignificant.

- **Combination therapy:** Combining an anti-inflammatory medication with a long-acting bronchodilator has proven particularly effective for control of moderate or severe asthma. For persons with moderate asthma needing additional controller therapy beyond low-to-medium doses of inhaled steroids, it was felt that first-choice therapy is addition of a long-acting inhaled beta-agonist bronchodilator (salmeterol [Serevent] or formoterol [Foradil]). This combination was recommended for adults and children over 5.

- **Antibiotics for acute asthmatic attacks:** Respiratory infections often trigger severe asthma attacks. Most often, the cause of the respiratory infection is a virus, not a bacterium. As you know, antibiotics are ineffective against viral infections. As a result, the expert panel indicated that antibiotics are *not* recommended for routine treatment of severe asthma attacks—unless fever and discolored sputum or nasal drainage point to pneumonia or bacterial sinusitis in addition to the attack of asthma.

MONITORING

- **Asthma Action Plans:** The experts recommended that the "use of written action plans as part of an overall effort to educate patients in self-management is recommended, especially for patients with moderate or severe persistent asthma and patients with a history of severe exacerbations." The experts found that there was supportive but not conclusive evidence for the value of asthma action plans.

  In Massachusetts a major initiative launched to improve asthma care among children includes the use of written Asthma Action Plans. This project, sponsored by Massachusetts Health Quality Partners, has made a standardized Asthma Action Plan available to pediatricians, parents, and school nurses throughout the state. Use of these written Asthma Action Plans is thought to improve communication among caregivers so they can provide better daily disease management and can respond more quickly and appropriately to asthmatic flare-ups.

- **Use of peak flow meters:** Members of the expert panel also addressed the question of whether Asthma Action Plans should use peak flow measurements as part of the decision-making process or whether action plans should be based solely on symptoms of asthma. Again they found that scientific study was lacking: only four published studies address this question, none adequate to give a reliable answer. They had to rely on their best judgment, which was that "peak flow monitoring for patients with moderate or persistent asthma should be considered because it may enhance clinician-patient communication and may increase patient and caregiver awareness of the disease status and control."

PREVENTION

- **Do medicines that treat asthma also prevent asthma from getting worse?** Preventive medicines for asthma, such as inhaled steroids and the leukotriene blockers, improve your breathing, quiet your asthma, and help protect you against serious asthma attacks. Members of the expert panel wondered whether there was also evidence, as some physicians had suggested, that treating children at a young age with preventive medicines might prevent worsening of asthma over time. Might early use of inhaled steroids protect against deterioration of lung function or worsening of symptoms as a child grows older? Based on their review of the evidence, they concluded that early use of controller medicines does not alter the course of asthma over time.

  Some people with asthma, probably a small minority, suffer a permanent loss of lung function as they grow older. The questions remain: Is there a treatment that can prevent this decline in breathing capacity, and if so, how soon after the diagnosis of asthma does it need to be begun? Future research studies will be needed to answer these questions.

Adhesion molecules: special chemicals involved in allergic reactions that help allergy cells in the circulating blood to stick to blood vessel walls and to migrate out of the blood vessels and into areas of allergic inflammation. Future asthma therapies may someday suppress allergic reactions by blocking the action of adhesion molecules.

Adrenal insufficiency: inadequate amounts of the hormone **cortisol** (see below), which result in low blood pressure, weakness, light-headedness, and nausea. Adrenal insufficiency is a potential complication in people who suddenly stop taking steroid tablets or liquid (oral steroids) after weeks or months of use.

Adrenaline: a hormone produced by the adrenal glands in response to sudden stress or fright. Adrenaline makes our hearts pound when we are frightened and prepares us for physical exertion by stimulating our air passageways to open as wide as possible. In purified form, adrenaline (also known as epinephrine) is a quick-acting bronchodilator medication administered by inhalation or injection.

Airway remodeling: This term is used to describe the permanent structural changes in the walls of the bronchial tubes caused by persistent asthmatic inflammation. In a small percentage of people with asthma, it is a cause of permanent, irreversible narrowing of the breathing tubes.

Allergen: a substance that stimulates the immune system to make an allergic reaction. In asthma, this substance is almost always breathed in. Only things of a certain shape and size can function as an allergen. For example, pollens from grasses and trees can act as allergens; ozone, lead paint, and perfumes cannot.

Allergic bronchopulmonary aspergillosis: a unique type of allergic reaction to the common fungus *aspergillus*. In this condition, which affects a very small percentage of people with asthma, the fungus lives superficially on the inner surface of the bronchial tubes. The allergic reaction to the fungus is intense, characterized by allergic-type pneumonia (eosinophilic pneumonia) and bronchial wall damage (bronchiectasis).

Allergic conjunctivitis: allergies of the lining of the eyes.

Allergic dermatitis (eczema): allergic reaction involving the skin.

Allergic rhinitis: allergies of the nose, such as hay fever.

Allergy: a specific type of reaction made by the body to certain substances that are foreign to it. Some people are genetically programmed to make allergic reactions; others are not. The allergic reaction in asthma serves no known beneficial purpose. It is probably a misdirected application of the part of the immune system designed to fight worms and parasites.

Allergy shots: the practice of injecting incrementally larger amounts of an allergen into the skin over time for the purpose of reducing one's sensitivity to that allergen. Also called allergen desensitization or allergen immunotherapy.

Allergy skin tests: These tests for allergic sensitivities involve scratching, pricking, or injecting small amounts of specific allergens into the skin to see if allergic reactions develop.

Alveoli: the tiny air sacs in our lungs through which oxygen enters into the blood and carbon dioxide is removed from the blood. The **bronchial tubes** (see below) function as the passageways for air leading to and from these air sacs.

Anaphylaxis: a very severe, potentially life-threatening generalized allergic reaction characterized by low blood pressure due to dilation of blood vessels throughout the body.

Antibodies: proteins that have a special ability to recognize and attach to "foreign invaders" in the body, including allergens.

Anticholinergics: medications that block the **cholinergic** (see below) constrictors of the bronchial tubes.

Antihistamines: a family of medications that block the effects of histamine, a chemical involved in allergy. Antihistamines are effective treatment for hives and allergic rhinitis, conjunctivitis, and dermatitis, but not for asthma.

Anti-IgE therapy: a new asthma therapy recently approved for use in allergic asthma. It involves injection of a genetically engineered antibody that interrupts the allergic process early by removing most of the allergy antibody immunoglobin E (IgE) from the blood.

Arterial blood gas: a blood test used to determine the levels of oxygen and carbon dioxide in the blood within arteries. Taking a sample of arterial blood for blood gas analysis may be necessary in a very severe flare-up of asthma, when it is possible for the level of carbon dioxide to rise dangerously high and the level of oxygen to fall dangerously low.

Aspirin sensitivity: sensitivity to aspirin characterized by a flare-up of asthma and nasal congestion following ingestion of aspirin or any of the nonsteroidal anti-inflammatory drugs, such as ibuprofen and naproxen. Aspirin sensitivity affects only a small percentage of people with asthma (3 to 5 percent). It is often found in association with nasal polyps.

Atopy: the inherited tendency to make the specific type of allergic reaction seen in hay fever, eczema, and asthma. Common to these atopic diseases are the allergy antibodies (IgE) and the allergy cells (mast cells and eosinophils).

Beta-agonist bronchodilators: a family of bronchodilator medicines that share a common pathway for stimulating the bronchial tubes. They are all derived originally from **adrenaline** (see above), which is also called epinephrine.

Beta-blockers: medications used to treat a variety of illnesses, including heart disease, high blood pressure, migraine headaches, hyperthyroidism, cirrhosis, and tremors. They can worsen asthma control and cause asthma flare-ups. They have the opposite effect of **beta-agonist bronchodilators** (see above).

Bone densitometry: an X-ray test that measures bone density, usually in the spine and the bones around the hip. Periodic bone densitometry is recommended for people who have taken high doses of inhaled steroids for several years (or those who regularly take oral steroids at any dose) to check for bone thinning, or **osteoporosis.**

Bronchial tubes: the system of branching tubes that carry air to the tiny air sacs (**alveoli**) of the lungs. The bronchial tubes are organized like a branching tree, with the windpipe (trachea) corresponding to the trunk of the tree.

Bronchioles: the smaller branches of the **bronchial tubes.**

Bronchoconstriction: contraction of the bronchial tubes, such as occurs in response to an asthma trigger. Strictly speaking, this term refers to narrowing of the bronchial tubes caused by contraction of the muscles that surround the tubes.

Bronchodilation: widening of the bronchial tubes, brought about by relaxation of the muscles that surround the tubes.

Bronchodilator: a type of medication that acts to open the breathing passages, primarily by causing the muscles surrounding the bronchial tubes to relax.

Bronchomalacia: a congenital or acquired condition in which the airways (**bronchial tubes**) are floppy and prone to collapse. Narrowing of the bronchial tubes due to bronchomalacia can cause wheezing and breathing difficulty that mimic asthma.

Bronchospasm: synonymous with **bronchoconstriction.**

CAM therapies: Complementary and Alternative Medicine, or CAM, is the name used by the National Institutes of Health to describe therapies considered unconventional by most Western medical practitioners, and thought by some to "complement" more conventional Western therapies.

Candidiasis: oral candidiasis, also called thrush, is an overgrowth of yeast (*Candida*) in the mouth. It is a potential side effect of the inhaled steroids, especially when they are used in combination with antibiotics (that kill the normal bacteria living in the mouth). It is marked by white spots at the back of the throat and on the roof of the mouth.

Cataract: clouding of the lens of the eye that can interfere with vision. It is a potential complication of steroid therapy (oral steroids or inhaled steroids in high doses).

Cell: the smallest individual living unit within the body. Each cell is microscopic in size, like a bacterium or an amoeba. Many different, specialized types of cells group together to form different parts of our bodies (for example, skin cells) and to perform various functions throughout the body (for example, blood cells).

Chlorofluorocarbons (CFCs): chemicals used to propel medicine out of many **metered-dose inhalers.** These chemicals are known to destroy the layer of ozone, located high in the atmosphere, that protects us from harmful ultraviolet rays. Chlorofluorocarbons are gradually being phased out of use.

Cholinergic: the term describing a group of nerve pathways, some of which have endings near bronchial muscles. When stimulated, these nerves release the chemical acetylcholine, which causes these bronchial muscles to constrict.

Chromosomes: the structures in our cells that contain our **genes** (see below) and the **DNA** (deoxyribonucleic acid, see below) of which they are composed. Human beings have 23 paired chromosomes; half of each pair is inherited from one parent.

Chronic bronchitis: a persistent inflammation of the bronchial tubes that is almost always caused by cigarette smoking and is characterized by daily cough and sputum production.

Chronic obstructive pulmonary disease (COPD): a term often used to describe **emphysema** (see below) and/or **chronic bronchitis** (see above). Another synonym is chronic obstructive lung disease (COLD).

Churg-Strauss syndrome: a very rare condition in which there is a generalized outpouring of allergy cells called **eosinophils** (see below), involving blood vessels throughout the body. It can cause disease of the heart, lungs, nerves, kidneys, and skin and has on rare occasions been associated with use of the leukotriene blockers montelukast (Singulair) and zafirlukast (Accolate).

Congestive heart failure: failure of the heart muscle to pump efficiently (such as when it has sustained multiple heart attacks), with resulting fluid buildup in the lungs. Congestive heart failure causing shortness of breath and wheezing similar to asthma has been referred to as cardiac asthma.

Controllers: asthma medications that are taken on a daily basis to prevent or control asthma symptoms.

Corticosteroids: a family of medications that are designed to reduce inflammation. They are often referred to simply as steroids, and as such need to be distinguished from the very different muscle-building steroids used by some weight lifters and competitive athletes. Corticosteroids are the anti-inflammatory steroids.

Cortisol: a hormone released by our adrenal glands that influences numerous bodily processes, including sugar metabolism, blood pressure, and energy level. **Corticosteroids** used to treat asthma (see above) are derived from cortisol.

Cyanosis: the turning blue of the skin and lips due to low blood oxygen.

Cystic fibrosis: a genetic disease characterized by infection and inflammation of the airways, potentially confused with asthma. Most children with cystic fibrosis also have digestive problems (chronic diarrhea), making it difficult for them to gain weight.

Dander: tiny particles from animal hair, feathers, or skin that may cause allergic reactions.

Decongestants: medications that narrow the blood vessels in the nose, thereby reducing leakage of fluids from the blood and the swelling and discharge caused by such leakage. Decongestants can help clear up a runny, stuffy nose caused by viruses (such as the common cold), as well as a congested nose caused by allergies.

DNA (deoxyribonucleic acid): Made up of four nucleotides, or building blocks, that are like a four-letter alphabet, DNA directs the manufacture of amino acids and proteins, on which all life depends.

Dry-powder inhaler: an alternative medication delivery system to metered-dose inhalers. With dry-powder inhalers, an aerosol of medicine is created by the force of one's inhalation rather than by chemical propellants.

Dust mite: a tiny animal visible only under the microscope. There are proteins in its droppings to which many people worldwide make allergic reactions. These mites are found living in dust particles; they thrive best in warm and moist climates.

Emphysema: a disease of the lungs almost always caused by long-term cigarette smoking. In emphysema, the lungs lose their normal springiness. As a result, it becomes difficult to exhale air quickly.

Eosinophils: allergy cells that linger in the walls of the breathing tubes even when asthma is quiet. Like **mast cells** (see below), they contain chemicals that contribute to the allergic reaction.

Epinephrine: another name for **adrenaline,** see above.

Exercise-induced asthma: asthma in which the major trigger of symptoms is exercise. Virtually everyone with asthma will develop exercise-induced bronchoconstriction if they exercise hard enough, especially while breathing cold air.

Extrinsic asthma: an old-fashioned expression used to describe asthma accompanied by identifiable allergies (and distinguished from **intrinsic asthma,** in which no allergic sensitivities can be identified).

Gastroesophageal reflux: the regurgitation of stomach contents into the esophagus, where they can cause a burning pain behind the breastbone, known as heartburn. Gastroesophageal reflux disease (abbreviated GERD) can also cause a hoarse voice, sore throat, sour taste in the mouth, and cough.

Genes: segments of our DNA that transmit inherited characteristics—everything from our height, eye color, and the shape of our noses to whether or not we are predisposed to develop asthma.

Gestational diabetes: diabetes (abnormally high levels of sugar in the blood) that develops during pregnancy and frequently goes away when hormones return to their prepregnancy levels.

glaucoma: a condition involving the buildup of fluid and pressure inside the eyes that if untreated can eventually lead to loss of vision. Oral and high-dose inhaled steroids can cause susceptibility to the development of glaucoma.

Histamine: one of the chemicals released by allergy cells in an allergic reaction. Histamine causes bronchial muscles to contract, bronchial mucous glands to secrete mucus, and blood vessels in the bronchial walls to leak fluid, causing localized swelling.

Hives: red, itchy welts that appear on the skin of susceptible people in an allergic reaction, triggered by certain substances or conditions.

Hydrofluoroalkanes (HFAs): chemicals used to propel medications from some of the newer metered-dose inhalers. Unlike the traditional propellants, **chlorofluorocarbons** (see above), they do not contribute to destruction of the ozone layer in the earth's atmosphere.

Hyperreactivity or hyperresponsiveness: the tendency of the bronchial tubes to narrow too much and too easily in response to certain stimuli. This is the fundamental property of asthmatic airways, present even when one is feeling well.

Immunoglobulin E (IgE): protein molecules (antibodies) made as part of our immune response to parasites and allergens. These molecules stick to the surface of **mast cells** (see below), where they sit like sentinels awaiting reexposure to specific allergens. When IgE antibodies recognize these allergens, they signal the **mast cells** (and other cells) to release their arsenal of chemicals (including histamine), as though defending against harmful invaders.

Immunotherapy: See **Allergy shots.**

Inflammation: a reaction made by the body that is characterized by swelling and the accumulation of inflammatory cells. Many different processes can cause inflammation in the body, as you probably know from having had a sunburn or a skinned knee. *Inflammation* in asthma refers to swelling and abnormal cellular infiltration of the bronchial tubes. Unlike a sunburn or a skinned knee, you cannot feel the allergic inflammation of the bronchial tubes.

Inhaled corticosteroids: anti-inflammatory steroids available by inhalation from a metered-dose inhaler, dry-powder inhaler, or nebulizer. Examples include beclomethasone (QVAR), budesonide (Pulmicort), flunisolide (Aerobid), fluticasone (Flovent), and triamcinolone (Azmacort). Advair contains an inhaled corticosteroid (fluticasone) in combination with a long-acting bronchodilator.

Interleukin: Released by allergy-related **lymphocytes** (see below), interleukins are chemical signals that direct crucial processes in the allergic response. They are one of the ways that cells communicate with one another.

Interleukin-4: Interleukin-4, among other functions, signals the increased production of **immunoglobulin E** proteins (see above), which are made by certain lymphocytes and directed at specific allergens.

Interleukin-5: an interleukin that draws the **eosinophils** (allergy cells) out of blood vessels and into the tissues in the bronchial tubes, and also enables them to survive longer there.

Intrinsic asthma: an old-fashioned term used to describe asthma in the absence of any identifiable allergies.

Laryngospasm: a brief and frightening spasm of the larynx, or vocal cords, that prevents any air at all from passing in and out of the lungs for a few seconds. Spasm of the larynx is probably triggered by saliva, mucus, or coughed liquid hitting the densely packed nerve endings in the area of the vocal cords.

Leukotriene blockers: asthma medications that work by blocking the production or action of a group of chemicals in the body called **leukotrienes** (see next page). The leukotriene blockers include montelukast (Singulair), zafirlukast (Accolate), and zileuton (Zyflo). The former two medications block the action of the leukotrienes, the last blocks their formation.

Leukotrienes: one family of chemicals made in the body as part of an allergic reaction. Many chemicals are released in an allergic reaction: histamine is one that has been known for many years; leukotrienes are another, very powerful group of such chemicals.

Lipoxins: recently discovered molecules made in the human body that seem to dampen the inflammatory response. Their discovery may lead to future asthma therapies designed to mimic the action of these natural anti-inflammatory chemicals.

Long-acting beta-agonist bronchodilators: asthma medications that cause the muscles around the bronchial tubes to relax for 12 or more hours after each dose. They tend to have minimal side effects because they act primarily on the beta-2 receptors in the bronchial tubes rather than on the beta-1 receptors in the heart. Examples are salmeterol (Serevent) and formoterol (Foradil).

Lymphocytes: cells that act as commanders to direct our bodies' immune reactions. Lymphocytes have many important functions in the body, including fighting infections, making antibodies, and identifying and eliminating cancerous cells. A specific group of lymphocytes has the capacity to direct the allergic response.

Mast cells: Key players in the allergic immune response, these cells are located mainly in parts of the body that routinely encounter substances from the outside world. They are present normally in our skin, our intestinal tract, and in the lining of our eyes, nose, and breathing tubes. Mast cells produce chemicals such as histamine and leukotrienes that are meant to interfere with the function of foreign invaders (for example, worms) but that also cause unpleasant allergic reactions.

Mast cell stabilizers: nonsteroidal anti-inflammatory medications that seem to work by preventing the allergy cells called **mast cells** (see above) from breaking open and releasing histamine and other chemicals that contribute to inflammation. Examples of mast cell stabilizers are cromolyn (Intal) and nedocromil (Tilade). The latter drug is no longer marketed in the United States.

Metered-dose inhaler: a type of delivery device for the administration of inhaled asthma medications. Multiple doses of medication are held within a pressurized canister. With each use, the exact, "metered," dose is released in the form of a spray.

Monoclonal antibodies: antibodies of exactly the same structure that come from a single clone (that is, a genetically identical type) of antibody-producing cells. Monoclonal antibodies that interfere with specific steps in the allergic immune response are being produced and tested for the treatment of asthma. Monoclonal antibodies have already proved highly successful in the treatment of other inflammatory diseases, specifically rheumatoid arthritis and ulcerative colitis.

Mucus: gelatinous secretions made by glands such as those along the walls of the bronchial tubes and the nose. Mucus helps trap inhaled germs and particles that can then be removed by coughing or blowing the nose. Excess mucus production, often part of the allergic reaction in the bronchial tubes and the nose, can lead to blockage of these breathing passageways.

Nasal polyps: protuberant growths along the lining of the nose. These growths can block the nasal passageways, leading to a constantly stuffy, plugged nose and often to the loss of one's sense of smell.

Nebulizer: a machine that takes a liquid form of medicine and converts it into a mist to be breathed in. Both quick-acting bronchodilators and asthma controller medicines are available for administration by nebulizer.

Nocturnal asthma: asthma with a tendency to have episodes that occur at night and cause awakening from sleep.

Nonsteroidal anti-inflammatory drugs (NSAIDs): medicines, such as ibuprofen and naproxen, that are used to treat the inflammation of arthritis and are routinely taken as painkillers. NSAIDs do *not* treat the inflammation of asthmatic airways. Persons with aspirin-sensitive asthma suffer flare-ups of their asthma after taking most of the NSAIDs.

Occupational asthma: asthma caused by substances inhaled in the workplace. Over 250 airborne substances found in the workplace, including metals, organic chemicals, and animal- and plant-derived proteins, have been identified as potential causes of occupational asthma.

Oral steroids: corticosteroids in tablet or liquid form—for example, prednisone (Orasone, Deltasone), prednisolone (Prelone, Pediapred), and methylprednisolone (Medrol). Oral steroids are often prescribed for a period of days to a few weeks to bring severe or stubborn asthma flare-ups under control.

Osteoporosis: thinning of the bones, making them fragile and vulnerable to breaks. Oral and high doses of inhaled steroids predispose one to the development of osteoporosis.

Peak flow: a measure of how fast you can blow air out of your lungs. In asthma, your peak flow reflects the extent to which your bronchial tubes are normally open or abnormally narrowed. It measures how close to normal your breathing is at any given moment.

Peak flow meter: a simple handheld device used to measure **peak flow** (see above).

Placebo: an "inactive" treatment made to look, taste, or feel like the "active," or real, treatment. Placebos are frequently used when a new treatment is being tested. Often, half of the experimental subjects are given the placebo, while the other half receive the active treatment. In many of these experiments, neither the subjects nor the experimenters know who received the placebo and who the real treatment until completion of the study and analysis of the results. Such experiments are referred to as placebo-controlled, double-blind studies. They protect against biases the investigators or subjects might have as to the likely outcome of the experiment.

Premenstrual (or perimenstrual) asthma: a worsening of asthma experienced by some women that is related to the menstrual cycle.

Pulse oximeter: a device designed to measure the level of oxygen in the blood and also your heart rate. The oxygen detector (or probe) clips painlessly onto a finger or earlobe. The pulse oximeter provides a continuous readout of your heart rate and blood oxygen level.

Quick relievers: medications that quickly open the bronchial tubes by relaxing the muscles surrounding these airways. Most effective are the **beta-agonist bronchodilators** taken by inhalation. They begin to work within five minutes of inhalation.

RAST: short for radioallergosorbent test. This blood test measures the amount of immunoglobin E (IgE) antibody directed at specific antigens, for example RAST for cat allergen or RAST for dust mite allergen. RASTs offer an alternative to allergy skin tests for assessing specific allergic sensitivities.

Reactive airways dysfunction syndrome (RADS): a form of **occupational asthma** (see above) caused by a one-time, intense, usually accidental exposure to noxious fumes that leads to persistent cough, wheezing, and breathlessness. People with this form of occupational asthma frequently recover spontaneously over time.

Sinusitis: inflammation of the sinus cavities. Common causes are allergy and infection.

Spacer: a hollow chamber into which inhaled medicines can be squirted before they are breathed in. Spacers are used to help deliver inhaled medicines more effectively to the bronchial tubes and to reduce the amount of medicine left behind on the tongue and throat.

Spirometer: the equipment used in spirometry, a simple, painless breathing test that measures how fast you can force air from your lungs and the total amount of air that you can empty from your lungs. Spirometry is a useful diagnostic test for asthma.

Steroid-dependent asthma: severe persistent asthma that requires the regular use of oral steroids for control.

Steroids: See **Corticosteroids.**

Tracheoesophageal fistula: a fistula, or small open pathway, between the windpipe (trachea) and the swallowing tube (esophagus), which runs directly behind it. Tracheoesophageal fistulas may be present at birth or develop as complications of surgery or prolonged dependence on a breathing machine (ventilator). They allow swallowed liquid to pass into the windpipe, causing symptoms such as coughing, wheezing, and shortness of breath, which can occasionally be confused with asthma.

Tracheomalacia: a congenital or acquired condition in which the wall of the windpipe (trachea) is weakened and has a tendency to collapse. Narrowing of the windpipe due to tracheomalacia can cause breathing difficulty and wheezing.

Trigger (of asthma): anything that can set off asthma symptoms. Many different categories of things can stimulate asthmatic symptoms, including allergens, inhaled irritants, strong odors, medications, respiratory tract infections, exercise, and strong emotions.

Twitchy: a nonmedical term used to describe the sensitive airways of people with asthma.

Vascular rings and slings: rare abnormalities, present at birth, involving blood vessels that may squeeze the trachea, or windpipe, from the outside, causing narrowing of the breathing passageway.

Vocal cord dysfunction: a disorder characterized by unknowingly drawing together the vocal cords during breathing. This action, which leaves only a narrow opening through which air can flow, causes symptoms similar to those of asthma.

Asthma Timeline

450 B.C.	Hippocrates, a Greek physician, provides an early description of asthmatic symptoms.
150 A.D.	Galen, a Roman physician, identifies narrowing of the bronchial tubes as the problem in asthma.
1000	Avicenna, a Persian physician, writes *The Canon of Medicine* and describes herbal remedies for asthma.
1160	Maimonides, a Jewish physician practicing in Egypt, writes the first book specifically about asthma, in which he advises, among other things, maintaining general fitness, moderation in diet, and chicken soup.
1698	Sir John Floyer, an English physician, publishes *A Treatise of the Asthma,* with detailed observations of his own and his patients' asthmatic symptoms.
Early 1800s	Inhaling the smoke of the burning leaves of *Datura stramonium* is used as a treatment for asthma.
1819	Rene Laënnec, a French physician, invents the stethoscope.
1846	An early spirometer is developed by Dr. John Hutchinson, an English surgeon.
1869	Tincture of belladonna (atropine) is used to treat asthma.
1877	Mast cells are described.
1903	Adrenaline (epinephrine) is administered by injection for the treatment of asthma.
1911	Desensitization is first used for the treatment of allergies.
1912	Scratch testing (allergy skin testing) is developed for the assessment of allergic sensitivities.
1920s	Ephedrine is purified from the ancient Chinese herbal remedy ma huang.
1922	Intravenous aminophylline is used to treat asthma.
1929	Epinephrine is administered by bulb nebulizer.
1944	Oral aminophylline/theophylline is used to treat asthma.
1948	Isoproterenol is administered by bulb nebulizer.
1948	The distinction between alpha- and beta-adrenergic receptors is made.
1950	Cortisone is first used in the treatment of asthma.
1954	The cortisone derivative prednisone is developed.
1956	The metered-dose inhaler is used to administer inhaled bronchodilators.
1966	Immunoglobulin E is identified.
1967	House dust mites are identified as the principal source of allergen in house dust.
1967	The distinction is made between beta-1 and beta-2 adrenergic receptors.
1968	The mast cell stabilizer cromolyn is introduced.
1968	Albuterol is introduced as an inhaled bronchodilator selective for beta-2 receptors.

1972	Ipratropium, an anticholinergic bronchodilator derived from atropine, is introduced.
1972	The first of the locally active inhaled steroids, beclomethasone, is introduced.
1982	The Nobel Prize in Physiology or Medicine is awarded to Bengt I. Samuelsson, Sune K. Bergström, and John R. Vane for their discoveries regarding the chemical structure and activity of leukotrienes and related compounds.
1987	The Montreal Protocol on Substances That Deplete the Ozone Layer is adopted, committing nations worldwide to the goal of eliminating production and use of ozone-depleting chemicals, including the chlorofluorocarbons (CFCs) used as propellants in metered-dose inhalers.
1990	The first long-acting inhaled beta-agonist bronchodilator, salmeterol (Serevent), is introduced in the United Kingdom. It is approved for use in the United States in 1994.
1996	The first of the leukotriene blockers is released (zafirlukast [Accolate]).
1999	The first metered-dose inhaler using a non-chlorofluorocarbon (CFC) propellant is introduced.
1999	The single-isomer form of albuterol (levalbuterol [Xopenex]) is released for administration by nebulizer.
2001	Identification of first asthma-associated gene.
2003	Anti-IgE monoclonal antibody omalizumab (Xolair) is approved for treatment of moderate and severe persistent allergic asthma.

Resources

ORGANIZATIONS AND WEB SITES

Allergy and Asthma Network / Mothers of
Asthmatics
2751 Prosperity Avenue, Suite 150
Fairfax, VA 22031
Phone: 800-878-4403
www.aanma.org

American Academy of Allergy, Asthma, and
Immunology
611 East Wells Street
Milwaukee, WI 53202
Phone: 414-272-6071
www.aaaai.com

American Academy of Pediatrics
141 Northwest Point Boulevard
Elk Grove Village, IL 60007-1098
Phone: 847-434-4000
www.aap.org

American College of Allergy, Asthma &
Immunology
85 West Algonquin Road, Suite 550
Arlington Heights, IL 60005
Phone: 847-427-1200
www.acaai.org

American College of Obstetricians and
Gynecologists
409 12 Street, SW
P.O. Box 96920
Washington, DC 20090-6920
Phone: 202-863-5400
www.acog.org

American Lung Association
1740 Broadway
New York, NY 10019
Phone: 800-LUNG-USA or 212-315-8700
www.lungusa.org

Americans with Disabilities Act Web site:
www.ada.gov

Asthma and Allergy Foundation of America
1233 20 Street, NW, Suite 402
Washington, DC 20036
Phone: 800-7-ASTHMA or 202-466-8940
www.aafa.org

Environmental Protection Agency
www.epa.gov

National Asthma Education and Prevention
Program
NHLBI Health Information Center
P.O. Box 30105
Bethesda, MD 20824-0105
Phone: 301-592-8573
For the National Asthma Education and
Prevention Program's *Expert Panel Report
II: Guidelines for the Diagnosis and
Management of Asthma,* issued in 1997,
and supplemental *Update on Asthma
2002,* go to www.nhlbi.nih.gov/
guidelines/asthma.

National Center for Complementary and
Alternative Medicine
P.O. Box 7923
Gaithersburg, MD 20898-7923
Phone: 888-644-6226 or 301-519-3153
www.nccam.nih.gov

National Collegiate Athletic Association
6201 College Boulevard
Overland Park, KS 66211-2422
Phone: 913-339-1906
www.ncaa.org

National Jewish Medical and Research Center
1400 Jackson Street
Denver, CO 80206
Phone: 800-222-LUNG or 303-388-4461
www.nationaljewish.org

Partners Asthma Center
15 Francis Street
Boston, MA 02115
Phone: 800-9PARTNERS or 617-732-7419
www.asthma.partners.org

BOOKS

Adams, F. V., M.D. *The Asthma Sourcebook.* Chicago: McGraw-Hill/Contemporary Books, 1998.

Benson, H., M.D. *The Relaxation Response.* New York: Avon Books, 2000.

Edelman, N. H. *The American Lung Association Family Guide to Asthma and Allergies.* Boston: Little, Brown, 1998.

Hannaway, P. J., M.D. *The Asthma Self-Help Book.* Roseville, Calif.: Prima, 1992.

Hannaway, P. J., M.D. *Asthma—An Emerging Epidemic.* Marblehead, Mass.: Lighthouse Press, 2002.

Kemper, K. *The Holistic Pediatrician.* New York: Harper Perennial, 1996.

Perry, A. R., ed. *American Medical Association's Essential Guide to Asthma.* New York: Pocket Books, 1996.

Plaut, T. F., M.D. *Children with Asthma: A Manual for Parents.* Amherst, Mass.: Pedipress, 1998.

Plaut, T. F., M.D. *Asthma Guide for People of All Ages.* Amherst, Mass.: Pedipress, 1999.

Polk, I. J., M.D. *All About Asthma: Stop Suffering and Start Living.* Cambridge, Mass.: Perseus, 1997.

Sander, N., and A. M. Weinstein. *A Parent's Guide to Asthma: How You Can Help Your Child Control Asthma at Home, School, and Play.* New York: Plume, 1994.

Welch, M. J., ed. *American Academy of Pediatrics Guide to Your Child's Allergies and Asthma: Breathing Easy and Bringing Up Healthy, Active Children.* New York: Villard, 2000.

Young, M. C., M.D. *The Peanut Allergy Answer Book.* Gloucester, Mass.: Fair Winds Press, 2001.

VIDEOS ABOUT ASTHMA FOR CHILDREN AND THEIR PARENTS

"A" is for Asthma
Sesame Street Childhood Asthma Awareness Project
Health Videos for Children
www.cecpd.org/videolibrary/HealthVideos.html

Classmates with Asthma
Learner Managed Designs, Inc.
Lawrence, KS
1-800-467-1664
www.lmdusa.com

Roxy to the Rescue
New England Research Institutes
617-923-7747
www.neri.org

So You Have Asthma Too
www.coloradohealthsite.org

WHERE TO PURCHASE ALLERGY-RELATED PRODUCTS

Allergy Control Products, Inc.
Phone: 1-800-422-DUST
www.allergycontrol.com

National Allergy Supply
Phone: 1-800-522-1448
www.natlallergy.com

Index

Page numbers in *italics* refer to illustrations.

Illustration Credits

Art on the following pages is by Scott Leighton: Figure 1, page 5; Figure 5, page 29; Figure 10, page 83; Figure 11, page 101; Figure 12, page 118; Figure 13, page 120.

Figure 2 on page 6 is by Jesse Tarantino.

Figure 3 on page 7 is by Hilda Muinos, from the *Harvard Medical School Family Health Guide* (Simon & Schuster, 1999), page 506.

Figure 4 on page 14 is copyright © Harriet R. Greenfield, West Newton, MA.

Figure 6 on page 57 appears courtesy of the American Academy of Allergy, Asthma, and Immunology.

Figure 8 on page 79 is from Nelson, H. S. "Drug Therapy: ß-Adrenergic Bronchodilators," *New England Journal of Medicine* 333 (Aug. 24, 1995): 499–507.

Figure 9 on page 81 is by Heather Foley.

The Partners Asthma Center Action Plan card on pages 271 and 272 is by Christopher Fanta, M.D.

The Massachusetts Asthma Action Plan on pages 273 and 275 was developed by a consortium of health care groups and appears courtesy of the Massachusetts Health Quality Partners.

About the Authors

Christopher H. Fanta, M.D., is the director of Partners Asthma Center and one of its co-founders. He is a member of the Pulmonary and Critical Care Division at Brigham and Women's Hospital and an associate professor of medicine at Harvard Medical School and has written more than 100 articles on asthma and related subjects for medical journals and books. Dr. Fanta served as a member of the first expert panel of the National Asthma Education and Prevention Program of the National Institutes of Health. Cited in *Best Doctors in the United States* and *America's Top Doctors,* 2002, and named one of *Boston Magazine*'s *best doctors in 2003,* he has been recognized for his clinical care of people with asthma.

Lynda M. Cristiano, M.D., is an instructor in medicine at Harvard Medical School. She is a member of the Pulmonary and Critical Care Division and an associate physician at Brigham and Women's Hospital. As an active member of Partners Asthma Center, she cares for individuals with a wide range of pulmonary diseases, including asthma; she has a special interest in lung disease in women. Dr. Cristiano has been recognized for her clinical care of people with pulmonary diseases, cited as a Physician Leader in Women's Lung Health by the American Lung Association of Greater Norfolk County, 2000, and named one of *Boston Magazine*'s *best doctors in 2003.*

Kenan Haver, M.D., is a member of the Pediatric Pulmonary Division at Massachusetts General Hospital, where he directs the Pediatric Pulmonary Fellowship Program, and an instructor of pediatrics at Harvard Medical School. Dr. Haver developed and directs Partners Asthma Center's annual Pediatric Asthma Update for Primary Care Providers course in Boston. He is also the director and cofounder of the Flying Fish Asthma Education and Swimming Program, which combines asthma education and exercise for children.

ABOUT THE WRITER
Nancy Waring, Ph.D., is an assistant professor at Lesley University and has 30 years' experience writing on health issues.

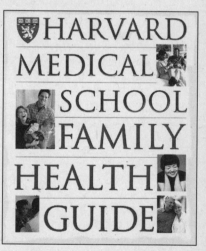